HQ
759.4   Teenage pregnancy:
.T46   opposing
1997   viewpoints

2 DAYS

AP 2 '98			
AP 16 '98			
MY 11 '98			
JU 20 '98			
NO 30 '98			
MR 3 '99			
AP 23 '99			
AP 30 '99			
MY 03 '99			
SE 24 '99			
AP 24 '00			

STAFF

teenage pregnancy

OPPOSING VIEWPOINTS®

OTHER BOOKS OF RELATED INTEREST

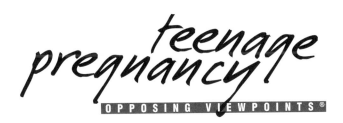

teenage pregnancy

OPPOSING VIEWPOINTS®

David L. Bender, *Publisher*

Bruno Leone, *Executive Editor*

Scott Barbour, *Managing Editor*

Brenda Stalcup, *Senior Editor*

Stephen P. Thompson, *Book Editor*

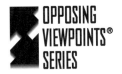

OPPOSING VIEWPOINTS® SERIES

Greenhaven Press, Inc., San Diego, California

Cover photo: Brent Peterson

Library of Congress Cataloging-in-Publication Data

Teenage pregnancy : opposing viewpoints / Stephen P. Thompson,
   book editor.
      p.   cm. — (Opposing viewpoints series)
   Includes bibliographical references and index.
   ISBN 1-56510-562-1 (lib. bdg. : alk. paper). —
ISBN 1-56510-561-3 (pbk. : alk. paper)
   1. Teenage Pregnancy—United States. 2. Teenage mothers—United
States. I. Thompson, Stephen P., 1953–   . II. Series: Opposing view-
points series (Unnumbered)
HQ759.4.T46 1997
304.6'32'08352—dc21
                                                          96-48031
                                                              CIP

Greenhaven Press, Inc., P.O. Box 289009
San Diego, CA 92198-9009

"CONGRESS SHALL MAKE NO LAW...ABRIDGING THE FREEDOM OF SPEECH, OR OF THE PRESS."

First *Amendment* to the U.S. Constitution

The basic foundation of our democracy is the First Amendment guarantee of freedom of expression. The Opposing Viewpoints Series is dedicated to the concept of this basic freedom and the idea that it is more important to practice it than to enshrine it.

CONTENTS

WHY CONSIDER OPPOSING VIEWPOINTS?

> "The only way in which a human being can make some approach to knowing the whole of a subject is by hearing what can be said about it by persons of every variety of opinion and studying all modes in which it can be looked at by every character of mind. No wise man ever acquired his wisdom in any mode but this."
>
> John Stuart Mill

In our media-intensive culture it is not difficult to find differing opinions. Thousands of newspapers and magazines and dozens of radio and television talk shows resound with differing points of view. The difficulty lies in deciding which opinion to agree with and which "experts" seem the most credible. The more inundated we become with differing opinions and claims, the more essential it is to hone critical reading and thinking skills to evaluate these ideas. Opposing Viewpoints books address this problem directly by presenting stimulating debates that can be used to enhance and teach these skills. The varied opinions contained in each book examine many different aspects of a single issue. While examining these conveniently edited opposing views, readers can develop critical thinking skills such as the ability to compare and contrast authors' credibility, facts, argumentation styles, use of persuasive techniques, and other stylistic tools. In short, the Opposing Viewpoints Series is an ideal way to attain the higher-level thinking and reading skills so essential in a culture of diverse and contradictory opinions.

In addition to providing a tool for critical thinking, Opposing Viewpoints books challenge readers to question their own strongly held opinions and assumptions. Most people form their opinions on the basis of upbringing, peer pressure, and personal, cultural, or professional bias. By reading carefully balanced opposing views, readers must directly confront new ideas as well as the opinions of those with whom they disagree. This is not to simplistically argue that everyone who reads opposing views will—or should—change his or her opinion. Instead, the series enhances readers' understanding of their own views by encouraging confrontation with opposing ideas. Careful examination of others' views can lead to the readers' understanding of the logical inconsistencies in their own opinions, perspective on why they hold an opinion, and the consideration of the possibility that their opinion requires further evaluation.

Evaluating Other Opinions

To ensure that this type of examination occurs, Opposing Viewpoints books present all types of opinions. Prominent spokespeople on different sides of each issue as well as well-known professionals from many disciplines challenge the reader. An additional goal of the series is to provide a forum for other, less known, or even unpopular viewpoints. The opinion of an ordinary person who has had to make the decision to cut off life support from a terminally ill relative, for example, may be just as valuable and provide just as much insight as a medical ethicist's professional opinion. The editors have two additional purposes in including these less known views. One, the editors encourage readers to respect others' opinions—even when not enhanced by professional credibility. It is only by reading or listening to and objectively evaluating others' ideas that one can determine whether they are worthy of consideration. Two, the inclusion of such viewpoints encourages the important critical thinking skill of objectively evaluating an author's credentials and bias. This evaluation will illuminate an author's reasons for taking a particular stance on an issue and will aid in readers' evaluation of the author's ideas.

As series editors of the Opposing Viewpoints Series, it is our hope that these books will give readers a deeper understanding of the issues debated and an appreciation of the complexity of even seemingly simple issues when good and honest people disagree. This awareness is particularly important in a democratic society such as ours in which people enter into public debate to determine the common good. Those with whom one disagrees should not be regarded as enemies but rather as people whose views deserve careful examination and may shed light on one's own.

Thomas Jefferson once said that "difference of opinion leads to inquiry, and inquiry to truth." Jefferson, a broadly educated man, argued that "if a nation expects to be ignorant and free . . . it expects what never was and never will be." As individuals and as a nation, it is imperative that we consider the opinions of others and examine them with skill and discernment. The Opposing Viewpoints Series is intended to help readers achieve this goal.

David L. Bender & Bruno Leone,
Series Editors

INTRODUCTION

"The welfare check . . . sustains a deranged social structure
of children having children and raising them alone and
abandoned by their men."

—Charles Krauthammer

"The conservative answer—abolishing welfare—is simplistic
and wrong. . . . Such strategies would harm the children we seek
to protect and undermine the family values we claim to revere."

—Kathleen Sylvester

In its 1996 report *Kids Having Kids: Economic Costs and Social Consequences of Teen Pregnancy*, the Robin Hood Foundation concludes
that adolescent childbearing has bleak consequences for teenage
mothers, for their children, and for society as a whole. Sum-
ming up the work of many scholars, the foundation, a New York
city organization that helps fund local antipoverty projects, observes that the teenage birthrate in the United States is the highest of all industrialized countries; it is twice as high as the next
highest rate, that of the United Kingdom. The report claims that,
of the 500,000 teenagers giving birth each year, "more than 80
percent end up in poverty and reliant on welfare, many for the
majority of their children's critically important developmental
years." Compared with children born to mothers between the
ages of twenty and twenty-one, the children of teenage mothers
are much more likely to suffer poor health, perform poorly in
school, live in poverty, be neglected or abused, and engage in
criminal activity. The economic burden to society of mothers
under the age of seventeen, in terms of welfare, medical care,
increased foster care, and other costs, is $6.9 billion a year.
Although some experts insist that the problem of teenage
pregnancy has been overstated, recent studies such as *Kids Having
Kids* have led many people to believe that something must be
done to address what they view as a disturbing trend. Numerous
approaches—including various types of sex education, increased
availability of contraceptives, and the enforcement of statutory
rape laws—have been proposed and tried in an effort to bring
down the teen pregnancy rate. One measure that has generated a
great deal of controversy is the proposal to limit welfare benefits
as a means of reducing the rate of teenage pregnancy.
Many commentators—especially conservatives—believe that

welfare encourages teenage pregnancy both directly and indirectly. By providing cash payments to unwed teenage mothers, they argue, the welfare system offers a direct incentive for teenage girls to have babies. In addition, critics contend, by supporting teenage mothers and their children, the system creates an environment where teen pregnancy and childbearing are implicitly condoned. Welfare opponents maintain that because teenagers who get pregnant and give birth do not suffer negative consequences, but are instead essentially rewarded with cash payments, teenage girls get the message that pregnancy and childbearing are acceptable.

Most liberals challenge the argument that welfare is a cause—either directly or indirectly—of teenage pregnancy. These commentators argue that the sexual activity of teenage girls is influenced by a variety of conditions and motivations; it is seldom driven solely by the confidence that they and their future babies will be taken care of by the welfare system. Pointing out that 80 percent of unwed teenage mothers grow up in extreme poverty, critics maintain that teenage childbearing is a response to poverty and to an environment lacking in educational and economic opportunities and expectations. Kristin Luker, the author of *Dubious Conceptions: The Politics of Teenage Pregnancy*, contends: add

> Even as we amass evidence showing that early childbearing is not a root cause of poverty in the United States, we are also realizing more clearly that the high rate of early childbearing is a measure of how bleak life is for young people who are living in poor communities and have no obvious arenas for success.

Luker and others argue that for poverty-stricken teenage girls, pregnancy and motherhood often provide a sense of purpose and meaning that are otherwise absent from their lives.

The debate over welfare's role in causing teenage pregnancy attracted public attention in August 1996, when Congress passed a welfare reform bill, subsequently signed by President Bill Clinton, that contained provisions designed to reduce teenage pregnancy. The law stipulated that teenage mothers who wish to receive federal welfare benefits must both live at home and continue their education. It also gave states the option to reduce or entirely eliminate welfare benefits to unwed teenage mothers.

The approach adopted by Congress effectively endorses the conservative response to teenage pregnancy. Teenage mothers are now subject to more restrictions than they were before the passage of the welfare legislation, including the possible reduction or loss of all welfare benefits. "The federal government has made it possible through welfare for unwed women to have babies without having to suffer," maintains Steve Boriss, press secretary for James Talent, a Republican congressman who supported the bill. "Our plan provides uncomfortable, survival living." The strategy aims to make teenage childbearing so "uncomfortable" a proposition that teenagers will take extra precautions or avoid sexual activity entirely in order to prevent pregnancy. As Douglas J. Besharov of the American Enterprise Institute says, "A decade-long commitment to making welfare 'inconvenient' could change the reproductive behavior of disadvantaged teens—as the implications of the new regime begin to sink in."

Critics of this approach contend that removing the safety net from struggling teenage mothers and their children will only result in more suffering and poverty. Many argue that requiring teenage welfare recipients to live at home and to continue in school will prove problematic. Kathleen Sylvester, vice president of domestic policy at the Progressive Policy Institute, contends that as many as 62 percent of teenage mothers have suffered sexual abuse, often by stepfathers or other adults residing in the home, and 44 percent report having been raped. Mike Males, a writer on youth issues, observes that 60 percent of teenage mothers say that they have experienced severe physical violence at home. Based on these statistics, opponents of the new welfare provisions suggest that home may not be the best environment for a sizable percentage of teenage mothers. Further, they maintain, requiring school attendance by teenage mothers presumes that someone else is available to take care of the child. Noting that the majority of teenage mothers are the primary care provider for their child, critics point out that the new legislation does not address who will pay for child care for these children if their mothers are required to attend school.

The policy choices codified in the welfare reform bill of 1996 may succeed in reducing some of the financial burden imposed on society by the welfare system. But as the viewpoints that follow reveal, the effect of these decisions on the teenage pregnancy rate and on the problems faced by teenage mothers and their children remains open to debate. *Teenage Pregnancy: Opposing Viewpoints* presents these and related issues in the following chapters: Is Teenage Pregnancy a Serious Problem? What Factors Contribute to Teenage Pregnancy? How Can Teenage Pregnancy Be Prevented? What New Initiatives Might Reduce Teenage Pregnancy? Throughout this anthology, authors discuss the extent of the problem of teenage pregnancy and what measures would most effectively balance the needs of teenage parents, their children, and society as a whole.

CHAPTER 1

IS TEENAGE PREGNANCY A SERIOUS PROBLEM?

CHAPTER PREFACE

In recent years, teenage pregnancy has been discussed in Congress and in the media as a serious crisis, even an "epidemic." According to Kathleen Sylvester of the Progressive Policy Institute, teenage pregnancy is

> a calamity for these young mothers because early motherhood denies them opportunities and choices. It is a calamity for their children because most will grow up poor and fatherless. And it is a calamity for this nation because these children are likely to repeat the tragic cycle of poverty and dysfunction into which they were born.

Some social commentators hold teenage pregnancy directly responsible for a host of society's ills. Charles Murray, author of *Losing Ground*, believes that the rising illegitimacy rate—including a growing number of births to unwed teenagers—is creating a vast "underclass" characterized by poverty, crime, and hopelessness. Columnist Suzanne Fields agrees that the increasing teenage pregnancy rate translates directly into increasing rates of "school failure, early behavioral problems, drug abuse, child abuse, depression, and crime." Therefore, these critics conclude, many social problems can be directly attributed to the poor choices of teenage girls.

Not all commentators agree that labeling the situation an "epidemic" is helpful or even accurate. Although most agree that a teen pregnancy problem exists, many social critics believe that the severity of the problem has been exaggerated and that the role of teenage pregnancy in causing other social problems has been misconstrued. Teenage pregnancy, to these critics, is not so much the cause of social problems as a symptom or reflection of larger social conditions, especially poverty and a lack of economic opportunity. These commentators argue that rather than blaming teenage mothers for contributing to various social pathologies, society should instead focus on eliminating the poverty and hopelessness that pervade the environments in which most teenage mothers live.

The viewpoints in the following chapter cover the spectrum of perspectives on the seriousness of the teen pregnancy problem, from the view that teenage pregnancy is society's most pressing and fundamental problem to the opinion that teenage pregnancy is a symptom of larger maladies.

> "Teen-age sex is dangerous not only for a young person's health but the health of our society because trouble is reproducing trouble."

TEENAGE PREGNANCY IS A SERIOUS PROBLEM

Suzanne Fields

Conservative columnist Suzanne Fields writes on many aspects of the family and U.S. society. In the following viewpoint, Fields suggests that a growing number of sexually active teens is causing an increase in teenage pregnancy. She sees a definite link between teenage pregnancy and many of society's most serious problems, such as failure in school, child abuse, drug abuse, and crime. According to Fields, the quest for instant gratification among both girls and boys is the heart of the problem of teenage pregnancy.

As you read, consider the following questions:

1. How does Fields describe "super predators"?
2. What coercive responses to the problem of teenage pregnancy does the author describe? Does she think they will succeed?
3. How does Fields propose to solve the problem of teenage pregnancy?

Suzanne Fields, "The Crime of Children Having Children," *Washington Times*, April 15, 1996. Reprinted by permission of the author.

The teen-age birth rate in the United States declined for two years in 1993 and 1994. That's promising, for the record. The reductions are slight, but at least the numbers seem to be moving in the right direction.

But then you see the fine print. The number of births decreased only to older teens, ages 18 and 19. Babies born to teens younger than 17 actually increased, reflecting a growing population of younger girls who are what we now euphemistically call "sexually active."

If your eyes glaze over at the subject of teen-age pregnancies, other numbers might wake you up to a special alarm. The number of girls aged 14–17 will increase by more than a million between 1996 and 2005, and sexually active unmarried teen-age girls are less likely than married women to use contraceptives, according to Child Trends Inc., a non-profit research organization in Washington, D.C.

SUPER PREDATORS

That means that the increasing numbers of children born to children are likely to repeat the devastating cycles of almost everything bad—teen-age pregnancy, school failure, early behavioral problems, drug abuse, child abuse, depression and crime. As the numbers of girls increase, so do the number of teen-age boys. Many of them will be what John DiIulio, Princeton professor and intellectual crime-fighter, calls "loveless, godless and jobless." These young men, says Mr. DiIulio, are likely to become "super predators," violent young men without the slightest conscience. No neighborhood will be safe from such foul children.

One such teen-ager recently stole my neighbor's pocketbook. He didn't have a knife or a gun; he merely cracked her jaw with his fist and knocked her out. He did not seem to think he was doing anything "wrong."

RAGING HORMONES

Teen-age sex is dangerous not only for a young person's health but the health of our society because trouble is reproducing trouble. Such raging hormones seeking immediate gratification may even be addictive (without artificial additives). But no rich tobacco corporation is available to pay the costs of sexual irresponsibility. One generation's sexual promiscuity becomes the next generation's crime wave.

Social predators often become sexual predators. The majority of the fathers of babies born to teen-age girls are more than three years older than the girls they get pregnant. The Urban Institute reports that three-quarters of the girls under the age of 14 who are sexually active say they were forced by their first partner to have sex relations. This is statutory rape, but who's around to say so?

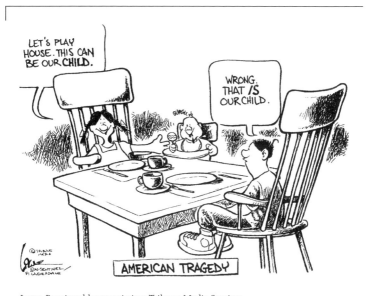

Lowe. Reprinted by permission: Tribune Media Services.

When Jerry Lee Lewis, the rock-and-roll pioneer, married his 13-year-old cousin in 1958, he created an international scandal that might have cost him the lasting fame that fell to Elvis; many music historians think Elvis hit the jackpot with Jerry Lee's nickel. He was ostracized even though he married the young girl he "got in trouble." So quickly has the culture changed that now we keep statistical tables to demonstrate how many teen-age girls get pregnant by older men.

CUSTOM OR COERCION?

How did this come about? Obviously there are many cultural streams that swell the running river of teen-age sexuality. Custom rather than coercion is probably a likelier force to rein in sexual drives, but custom proscribing sexual activity for teenagers has gone with the winds of personal liberation and media-saturated sex desire. "If it feels good do it" has become "do it and see if it feels good."

So that leaves coercion. Prosecutors in California, where more than 70,000 babies were born to teen-age mothers in 1993 (nearly 28,000 were 17 and younger), are now charging men in their 20s who get underage girls pregnant with either statutory rape or lewd sexual activity with a minor. This may frighten a few young men who pursue what an earlier generation called "jail bait" or "San Quentin quail," but it's not likely to have a great impact on out-of-control male behavior. Requiring teen-age girls with babies on welfare to stay in their parents' home, or cutting off welfare if a woman has more than one or two illegitimate babies may coax some teen-agers to restrain themselves, but I wouldn't bet on that, either.

John Updike, in an essay on lust, colorfully describes medieval prohibitions against sex as "patchwork attempts to wall in the polymorphous-perverse torrents." We've replaced those prohibitions with a patchwork of laws to curtail children from having children. Maybe we ought to revive medieval patches.

| "[The media are] casting the unmarried teenaged mother as the source of virtually all of society's ills."

THE PROBLEM OF TEENAGE PREGNANCY IS EXAGGERATED BY THE MEDIA

Janine Jackson

In the following viewpoint, Janine Jackson argues that the media have sensationalized the issue of teenage pregnancy and have unfairly blamed teenage mothers for society's problems. She contends that, contrary to popular perceptions, pregnant teenage girls are more often victims than perpetrators of immoral behavior. According to Jackson, the media wrongly assess blame on teenage mothers while ignoring objective research that counters their claims. Jackson is the research director for EXTRA!, the magazine of Fairness and Accuracy in Reporting, a liberal media watchdog organization.

As you read, consider the following questions:

1. What is Jackson's reasoning in claiming that single motherhood does not cause poverty?
2. According to the author, what factors contribute more to teenage pregnancy than the availability of welfare benefits?
3. In Jackson's opinion, why is calling teenage mothers "children" unfair and insulting?

From Janine Jackson, "The 'Crisis' of Teen Pregnancy: Girls Pay the Price for Media Distortion," Extra! March/April 1994. Reprinted by permission of the publisher.

A recent round of media attention focused on the "tragedy" of teenage pregnancy, casting the unmarried teenaged mother as the source of virtually all of society's ills. Papers and pundits were moved to florid prose on teen mothers' "world of warped morals and wasted lives that affects the quality of life for all of us." (*Cleveland Plain Dealer*)

Various indicators on birth rates and poverty rates were tossed around to document the "social catastrophe." (*Detroit News*) No serious analysis was needed, since it was obvious to bipartisan politicians and media alike that the "soaring birth rate among welfare mothers" (*Chicago Sun-Times*) is "the smoking gun in a sickening array of pathologies—crime, drug abuse, physical and mental illness, welfare dependency." (*Newsweek*) *USA Today* reported in a near-panic: "Beyond the drugs and the gunfire lies what is perhaps the most shocking of social pathologies: rates of out-of-wedlock births."

The most recent round of finger-pointing was largely touched off by a *Wall Street Journal* op-ed by the American Enterprise Institute's Charles Murray, which contended that "illegitimacy is the single most important social problem of our time—more important than crime, drugs, poverty, illiteracy, welfare or homelessness, because it drives everything else."

Murray's call for denial of all government support to any unmarried woman who has a child (and orphanages for children whose parents can't support them) fits a familiar conservative pattern of blaming poverty on the character faults and bad decisions of the poor themselves. He hearkens back to "the old way, which worked," and calls for making "illegitimate birth the socially horrific act it used to be."

What was chilling was how easily the mainstream media latched on to Murray's ideology-laden notions, presenting the condemnation of poor unwed mothers as a fresh policy approach—"given the failure of all other remedies." (*Detroit News*)

In fact, the conservative argument's assumptions are demonstrably false, but it successfully plays on cultural (and racial) tensions and fears, along with the need for scapegoats in times of economic strain. Unfortunately, mainstream media have done a poor job of separating moralistic arguments from economic ones.

TEENAGE MOMS AND POVERTY

Journalists speak of "teen pregnancies and the underclass" as "entwined social pathologies." (*Atlanta Journal and Constitution*) But few question *why* this should be.

Substantial evidence shows that while single motherhood is

associated with poverty, it does not *cause* poverty. First, most teenagers who give birth were living at or below poverty levels to begin with. Explaining their choice to researchers, these women speak of factors associated with socio-economic status: educational failure, low self-esteem (often connected with sexual abuse) and a lack of job opportunities. These factors, not "the sex-me-up songs on radio and television" (*Plain Dealer*), can make early motherhood appear to be a rational option.

WELFARE AND BABIES

Conservatives know where babies come from: welfare. They are under the impression that nubile 14-year-olds produce babies to collect cash and food stamps at the welfare office. Cut off welfare and you will stem the flow of babies. That's the theory.

It is a bizarre theory. Most 14-year-olds can't figure out that leaving their clothes in a pile makes them wrinkled, let alone that surrendering to one's glands has unintended consequences.

Cutting off welfare might have some effect on the birth rate if it were combined with some sort of birth control program, but conservatives are against passing out condoms to kids or even informing them about birth control. As for abortion counseling: immoral.

So, apparently, they intend to stop teenage sex by cutting off welfare benefits. This is like trying to stop drunken driving by raising the price of gasoline.

Donald Kaul, *Liberal Opinion Week*, March 6, 1995.

After becoming mothers, young women are confronted with a lack of affordable childcare and a job market that pays women (especially minority women) inadequate, disproportionately low wages. That many are pushed below the poverty level is not surprising. Nor is it surprising that single fathers are less than half as likely to live in poverty as single mothers.

In an earlier round of the "unwed mothers" discussion, this overlooked economic context was pointed out by family historian Stephanie Coontz in a *Washington Post* op-ed. Most poverty in the U.S., Coontz wrote, is related not to family structure, but to workforce and wage structures, including the "growth of low-wage work that makes one income inadequate to support a family."

"The United States tolerates higher levels of child poverty in *every* family form than any other major industrial democracy," Coontz wrote. "The fastest growing poverty group in America since 1979 has been married-couple families with children."

Nevertheless, the notion that cutting women's welfare benefits will discourage them from having children is finding new receptivity among the press and policymakers, including President Clinton, who called Murray's idea "essentially right."

"What many experts suspect, and fear," Newsweek's Joe Klein told readers, "is that nothing short of [Murray's] draconian solution . . . will change the culture of chronic dependency." The Milwaukee Sentinel called it "the only real way to send the message that illegitimacy doesn't pay."

Murray's basic theory—that women have children because of the "economic incentive" of welfare—has been thoroughly disproven by research, most recently in a study by the Urban Institute (Urban Institute Policy and Research Report, Fall/93). The study found that "generosity [of welfare payments] has at best a very modest impact on a woman's initial childbearing decision and virtually no effect on subsequent births."

What did have significant impact, the researchers found, were education, race and income. Fairness and Accuracy in Reporting (FAIR) saw no major media reporting on these findings.

CONTROLLING TEENAGE MOTHERS

The ubiquitous media label for teen motherhood, "children having children"—or even "babies having babies," as syndicated columnist Charles Krauthammer put it (Washington Post)—evokes the cultural discomfort the phenomenon stirs, but it's more evocative than accurate, since about two-thirds of teenage births are to women 18 and 19, not 13 or 14.

Many welfare rights and women's advocates also believe the "children having children" label infantilizes adolescent mothers, helping to justify policies that treat them as incapable of making decisions. Punitive proposals that compel teenage mothers to live with their families and stay in school in order to receive public assistance (no analogous rules are suggested for fathers) are justified by the press because unwed mothers are, "especially if they're teenagers, plain ignorant." (New York Times editorial)

But as Mike Males has pointed out, labeling pregnancies of women under 20 a "teen" problem is itself questionable, since 70 percent of such pregnancies result from sex with a man over 20. Some 50,000 teen pregnancies a year are the result of rape, and two-thirds of teen mothers have a history of rape or sexual molestation, with a perpetrator averaging 27 years of age (In These Times). You won't find mention of this in editorials decrying "teenagers shouting about their 'right' to become mothers." (Plain Dealer)

Some in the press mourned the loss of the "stigma" of teen pregnancy. *Newsweek* asked, in an interview with President Clinton: "Should we reattach a stigma to those who are having children out of wedlock?" In an NBC *Nightly News* report, Betty Rollin announced, "The stigma of being an unwed mother is history." She then went on to harangue teenage girls about their pregnancies: "Did you feel any shame about this?"

The nostalgia for "stigma" suggests that what many politicians and their supporters in the media find troubling is not so much teen pregnancy as teen sexuality, and that their intention is not so much to offer young women better choices as to socially engineer the "right" kind of families.

VOICES DROWNED OUT

While they hype the urgency of the crisis, mainstream media simultaneously constrict the range of debate, such that simplistic "solutions" crowd out years of relevant research.

Charles Murray was cited in 55 major dailies and newsweeklies in the two months following his *Wall Street Journal* column; his ideas appeared in many more. . . .

On the other hand, social service agencies and research groups that actually work with pregnant teens and young mothers, who might point out the fallacies and omissions in conservative proposals, were largely missing from stories concerned with moralizing and "New Democrat" rhetoric.

Of the many newspaper and magazine articles on the topic of teen pregnancy, only a handful contained comments from actual teen mothers, whose motivations and beliefs are the subject of so much speculation. The object of high-minded harangues and the target of endless programs, their voices are easily drowned out in both the media and the policy debate.

GETTING TOUGH

The talk about Clinton's stand on teenage pregnancy as proof that he'll "get tough on entitlements" is evidence of another distressing media trend: the tendency to see complex socioeconomic issues primarily as political footballs. *Time* magazine confronted President Clinton: "There's a story in the paper today saying that the stigma has been removed from teenage pregnancy and that Democrats are responsible."

The *Cleveland Plain Dealer* summed up the significance of welfare "reform" proposals that may disrupt the lives of millions of people: "Riding on the outcome are Clinton's claim to be a 'new Democrat' and the hopes of dozens of moderate and conservative House Democrats hoping to pocket a politically popular vote in time for next year's elections."

By allowing symbolic politics to outweigh reasoned research, and by focusing attention on individual teens and their morals, media accounts of teen pregnancy sidestep just the issues politicians of both parties want to avoid: the role of structural economic forces that condemn single mothers—and many others—to poverty.

"Illegitimacy is the single most important social problem of our time—more important than crime, drugs, poverty, illiteracy, welfare or homelessness because it drives everything else."

ILLEGITIMACY IS SOCIETY'S MOST SERIOUS PROBLEM

Charles Murray

In the following viewpoint, Charles Murray contends that illegitimacy is the main underlying cause of society's most serious problems. Although Murray does not focus exclusively on teenagers, unwed teenage mothers are clearly included among the growing number of women he identifies as having children out of wedlock. Murray calls for radical changes in the way society deals with illegitimacy, including the elimination of all government support for unwed mothers. Murray is the author of *Losing Ground: American Social Policy, 1950–1980*, coauthor of *The Bell Curve: Intelligence and Class Structure in American Life*, and a fellow at the American Enterprise Institute.

As you read, consider the following questions:

1. What does Murray mean by the "white underclass"?
2. How should adoption policies be reformed, according to the author?
3. How does Murray propose to increase the appeal and rewards of marriage as a way of combating illegitimacy?

Charles Murray, "The Coming White Underclass," *Wall Street Journal*, October 29, 1993. Reprinted with permission of the *Wall Street Journal*, ©1993 Dow Jones & Company, Inc. All rights reserved.

Every once in a while the sky really is falling, and this seems to be the case with the latest national figures on illegitimacy. The unadorned statistic is that, in 1991, 1.2 million children were born to unmarried mothers, within a hair of 30% of all live births. How high is 30%? About four percentage points higher than the black illegitimacy rate in the early 1960s that motivated Daniel Patrick Moynihan to write his famous memorandum on the breakdown of the black family.

The 1991 story for blacks is that illegitimacy has now reached 68% of births to black women. In inner cities, the figure is typically in excess of 80%. Many of us have heard these numbers so often that we are inured. It is time to think about them as if we were back in the mid-1960s with the young Moynihan and asked to predict what would happen if the black illegitimacy rate were 68%.

Impossible, we would have said. But if the proportion of fatherless boys in a given community were to reach such levels, surely the culture must be *Lord of the Flies* writ large, the values of unsocialized male adolescents made norms—physical violence, immediate gratification and predatory sex. That is the culture now taking over the black inner city.

WHITE ILLEGITIMACY

But the black story, however dismaying, is old news. The new trend that threatens the U.S. is white illegitimacy. Matters have not yet quite gotten out of hand, but they are on the brink. If we want to act, now is the time.

In 1991, 707,502 babies were born to single white women, representing 22% of white births. The elite wisdom holds that this phenomenon cuts across social classes, as if the increase in Murphy Browns were pushing the trendline. Thus, in 1993 a Census Bureau study of fertility among all American women got headlines for a few days because it showed that births to single women with college degrees doubled in the last decade to 6% from 3%. This is an interesting trend, but of minor social importance. The real news of that study is that the proportion of single mothers with less than a high school education jumped to 48% from 35% in a single decade.

A LOWER-CLASS PHENOMENON

These numbers are dominated by whites. Breaking down the numbers by race (using data not available in the published version), women with college degrees contribute only 4% of white illegitimate babies, while women with a high school education or less contribute 82%. Women with family incomes of $75,000 or more contribute 1% of white illegitimate babies, while women with family incomes under $20,000 contribute 69%.

The National Longitudinal Study of Youth, a Labor Department study that has tracked more than 10,000 youths since 1979, shows an even more dramatic picture. For white women below the poverty line in the year prior to giving birth, 44% of births have been illegitimate, compared with only 6% for women above the poverty line. White illegitimacy is over-whelmingly a lower-class phenomenon.

This brings us to the emergence of a white underclass. In raw numbers, European-American whites are the ethnic group with the most people in poverty, most illegitimate children, most women on welfare, most unemployed men, and most arrests for serious crimes. And yet whites have not had an "underclass" as such, because the whites who might qualify have been scattered among the working class. Instead, whites have had "white trash" concentrated in a few streets on the outskirts of town, some-times a Skid Row of unattached white men in the large cities. But these scatterings have seldom been large enough to make up a neighborhood. An underclass needs a critical mass, and white America has not had one.

But now the overall white illegitimacy rate is 22%. The figure in low-income, working-class communities may be twice that. How much illegitimacy can a community tolerate? Nobody knows, but the historical fact is that the trendlines on black crime, dropout from the labor force, and illegitimacy all shifted sharply upward as the overall black illegitimacy rate passed 25%.

DEGRADED NORMS

The causal connection is murky—I blame the revolution in social policy during that period, while others blame the sexual revolu-tion, broad shifts in cultural norms, or structural changes in the economy. But the white illegitimacy rate is approaching that same problematic 25% region at a time when social policy is more comprehensively wrongheaded than it was in the mid-1960s, and the cultural and sexual norms are still more degraded.

The white underclass will begin to show its face in isolated ways. Look for certain schools in white neighborhoods to get a reputation as being unteachable, with large numbers of disrup-tive students and indifferent parents. Talk to the police; listen for stories about white neighborhoods where the incidence of do-mestic disputes and casual violence has been shooting up. Look for white neighborhoods with high concentrations of drug activity and large numbers of men who have dropped out of the labor force. Some readers will recall reading the occasional news story about such places already.

Top Social Problem

As the spatial concentration of illegitimacy reaches critical mass, we should expect the deterioration to be as fast among low-income whites in the 1990s as it was among low-income blacks in the 1960s. My proposition is that illegitimacy is the single most important social problem of our time—more important than crime, drugs, poverty, illiteracy, welfare or homelessness because it drives everything else. Doing something about it is not just one more item on the American policy agenda, but should be at the top. Here is what to do:

In the calculus of illegitimacy, the constants are that boys like to sleep with girls and that girls think babies are endearing. Human societies have historically channeled these elemental forces of human behavior via thick walls of rewards and penalties that constrained the overwhelming majority of births to take place within marriage. The past 30 years have seen those walls cave in. It is time to rebuild them.

A Downward Spiral

According to the Alan Guttmacher Institute, only 70 percent of women who give birth as teen-agers finish high school, compared to more than 90 percent of women who postpone childbirth. The teen-age mother's chance of attaining any higher education is very slim. With little schooling and the extra responsibilities of being a parent, life is a downward spiral. By the time her child reaches grade school, a young mother is 2.5 times less likely to own a home and 50 percent less likely to have savings than mothers who started families after they were 24.

Suzanne Chazin, *Reader's Digest*, September 1996.

The ethical underpinning for the policies I am about to describe is this: Bringing a child into the world is the most important thing that most human beings ever do. Bringing a child into the world when one is not emotionally or financially prepared to be a parent is wrong. The child deserves society's support. The parent does not.

The social justification is this: A society with broad legal freedoms depends crucially on strong nongovernmental institutions to temper and restrain behavior. Of these, marriage is paramount. Either we reverse the current trends in illegitimacy—especially white illegitimacy—or America must, willy-nilly, become an unrecognizably authoritarian, socially segregated, centralized state.

REWARDS AND PENALTIES

To restore the rewards and penalties of marriage does not require social engineering. Rather, it requires that the state stop interfering with the natural forces that have done the job quite effectively for millennia. Some of the changes I will describe can occur at the federal level; others would involve state laws. For now, the important thing is to agree on what should be done.

I begin with the penalties, of which the most obvious are economic. Throughout human history, a single woman with a small child has not been a viable economic unit. Not being a viable economic unit, neither have the single woman and child been a legitimate social unit. In small numbers, they must be a net drain on the community's resources. In large numbers, they must destroy the community's capacity to sustain itself. *Mirabile dictu*, communities everywhere have augmented the economic penalties of single parenthood with severe social stigma.

END ECONOMIC SUPPORT

Restoring economic penalties translates into the first and central policy prescription: to end all economic support for single mothers. The AFDC (Aid to Families With Dependent Children) payment goes to zero. Single mothers are not eligible for subsidized housing or for food stamps. An assortment of other subsidies and in-kind benefits disappear. Since universal medical coverage appears to be an idea whose time has come, I will stipulate that all children have medical coverage. But with that exception, the signal is loud and unmistakable: From society's perspective, to have a baby that you cannot care for yourself is profoundly irresponsible, and the government will no longer subsidize it.

How does a poor young mother survive without government support? The same way she has since time immemorial. If she wants to keep a child, she must enlist support from her parents, boyfriend, siblings, neighbors, church or philanthropies. She must get support from somewhere, anywhere, other than the government. The objectives are threefold.

THE PROBABLE OUTCOMES

First, enlisting the support of others raises the probability that other mature adults are going to be involved with the upbringing of the child, and this is a great good in itself.

Second, the need to find support forces a self selection process. One of the most short-sighted excuses made for current behavior is that an adolescent who is utterly unprepared to be a mother "needs someone to love." Childish yearning isn't a good enough selection device. We need to raise the probability that a young single woman who keeps her child is doing so volitionally and thoughtfully. Forcing her to find a way of supporting the child does this. It will lead many young women who shouldn't be mothers to place their babies for adoption. This is good. It will lead others, watching what happens to their sisters, to take steps not to get pregnant. This is also good. Many others will get abortions. Whether this is good depends on what one thinks of abortion.

Third, stigma will regenerate. The pressure on relatives and communities to pay for the folly of their children will make an illegitimate birth the socially horrific act it used to be, and getting a girl pregnant something boys do at the risk of facing a shotgun. Stigma and shotgun marriages may or may not be good for those on the receiving end, but their deterrent effect on others is wonderful—and indispensable.

ENCOURAGING ADOPTION

What about women who can find no support but keep the baby anyway? There are laws already on the books about the right of the state to take a child from a neglectful parent. We have some 360,000 children in foster care because of them. Those laws would still apply. Society's main response, however, should be to make it as easy as possible for those mothers to place their children for adoption at infancy. To that end, state governments must strip adoption of the nonsense that has encumbered it in recent decades.

The first step is to make adoption easy for any married couple who can show reasonable evidence of having the resources and stability to raise a child. Lift all restrictions on interracial adoption. Ease age limitations for adoptive parents.

The second step is to restore the traditional legal principle that placing a child for adoption means irrevocably relinquishing all legal rights to the child. The adoptive parents are parents without qualification. Records are sealed until the chid reaches adulthood, at which time they may be unsealed only with the consent of biological child and parent.

Given these straightforward changes—going back to the old way, which worked—there is reason to believe that some extremely large proportion of infants given up by their mothers will be adopted into good homes. This is true not just for flawless blue-eyed blond infants but for babies of all colors and conditions. The demand for infants to adopt is huge.

Some small proportion of infants and larger proportion of older children will not be adopted. For them, the government should spend lavishly on orphanages. I am not recommending Dickensian barracks. Today, we know a lot about how to provide a warm, nurturing environment for children, and getting rid of the welfare system frees up lots of money to do it. Those who find the word "orphanages" objectionable may think of them as 24-hour-a-day preschools. Those who prattle about the importance of keeping children with their biological mothers may wish to spend some time in a patrol car or with a social worker seeing what the reality of life with welfare-dependent biological mothers can be like.

THE REWARDS OF MARRIAGE

Finally, there is the matter of restoring the rewards of marriage. Here, I am pessimistic about how much government can do and optimistic about how little it needs to do. The rewards of raising children within marriage are real and deep. The main task is to shepherd children through adolescence so that they can reach adulthood—when they are likely to recognize the value of those rewards—free to take on marriage and family. The main purpose of the penalties for single parenthood is to make that task easier.

One of the few concrete things that the government can do to increase the rewards of marriage is make the tax code favor marriage and children. Those of us who are nervous about using the tax code for social purposes can advocate making the tax code at least neutral.

A more abstract but ultimately crucial step in raising the rewards of marriage is to make marriage once again the sole legal institution through which parental rights and responsibilities are defined and exercised.

Little boys should grow up knowing from their earliest memories that if they want to have any rights whatsoever regarding a child that they sire—more vividly, if they want to grow up to be a daddy—they must marry. Little girls should grow up knowing from their earliest memories that if they want to have any legal claims whatsoever on the father of their children, they must marry. A marriage certificate should establish that a man and a woman have entered into a unique legal relationship. The changes in recent years that have blurred the distinctiveness of marriage are subtly but importantly destructive.

Together, these measures add up to a set of signals, some with immediate and tangible consequences, others with long-term consequences, still others symbolic. They should be supplemented by others based on a re-examination of divorce law and its consequences.

VIRTUE AND TEMPERANCE

That these policy changes seem drastic and unrealistic is a peculiarity of our age, not of the policies themselves. With embellishments, I have endorsed the policies that were the uncontroversial law of the land as recently as John Kennedy's presidency. Then, America's elites accepted as a matter of course that a free society such as America's can sustain itself only through virtue and temperance in the people, that virtue and temperance depend centrally on the socialization of each new generation, and that the socialization of each generation depends on the matrix of care and resources fostered by marriage.

Three decades after that consensus disappeared, we face an emerging crisis. The long, steep climb in black illegitimacy has been calamitous for black communities and painful for the nation. The reforms I have described will work for blacks as for whites, and have been needed for years. But the brutal truth is that American society as a whole could survive when illegitimacy became epidemic within a comparatively small ethnic minority. It cannot survive the same epidemic among whites.

> "Pregnant teens are an easy target:
> they are a young, impoverished, and
> largely disenfranchised segment of
> the U.S. public."

ILLEGITIMACY AND TEEN PREGNANCY ARE NOT SOCIETY'S MAIN PROBLEMS

Sue Woodman

Many social commentators contend that illegitimacy and teenage pregnancy are the most serious problems facing society, and that they contribute to other social ills such as poverty and crime. In the following viewpoint, Sue Woodman argues that politicians and social critics have seized on the issue not because it is a genuine crisis, but in order to advance their own agendas concerning the welfare system. According to Woodman, pregnant teens have been scapegoated by politicians who find it easier to blame pregnant teens for society's problems than to address the poor social and economic conditions such teenagers experience. Woodman is a freelance writer living in New York City.

As you read, consider the following questions:

1. Why does Woodman believe pregnant teens deserve protection rather than punishment?
2. According to the Alan Guttmacher Institute, as quoted by Woodman, by what measure are sex education programs successful?
3. According to Woodman, what is a better solution to teenage pregnancy than denying benefits to pregnant teens?

Sue Woodman, "How Teen Pregnancy Has Become a Political Football," Ms., January/February 1995. Reprinted by permission of Ms. magazine, ©1995.

As welfare reform moves to the top of Washington's legislative agenda, politicians from both sides wrangle for rights to the teen pregnancy issue, a debate that panders to an increasingly moralistic and patriarchal element in this country. Already a national obsession, teen pregnancy is tailor-made for the ideological fray, since it fuses some of the most difficult political problems of the day. In teen pregnancy, the specter of poverty meets the nation's most incendiary social preoccupations: sex, sexual and reproductive freedom, abortion, and the breakup of the traditional family.

The issue of rising pregnancy rates among U.S. teens is not a new one. But after a relatively steady decline through most of the 1980s, numbers over the past few years have inexplicably started to climb again. Today, more than half of all high school students are having sexual intercourse, and about one million teenagers—12 percent of all 15- to 19-year-olds—are getting pregnant each year; teenagers are responsible for 12 percent of all the births in the U.S. This rate is higher than that of any other country in the industrialized world.

"We all know it's not good for 14-year-olds to be raising kids," says Mimi Abramovitz, author of *Regulating the Lives of Women: Social Welfare Policy from Colonial Times to the Present*. "But the children-having-children issue has become a paradigm for moralistic scapegoating at a time when politicians badly need scapegoats."

AN EASY TARGET

The very politicians who are exploiting the issue of teen pregnancy are also ignoring the dangers of teen pregnancy itself. Instead they're using society's most vulnerable group to sidestep difficult decisions and advance their own agendas for such lightning rod issues as welfare reform. Pregnant teens are an easy target: they are a young, impoverished, and largely disenfranchised segment of the U.S. public. Because it involves poor, mostly unmarried young mothers, the teen pregnancy issue taps into a vengeful national mood that blames women and demands harsh, ideological solutions to complex and seemingly intractable problems.

To face the issue of teen pregnancy head-on, politicians would have to assume the unpopular stance of protecting rather than punishing. The agenda should be not to blame girls but to fight against sexual predators, violence and incest at home, and a merchandising ethos that capitalizes on sex.

According to Washington, D.C., researchers Debra Boyer and David Fine, authors of a detailed 1992 study of young women who became pregnant during adolescence, a significant number have been physically or sexually abused at home. Boyer and Fine found that of the young women they interviewed, two thirds had been raped or sexually abused, nearly always by fathers, stepfathers, or other relatives or guardians. Other studies also show that the younger the girl who has engaged in sexual intercourse, the more likely that the sexual encounter was not consensual, and the more likely that the encounter was with an adult male.

OUT OF WEDLOCK

Cashing in on the country's self-righteous mood, many politicians are insisting that pregnant adolescents should at least marry. For a large faction, the crisis is not just that young girls are having sex, not just that they're getting pregnant and giving birth as a result, but that they're doing so out of wedlock.

Today, some 29 percent of mothers are unmarried when they give birth—the highest number in this country's history. Among teenagers, the number who are unmarried when they give birth has risen from about 270,000 in 1980 to about 370,000 in 1991. The trend of out-of-wedlock births is increasing not just in the U.S. but throughout the industrialized world. And although there are more adult women giving birth outside marriage than young poor women, the rise in out-of-wedlock births, especially among teenagers, is what the *Wall Street Journal* recently called "one of the most destructive social ills of our time."

A SOCIALLY HORRIFIC ACT

Charles Murray, President Reagan's social policy guru and author of *The Bell Curve*, which links IQ to race, brought the issue of out-of-wedlock births to public attention in the mid-1980s. Murray labeled it "the single most important social problem of our time—more important than crime, drugs, poverty, illiteracy, welfare, or homelessness because it drives everything else." In his fervor, Murray even dusted off the word "illegitimacy," pulling it out of retirement with the hope of restoring its powers of stigmatization—to "make an illegitimate birth the socially horrific act it used to be." In his book *Losing Ground*, Murray suggests that the punishment for this "horrific" act should be an end to all government subsidies, including food stamps and subsidized housing. And now Congress is calling for just such Draconian measures.

All sides of the debate are latching on to statistics to advance their own views. Liberal institutions such as New York City's

Alan Guttmacher Institute can point to numbers suggesting that, in the last two decades, while more teenagers are having sex, 19 percent fewer of them are getting pregnant. These figures, says the institute's report, show that teenagers have been using contraception more effectively. And that is an important affirmation of the belief that sex education is a necessary element in reducing teen pregnancy. "If the goal is to prevent not teen sexuality but teen pregnancy, then these programs seem to be working," says Margaret Pruitt Clark, president of Advocates for Youth in Washington, D.C.

Those whose goal is preventing teen sexuality, however, fault

---

A Conservative Hoax

[One] of the great conservative hoaxes of our time is the idea of the illegitimacy epidemic. The conservative account of illegitimacy begins with a demonstrable fact: the number of births out of wedlock, as a percentage of all births, has risen dramatically in western democracies in recent decades. Within the black community, the increase in the proportion of births to single mothers has been particularly dramatic: from 23 percent in 1960 to 28 percent in 1969, to 45 percent in 1980, to 62 percent at the beginning of the 1990s. To this indisputable statistic, conservative policy experts join another conclusion which is contested by left-liberals, but which moderate liberals and centrists have every reason to accept—namely, that children in female-headed households tend to be worse off in economic terms, and perhaps in psychological terms as well, than the children of intact families. . . .

The increase in the proportion of illegitimate births in the black community is a result, not of a strikingly greater tendency in recent decades on the part of poor blacks to have more children out of wedlock, but of the striking tendency of middle-class and affluent blacks to have fewer children in wedlock. Poor black women have had illegitimate children at a rate during the age of post-1960s "liberalism" only slightly above the rate that prevailed for poor black women during the supposed Golden Age of pre-1960s social conservatism. According to a 1995 Census Bureau Report on Characteristics of the Black Population, "the rate of babies being born to unwed black teenagers—about 80 per 1,000 unmarried teenagers—remained virtually the same from 1920 through 1990." The rise in the number of illegitimate births from 23 percent in 1960 to 62 percent in 1990 reflects, not greater fertility by poor blacks, but a significant decline in the number of legitimate births among the non-poor black majority.

Michael Lind, *Up from Conservatism: Why the Right Is Wrong for America*, 1996.

Guttmacher's findings. The right-wing Family Research Council (FRC), putting ideology over data, blasted Guttmacher's conclusions for proffering "the largest myth of them all: that the government-subsidized, contraceptive/abortion approach to teenage sexuality . . . offers hope for progress." The FRC ignores corroborating evidence from a number of well-respected adolescent sex education programs that have already shown results in reducing teen pregnancy—both by encouraging abstinence or delay, and by teaching about contraception.

Teen pregnancy has been a troubling issue since the mid-1950s, when birthrates among teens were actually higher than they are today. "But more pregnant teenagers married in the fifties, and the economy was such that even a non–high school graduate could support a family," says Pruitt Clark. "What people are really concerned about today is teen pregnancy that results in welfare dependency."

THE WELFARE REFORM DEBATE

Teen pregnancy, because it exploits the issues of poverty and sexual control, plays nicely into the welfare reform debate. In his bid to "end welfare as we know it," President Clinton has zeroed in on teenage mothers, reinforcing the national perception that they regard having babies—and plenty of them—as their meal ticket to a life of indolence at the working nation's expense.

Clinton's plan [the Work and Responsibility Act] continues the erosion of welfare benefits that began with the federal Family Support Act of 1988. This act, the brainchild of Senator Daniel Patrick Moynihan (D.-N.Y.), added a mandatory work and training component to public assistance. Clinton's version, introduced in June 1994, intends to stop welfare payments after two years, regardless of whether the recipient has found work or not. Clinton has also given free rein to state legislatures to create their own variations on the theme: at present, 15 states already have or are considering proposals that advocate some form of "family cap." These proposals all involve limiting the amount of money welfare mothers receive and the length of time they're eligible to receive it. [Clinton's plan did not pass.]

The hope behind these policies is that if welfare is harder to get, teenagers will be discouraged from giving birth to babies they have no means of supporting. But numerous empirical studies have shown that girls and women are generally not motivated by welfare payments when they decide to have babies. "Research shows that even states with higher benefits don't, by and large, have higher birthrates," says Kristin Moore, a researcher at the private nonprofit research organization Child Trends in Washington, D.C.

Adds sociologist Ruth Sidel, author of *On Her Own: Growing Up in the Shadow of the American Dream*: "The quickest way to lessen the number of children women have is to give them real options. Women with the lowest birthrates are those who have other goals in life."

"The greatest suffering and
deprivation . . .—for both mothers
and children—comes about from
unmarried teenage pregnancy."

TEENAGE PREGNANCY CAUSES POVERTY AND POOR HEALTH

Lloyd Eby and Charles A. Donovan

Many recent commentators see a causal link between the decline of the traditional two-parent family and the rise of a host of social problems. In the following viewpoint, Lloyd Eby and Charles A. Donovan argue that the current high percentage of out-of-wedlock pregnancies, including teen pregnancies, has intensified poverty, poor health, crime, and other social pathologies. Eby is assistant senior editor of the *World & I* magazine. Donovan is senior policy consultant at the Family Research Council in Washington, D.C.

As you read, consider the following questions:

1. In assessing the impact of single-parent families on children, what do the authors mean by the term "pathologies"?
2. According to Eby and Donovan, how does welfare use by married women differ from that of unmarried women?
3. What do the authors mean by the "technological" approach to avoiding pregnancy?

From Lloyd Eby and Charles A. Donovan, "Single Parents and Damaged Children: The Fruits of the Sexual Revolution." This article appeared in the July 1993 issue and is reprinted with permission from the *World & I*, a publication of The Washington Times Corporation, copyright ©1993.

The social science evidence now available shows conclusively that children suffer when they grow up in any family situation other than an intact two-parent family formed by their biological father and mother who are married to each other. As recently as 1960, the biological two-parent family was the norm; in that year, about 75 percent of children in the United States lived with both of their biological parents, who had been married only once, to one another. By 1991 this percentage had declined to about 56 percent. Now, if the darker forecasts are accurate, fewer than 50 percent of children can expect to live continuously throughout their childhood in such families. . . .

Children who grow up in single-parent families invariably suffer. The greatest suffering and deprivation, however—for both mothers and children—comes about from unmarried teenage pregnancy.

AN ACCELERATING PROBLEM

Today, the United States has a very high and increasing rate of pregnancies to unmarried teenage girls, a much higher rate than any other country in the developed world. In 1950 there were 56,000 births to unmarried teenage girls aged 15 to 19 years, and the birthrate was 12.6 births per thousand such teenagers. In 1960 there were 87,000 such births, and the rate had climbed to 15.3. Between 1961 and 1962 the rate fell slightly, although the number of such births continued to rise. From that date on, the rate has continued to rise every year, and the rate of increase itself has risen—the problem is accelerating. In 1970 there were 190,000 births to unmarried teenage mothers aged 15 to 19, and the rate of such births was 22.4 per thousand unmarried teenagers. In 1980 the figures were 263,000 births and a rate of 27.6. In 1990 the rate was 42.5 and the number of births was nearly 350,000—361,000 if we include those children born to girls under 15.

In 1990, 4,158,212 babies were born in the United States to all women. This means that of all births in 1990, about 8.7 percent—or one out of every twelve—was born to an unmarried teenager between 15 and 19 years of age. One birth in twelve may seem relatively insignificant, but the total is for births to unmarried teenagers of all races, compared to all births to all women, of whatever age or race, married or unmarried. If the statistics are broken down by race and restricted to unmarried women, a strong trend appears. Of all births to white women of all ages, the percentage of births to unmarried women in 1990 was 20.35 percent. For all births to women of all races, 28.0 percent were to unmarried women. Of all births to black women of all ages, 66.5 percent were to unmarried women.

BIRTHS TO UNMARRIED TEENAGERS

The figures for nonmarital births to girls aged 15 to 19 are even more bracing. For white teens, 56.4 percent of births were non-marital in 1990; for black teens, 91.97 percent. Overall, 67.1 percent of teen births in 1990 were nonmarital—a mirror image of the situation as recently as 1970, when 70 percent of *all* teen births were to married women.

If anything, current figures may be worse: More than half the white teens giving birth are unmarried, and among young black mothers fewer than one in ten is married. In short, hardly any births to black teenagers are to married women, and two-thirds of births to all black women are to unmarried women. Each year, one in ten black teenagers will give birth. Nearly half will become unmarried mothers before the end of their teenage years—and many will have more than one child. Another conclusion is that in the United States a large number of children of all races—and the vast majority of black children—are growing up as children of single mothers, that is, as *fatherless* children. . . .

THE COSTS OF TEEN PREGNANCY

Teenage pregnancy has costs to the mothers, to the children, and to the larger society and nation. In 1987, more than $19 billion in public funds was spent for income maintenance, health care, and nutrition for support of families begun by teenagers. Babies born to teenagers have a high risk of being born with low birth weight, and low birth weight requires initial hospital care averaging $20,000 per infant. The total lifetime medical costs for each low-birth-weight infant average $400,000. For all adolescents (married and unmarried) giving birth, 46 percent go on welfare within four years, and 73 percent of unmarried teenagers giving birth go on welfare within four years. The costs of welfare are extremely high, especially for state budgets. The total state budget for Michigan in 1992, for example, was about $30 billion, and one-third of this—$10 billion—went to the state's social service (welfare) program. Michigan's plight is similar to that of other states—it has neither the lowest nor the highest such expenditure. Moreover, members of these single-parent-headed, welfare-receiving families are at very high risk of remaining poor and ill educated throughout their lives. When married women go on welfare, they tend to get off welfare within a few years. When unmarried women go on welfare, they tend to remain there permanently. We now have the phenomenon in every state of large numbers of families, made up of unmarried women and their children, being on welfare for three or more generations, with no end in sight.

Has anyone ever heard of a child who is happy because he does not know his father? Being a child of a single mother is a handicap, regardless of the wealth, maturity, or social status of that mother.

ILLEGITIMACY IS UNHEALTHY

Fifty years ago 5 percent of American births were to unmarried women. That began to change in the 1960s. By 1970 it was 10 percent. Since then the increasing rate has produced a virtually straight line—almost 1 percent a year for 21 years. . . .

Now, trends are not inevitabilities. However, rising illegitimacy is a self-reinforcing trend because of the many mechanisms of the intergenerational transmission of poverty. . . .

America is undergoing a demographic transformation the cost of which will be crushing. Why? Because poverty is, strictly speaking, sickening. The children of unmarried women are particularly apt to be poor. And poverty, with its attendant evils—ignorance, dropping out of school, domestic and other violence, drug abuse, joblessness—is unhealthy.

George F. Will, *Conservative Chronicle*, November 10, 1993.

Numerous studies of child development have shown that growing up as the child of a single parent is linked with lower levels of academic achievement (having to repeat grades in school or receiving lower marks and class standing); increased levels of depression, stress, and aggression; a decrease in some indicators for physical health; higher incidences of needing the services of mental health professionals; and other emotional and behavioral problems. All these effects are linked with lifetime poverty, poor achievement, susceptibility to suicide, likelihood of committing crimes and being arrested, and other pathologies. . . .

PREVENTING TEENAGE PREGNANCY

It is estimated that 41 percent of unintended pregnancies among teenagers could be avoided if all sexually active teenagers used contraception. But one-fourth of such teenagers use no contraceptive method or an ineffective one. Half of all teenage pregnancies occur within six months of first sexual intercourse, and more than 20 percent of all initial premarital pregnancies occur in the first month after the initiation of sex. But the use of contraception requires planning, and planned initiation of sexual intercourse among teens is rare. Only 17 percent of women and 25 percent of men report having planned their first intercourse. The contraceptives most widely used by teenagers are the pill and condoms.

Nature equips humans with two differing timetables for maturity; physical and sexual maturity comes first, and emotional and psychological maturity appears later. Teenagers, particularly younger ones, are poorly equipped with the ability to foresee the consequences of their acts and plan accordingly. Teens tend to see themselves as invulnerable to risks. Moreover, this is a time of life when peer pressure and media pressure for engaging in sex are especially acute.

There is reliable but anecdotal evidence that, at least for many inner-city and other poor unmarried teenage girls, their pregnancies are not actually unplanned but actively desired. These studies conclude that the girls are not ignorant about contraception; they do not use it because they actually yearn for babies. Their emotional and psychological immaturity, however, does not allow them to know or understand the real consequences of motherhood, especially teenage motherhood. This is the phenomenon commonly called "babies having babies." Typically, a poor girl who has a baby while unmarried is especially vulnerable to becoming pregnant again while still in her teens.

TECHNOLOGICAL SOLUTIONS

The primary goal of teenage pregnancy prevention programs since 1970 has been to educate teenagers about the risks of pregnancy and to get them to use contraceptives; this sometimes has been derided as "throwing condoms at the problem." But teenagers typically do not go to see the school nurse or to a health clinic until after they have become sexually active; girls often go for the first time because they think they may be pregnant.

The received approach to the problem of teenage pregnancy has been "technological," in that it has relied on providing teenagers with the technology for avoiding pregnancy, or, once pregnant, with abortions as a technological solution to the pregnancy. But rising rates of teenage pregnancy, abortion, and births to teenage mothers show that these technological solutions have been anything but effective. Advanced as the "realistic" answer to the out-of-wedlock pregnancy problem, these interventions have come athwart the reality of failure statistics. Abortion has reduced the overall adolescent birthrate, but the unmarried adolescent birthrate has gone up dramatically since 1970. Adolescents have become slightly more efficient users of contraception in recent years, but they remain dramatically less so than the adult married population. Moreover, the slight increase in efficiency has been overwhelmed by three factors that are not unrelated to contraceptive availability itself: (a) an increase in the percentage of adolescents in each age cohort having sex; (b) a decrease in the age of the first reported sexual experience; and (c) increases in the frequency of intercourse and the number of sexual partners among adolescents. In this environment, more intense contraceptive use and increased pregnancy rates coexist and may be mutually reinforcing. . . .

MORAL GROUNDS

Perhaps it is time to abandon technological solutions and return to teaching abstinence on moral grounds. Although it sometimes failed, teaching children to abstain was socially, psychologically, and medically far more effective than any of the methods introduced by the sexual revolution—a revolution that was supposed to offer us freedom but that seems instead to have failed us, threatening our livelihoods, our civil order, and perhaps even our liberty itself.

> "While privileged people may see a detriment in a teenager becoming a mother, these girls see it as a realistic improvement in their lives."

PREGNANCY IMPROVES SOME TEENS' LIVES

Mike Males

Mike Males is a reporter on youth issues for In These Times magazine and the author of The Scapegoat Generation: America's War Against Adolescents. In this viewpoint, he argues that, contrary to popular opinion, the lives of many pregnant girls may improve due to their pregnancy. Pregnancy sometimes enables teens to move out of abusive homes, provides an emotional centering, and brings the guidance and support of social service agencies.

As you read, consider the following questions:

1. According to Males, what conditions or experiences often make a pregnant girl's home a poor place for her pregnancy?
2. What does the author say is misleading about the popular posters depicting teen pregnancy?
3. In Males's opinion, how does pregnancy offer a "way out" for troubled and abused teen girls?

Mike Males, "In Defense of Teenaged Mothers," Progressive, August 1994. Reprinted by permission of the Progressive, 409 E. Main St., Madison, WI 53703.

At the Crittenton Center for Young Women near downtown Los Angeles, seventeen-year-old LaSalla Jackson sets down her tiny infant and shows the scars on her calves where her drug-addicted mother beat her with an extension cord. Jackson left home when she had her baby to live at the Crittenton Center. After she graduates from the Center's high school, she plans to marry her child's twenty-three-year-old father, who visits twice a week. "I was watching five little brothers, sisters, cousins at home," she says. "Here it's one, and I'm not getting hit around."

Almonica, another Crittenton resident, saw her mother set on fire and murdered by her stepfather during a drunken fight. At age sixteen, she got pregnant by a twenty-one-year-old man. "It was a way out," she says.

KEEPING FAMILIES TOGETHER

To President Clinton [*Bush*], these unwed teenaged mothers represent an assault on family integrity and public coffers. "Can you believe that a child who has a child gets more money from the Government for leaving home than for staying home with a parent or grandparent? That's not just bad policy, it's wrong," the President declared in his State of the Union address. "We will say to teenagers: If you have a child out of wedlock, we'll no longer give you a check to set up a separate household." Clinton has won praise from liberals and conservatives alike for his "family values" campaign, which includes welfare sanctions to force unwed teen mothers back into their parents' homes. Some Congressional Republicans have proposed cutting off welfare to all teen mothers to achieve the same end. "We want families to stay together," Clinton [*Bush*] says.

But the supervising social worker at the Crittenton Center, Yale Gancherov, takes a different view. "The parents of these young women were violent, were drug abusers, were sexually abusive, were absent or neglectful. While privileged people may see a detriment in a teenager becoming a mother, these girls see it as a realistic improvement in their lives."

DIFFICULT HOME CONDITIONS

Current rhetoric about sex, values, and teenaged parenthood in the United States ignores several crucial realities. Contrary to welfare reformers' contention, many teenaged mothers cannot return home. Washington researchers Debra Boyer and David Fine's detailed 1992 study of pregnant teens and teenaged mothers showed that two-thirds had been raped or sexually abused, nearly always by parents, other guardians, or relatives.

Six in ten teen mothers' childhoods also included severe physical violence: being beaten with a stick, strap, or fist, thrown against walls, deprived of food, locked in closets, or burned with cigarettes or hot water.

PUBLIC ENEMY NO. 1

I don't know how I missed it.

I wake up one day, and welfare mothers are Public Enemy No. 1. I'd been so busy keeping track of all the other Public Enemies that the insidiousness of poor women with babies just escaped me. Over 14 million people on welfare, and they snuck up on us, just like that. Incredible. They must have been wearing sneakers. . . .

"It's now clear," begins the *Wall Street Journal*, clearing its opinionated throat for a we-mean-business editorial, "that teen pregnancy among unmarried girls is one of the most destructive social ills of our time."

Excuse me; more destructive than the handgun manufacturer's lobby and the assault-weapon makers of the globe? More destructive than the *Exxon Valdez*?

How about those wholesalers of death who peddle plastic land mines at six bucks a crack, which cost a grand each to locate after war ends, and meantime maim thousands of peasants a year, every year? More destructive than the cigarette makers and their Wall Street handmaidens? More destructive to family intactness than, oh, say, the largest 100 U.S. corporations who've downsized so precipitately that millions of middle-class families lost paychecks?

More destructive than all that? Wow. Somebody phone the city desk. We got a helluva story here. . . .

Keep talking about poor women and sex, and everyone forgets about rich white people soaking up tax subsidies on milliondollar mortgages, and retired stockbrokers cashing in the max on Social Security checks, and the whole Medicaid thing for the pretty-well-off elderly, etc.

David Nyhan, *Liberal Opinion Week*, July 4, 1994.

Most teen mothers stay with their families even under difficult conditions. More than 60 per cent of the young mothers in Boyer and Fine's study lived with their parents, foster parents, or in institutions. Nearly all the rest lived with adult relatives, husbands, or friends, often with combinations of the above. "Very few live apart from adults," says Fine. Those who did, Fine says, are often escaping intolerable situations at home. "Young mothers who live away from home are significantly more likely to have been physically or sexually abused at home than those who live with parents."

Despite all the talk of "children having children" the large majority of births—as well as sexually transmitted disease, including AIDS—among teenaged girls is caused by adults. The most recent National Center for Health Statistics data show that only one-third of births among teenaged mothers involved teenaged fathers. Most were caused by adult men over the age of twenty.

BLAMING TEEN MOTHERS

In order to mold teenaged pregnancy into a safe, expedient issue, some uncomfortable facts have been suppressed—even by groups that know better. Child advocates such as the Children's Defense Fund might be expected to speak out against official distortions of "teen" parenthood. Not so. Despite its excellent research papers, which show the complexity of the problems teenaged mothers face, a popular poster campaign by the Children's Defense Fund promotes a two-dimensional—and misleading—picture of the issue. IT'S LIKE BEING GROUNDED FOR EIGHTEEN YEARS, says one poster, depicting teenaged mothers as naughty airheads. WAIT'LL YOU SEE HOW FAST HE CAN RUN WHEN YOU TELL HIM YOU'RE PREGNANT, says another, showing a stereotypical picture of a callous varsity jock.

"Teen-adult sex is not being dealt with," says Angie Karwan of Michigan's Planned Parenthood. Part of the reason, Karwan theorizes, is that the Federal preoccupation with teenaged sex influences programs that receive grant funding. "That's how the money is awarded," she told a reporter from Michigan's *Oakland Press*.

The spin put on teen pregnancy, in turn, has some serious consequences for social policy. Present policy blames teenaged mothers for causing a multi-billion-dollar social problem. Says Health and Human Services Secretary Donna Shalala, "We will never successfully deal with welfare reform until we reduce the amount of teenaged pregnancy."

THE ROLE OF POVERTY

In fact, the opposite seems to hold: Poverty causes early childbearing. The rapid increase in child and youth poverty, from 14 per cent in 1973 to 21 per cent in 1991, was followed—after a ten-year lag—by today's rise in teenaged childbearing. Like

Ronald Reagan's anecdotes about "welfare Cadillac" black mothers, the allegation by Clinton's welfare-reform task force and members of Congress that teens have babies to collect the "incentive" of $150 a month in AFDC benefits has been repeatedly disproven.

Recent studies show that, rather than "risking the future" (the title of a 1987 National Research Council report), most adolescent mothers may be exercising their best option in bleak circumstances when they latch onto older men who promise them a "way out" of homes characterized by poverty, violence, and rape.

"Troubled, abused girls who have babies become more centered emotionally," says social worker Gancherov.

"They often gain the attention of professionals and social services. Such girls are more likely to stay in school with a baby than without. Their behavioral health improves."

Teen Mothers Are Healthier

A 1990 study of 2,000 youths found that teenaged mothers show significantly lower rates of substance abuse, stress, depression, and suicide than their peers.

"Becoming a mother is not the ideal way to accomplish these goals," Gancherov emphasizes. But impoverished girls who get pregnant may not be the heedless, self-destructive figures politicians and the media portray.

To decrease the incidence of teen pregnancy, we must improve environments for teens, Gancherov argues. Girls who see a brighter future ahead have reason to delay childbearing. Dramatically lower rates of teenaged pregnancy in the suburbs, as opposed to the inner city, bear this out.

The Clinton Administration's budget and its rhetoric offer little to millions of youth subjected to poverty and physical, emotional, and sexual violence—conditions many girls form liaisons with older men to escape. Instead, the myth Clinton and those around him continue to foster is that of reckless teenaged mothers guilty of abusing adult moral values and welfare generosity. Female "survival strategies," in the words of sociologist Meda Chesney-Lind, are what the Government seeks to punish.

In an Administration led by the most knowledgeable child advocates ever, the concerted attack on adolescents has never been angrier, more illogical, or more potentially devastating to a generation of young mothers and their babies, who cannot fight back.

PERIODICAL BIBLIOGRAPHY

The following articles have been selected to supplement the diverse views presented in this chapter. Addresses are provided for periodicals not indexed in the *Readers' Guide to Periodical Literature*, the *Alternative Press Index*, the *Social Sciences Index*, or the *Index to Legal Periodicals and Books*.

Nan Marie Astone	"Thinking About Teenage Childbearing," *Report from the Institute for Philosophy and Public Policy*, Summer 1993. Available from University of Maryland, College Park, MD 20742.
William F. Buckley	"How to Deal with Illegitimacy," *Conservative Chronicle*, May 5, 1993. Available from PO Box 11297, Des Moines, IA 50340-1297.
Suzanne Chazin	"Teen Pregnancy: Let's Get Real," *Reader's Digest*, September 1996.
Ellen Goodman	"Teens, Sex, and Consequences," *Liberal Opinion Week*, February 27, 1995. Available from 108 E. Fifth St., Vinton, IA 52349.
D. Hollander	"Studies Suggest Inherent Risk of Poor Pregnancy Outcomes for Teenagers," *Family Planning Perspectives*, November/December 1995. Available from the Alan Guttmacher Institute, 120 Wall St., 21st Fl., New York, NY 10005.
Iris F. Litt	"Pregnancy in Adolescence," *Journal of the American Medical Association*, April 3, 1996. Available from 515 N. State St., Chicago, IL 60610.
Beth Maschinot	"After the Fall," *In These Times*, March 7–20, 1994.
National Catholic Reporter	"Teenage Mothers Are Not Cause of Nation's Woes," April 28, 1995. Available from 115 E. Armour Blvd., Kansas City, MO 64111.
Kim Phillips	"Taking the Heat Off Teen Moms," *In These Times*, March 4, 1996.
S. Rodenbaugh	"Better Dead Than Unwed? Straight Talk on the Stigma of Illegitimacy," *Utne Reader*, May 1995.
Carl Rowan	"Illegitimacy: Reflections of a Broad Moral Erosion," *Liberal Opinion Week*, January 22, 1996.
George Will	"Illegitimacy Approaches Crisis Proportions," *Conservative Chronicle*, November 10, 1993.

WHAT FACTORS CONTRIBUTE TO TEENAGE PREGNANCY?

CHAPTER PREFACE

There are many competing explanations for the high rate of teenage pregnancy in recent years, ranging from a general moral breakdown in American society to such specific sources as suggestive television shows and sex education programs that some people blame for encouraging teenagers to engage in sexual activity. This chapter presents several factors that are thought to contribute to high rates of teenage pregnancy, including poverty, sexual exploitation of teenage girls, lack of parental role models, and the availability of welfare benefits.

One area of debate is whether teenage pregnancy causes poverty or whether it is a response to poverty. There is no doubt that the two conditions are closely related. In fact, 80 percent of unmarried teenage mothers grew up in extreme poverty, and a very high percentage continue to live in poverty. A number of social analysts, including scholar Judith S. Musick, believe that the lack of economic and educational prospects associated with poverty leads to a kind of hopelessness in which the idea of bearing a child at a young age seems a positive, fulfilling option. As Musick writes, "What is available to disadvantaged young women that is as emotionally satisfying as the idea of motherhood? . . . What other pathways lead so directly to achievement, identity, and intimacy?"

Other social critics argue that teenage pregnancy should be viewed as a cause rather than a consequence of poverty. When a disadvantaged teen has a baby, many argue, she merely digs herself deeper into poverty and reduces her chances of improving her economic status. Many conservatives believe that this cycle of poverty associated with teenage mothers is exacerbated by the welfare system, which provides benefits for unwed teenage mothers as long as they do not marry or get a job. According to Robert Rector, a policy analyst for the Heritage Foundation, this system encourages poor teenage girls to have babies and prevents teenage mothers from working to lift themselves out of poverty. "By undermining the work ethic, and rewarding illegitimacy," Rector writes, "the welfare system thus insidiously generates its own clientele."

The connection between poverty, welfare, and teenage pregnancy remains a hotly contested issue. This and other factors contributing to teenage pregnancy are discussed in the following viewpoints.

"Early childbearing doesn't make
young women poor; rather it is
poverty that makes women bear
children at an early age."

POVERTY IS A CAUSE OF TEENAGE PREGNANCY

Ruth Rosen

Teenage pregnancy is often blamed for perpetuating poverty in
American society. In the following viewpoint, Ruth Rosen argues that the opposite is true: Severe poverty leads teenage girls
to accept rather than avoid pregnancy and to see childbearing as
a means of improving their lives. Rosen, who writes frequently
on political and social issues, is a professor of history at the University of California at Davis.

As you read, consider the following questions:

1. According to Rosen, what percentage of unwed mothers
   grew up in extreme poverty?
2. What evidence does Rosen present to refute the depiction of
   pregnant teenagers as welfare abusers?
3. What does Rosen identify as the dominant liberal response to
   teenage pregnancy since 1975?

Ruth Rosen, "Poverty Drives Girls into Early Motherhood," Los Angeles Times, July 21, 1996.
Reprinted by permission of the author.

Amanda Simsek, a junior in high school, didn't realize she had committed a crime when she made love with her boy-friend. But authorities in Emmett, Idaho, charged the pregnant teenager with criminal fornication by resurrecting a little-known 1921 state law that holds that "any unmarried person who shall have sex with an unmarried person of the opposite sex shall be found guilty of fornication." Simsek now has a criminal record.

Across the country, cities and states are trying to stem what they view as a national epidemic in teenage pregnancy. But is there really an epidemic?

DEBUNKING MYTHS

All societies create myths, but they are eventually debunked if they are not grounded in reality. In his new book, *Up from Conservatism:Why the Right Is Wrong for America*, former conservative Michael Lind describes the illegitimacy epidemic as one of "the great conservative hoaxes of our time."

Even more convincing is *Dubious Conceptions*, Kristin Luker's stunning new account of how both liberals and conservatives "constructed" an epidemic of teenage pregnancy. Luker's metic-ulous research challenges the myth of an epidemic and con-cludes that it is poverty that causes teen pregnancy and not the reverse.

Take into account these facts:

The birth rate among teenagers has not been rising.

Most unwed mothers are not teenagers.

Teenagers account for fewer than 10% of people on welfare.

The United States has the highest proportion of pregnant teens in the developed world, yet offers less assistance to un-married mothers—child care, health care—than any other in-dustrialized nation. Aid to Families With Dependent Children ac-counts for a mere 3% of the annual federal budget.

Eighty percent of unwed teenage mothers grew up in ex-treme poverty.

CALCULATING CREATURES

Despite conservative efforts to portray unwed teenage mothers as calculating creatures scheming how to get a government check, welfare cuts during the past 20 years have not resulted in a decline in teenage pregnancies.

If there is no epidemic, why have we devoted so much moral and political capital to the crisis of teenage pregnancy?

In part, it is because Americans are still reeling from the momentous sexual, economic and social changes of the last three decades. In the 1960s, birth control ruptured the connection between sex and procreation. In the '70s, the legalization of abortion decoupled pregnancy and birth. By the '80s, a skyrocketing divorce rate had created vast numbers of "post-modern" families.

A Cause of Poverty?

At the same time, liberals and conservatives began to build separate cases for pregnancy as a cause of poverty. It was Sen. Ted Kennedy (D-Mass.) who first brought the topic of teenage pregnancy to the public's attention. Arguing that teen pregnancy caused poverty, he sought legislation in 1975 that would provide publicly funded contraception and training programs to the "babies that were having babies."

Meanwhile, the growing conservative movement waged a campaign that blamed teenagers for their degraded values and justified punitive welfare cuts. Conservatives insisted that all teenagers must abstain from sex.

A Coping Mechanism

Unfortunately, many teen males and females do not have the good fortune of living in [stable family] situations and do not see much of a future for themselves. Most young people see little employment opportunity around them and will probably face a life of low economic status, ever-present racism, and inadequate opportunities for quality education. . . . Under such conditions, it is no wonder that some young people, instead of becoming industrious and hopeful, become sexually intimate for a short-term sense of comfort, and ultimately become profoundly fatalistic. In such cases, intercourse is used as a coping mechanism. Youth workers, teachers, and counselors must replace the use of that coping mechanism with concrete and hopeful (not rhetorical) alternatives such as decent employment, a bank account, improvement in school, a place in college, or a meaningful career or vocational track. These are the elements that produce desirable outcomes in young people and reduce teen pregnancy, teen violence, and teen substance abuse.

Michael A. Carrera, *Siecus Report*, August/September 1995.

Though they differed over the solution, liberals and conservatives agreed: Teenage pregnancy causes poverty.

Challenging this consensus, Luker argues that "early childbearing doesn't make young women poor; rather it is poverty that makes women bear children at an early age. Society should not worry about some epidemic of 'teenage pregnancy,' but about the hopeless, discouraged and empty lives that early childbearing denotes."

CREATING MEANING

Interestingly, it is not the behavior of teenagers that has changed. It is middle-class women who have broken with the traditional American pattern of early childbearing. Investing in their futures, middle-class women have begun to postpone having children. In contrast, teenagers growing up in severe poverty face a dearth of opportunities for personal and professional fulfillment. Teenage mothers view childbearing as the one thing they can do that is socially responsible, gives meaning to their lives and offers hope for the future.

If poverty causes teenage pregnancy, we should be considering the political and policy changes required to address the real epidemic of widespread destitution. Ah, but it's so much more fun to blame teenagers for their impulsive, immature sexual behavior.

> "Illegitimacy is the royal road to poverty and all its attendant pathologies."

TEENAGE PREGNANCY IS A CAUSE OF POVERTY

Charles Krauthammer

In the following viewpoint, Charles Krauthammer suggests that the prevailing sexual ethic of inner-city teenagers encourages boys to casually impregnate and abandon girls. In the author's view, this situation is made possible only by the safety net of welfare, which provides for the resulting children. Krauthammer, like other conservative social commentators, believes that welfare encourages illegitimacy and teenage pregnancy, which in turn lead to poverty for single teenage mothers and their children. Krauthammer is a columnist on social issues for the Washington Post Writers Group.

As you read, consider the following questions:

1. According to Krauthammer, what do inner-city males gain by impregnating teenage girls?
2. In the author's view, how has government welfare made fathers dispensable?
3. What does Krauthammer say will result if welfare is taken away from prospective teenage mothers?

Charles Krauthammer, "Welfare Mama," *San Diego Union-Tribune*, November 23, 1993, ©1993, Washington Post Writers Group. Reprinted with permission.

"**S**ex Codes Among Inner-City Youth" is the title of a remark-able paper presented in 1993 by University of Pennsylvania Professor Elijah Anderson to a seminar at the American Enterprise Institute. Its 40 pages describe in excruciating detail the sex and abandonment "game" played by boys and girls in an inner-city Philadelphia community, one of the poorest and most blighted in the country.

FAMILY BREAKDOWN

Anderson is a scrupulous and sympathetic student of inner-city life. *Streetwise*, his book on life in a ghetto community, is a classic of urban ethnography. Five years of intensive observation and interviews have gone into the sex code study. It is the story, as told by the participants, of family breakdown on an unprecedented scale.

It is the story of a place where "casual sex with as many women as possible, impregnating one or more, and getting them to 'have your baby' brings a boy the ultimate in esteem from his peers and makes him a man." As for the girl, "her dream (is) of a family and a home." But in a subculture where for the boy "to own up to a pregnancy is to go against the peer-group ethic of 'hit and run,'" abandonment is the norm.

The results we know. Illegitimacy rates of 70 percent, 80 percent. Intergenerational poverty. Social breakdown.

Toward the end of the seminar, I suggested that the only realistic way to attack this cycle of illegitimacy and its associated pathologies is by cutting off the oxygen that sustains the system: Stop the welfare checks. The check, generated by the first illegitimate birth, says that government will play the role of father and provider. It sustains a deranged social structure of children having children and raising them alone and abandoned by their men.

THE CHANGING DEBATE

It is a mark of how far the debate on welfare policy has come that my proposal drew respectful disagreement from only about half of the panel—including, I should stress, Professor Anderson himself, who argued that the better answer is giving the young men jobs and hope through training and education for a changing economy.

In fact, the idea I proposed is not at all original. A decade ago in his book *Losing Ground*, Charles Murray offered the cold turkey approach as a "thought experiment." In October 1993 in the *Wall Street Journal*, he proposed it as policy.

Nor is this idea coming only from conservatives. Neo-liberal journalist Mickey Kaus proposed a similar idea in his book, *The End of Equality*, though in a less Draconian variant: He would replace welfare with an offer of a neo-WPA jobs program.

A REASONABLE ALTERNATIVE

What is it about living in America and Britain that makes the disastrous decision to become an unwed teen mother so attractive? There are no firm answers, but there are some hints. . . .

In the U.S. and Great Britain, unwed mothers can rely on a dole that permits them (pace nominal workfare requirements) to stay home. When free time and health benefits are added to the secure, if low, income of welfare, teen motherhood may seem a reasonable alternative to a lonely independence eked out on the minimum wage.

This is an old and controversial argument. Many have disputed the suggestion that teenage mothers are much influenced by economic incentives. It is frequently pointed out that the number of unwed mothers has continued to rise despite declines in the real value of welfare grants. But while it is true that the value of cash grants has declined from a high in the mid-1970s, new calculations suggest that once the value of additional benefits, such as food stamps, Medicaid, and free school lunches, is calculated in, the total economic value of the welfare package has risen in tandem with the growth of welfare caseloads. Life on welfare may indeed be economically rational in countries such as the U.S., where the wages of unskilled women are relatively low.

Jessica Gress-Wright, *Public Interest*, Fall 1993.

And in 1992, candidate and "New Democrat" Bill Clinton gingerly approached the idea with his "two years and out" welfare reform plan.

But "two years and out," however well-intentioned, misses the point. The point is to root out at its origin the most perverse government incentive program of all: the subsidy for illegitimacy.

HEROISM IS NOT THE NORM

Why? Because illegitimacy is the royal road to poverty and all its attendant pathologies. The one-parent family is six times more likely to be poor than the two-parent family. The numbers simply translate common sense. In a competitive economy and corrupting culture, it is hard enough to raise a child with two parents. To succeed with only one requires heroism on the part of the young mother.

Heroism is not impossible. But no society can expect it as the norm. And any society that does is inviting social catastrophe of the kind now on view in the inner cities of America.

The defenders of welfare will tell you that young women do not have babies just to get the check. Yes, there are other reasons: a desire for someone to love, a wish to declare one's independence, a way to secure the love of these elusive young males, and a variety of other illusions.

But whether or not the welfare check is the conscious reason, it plays a far more critical role. As Kaus indicated at the seminar, the check is the condition that allows people to act on all the other reasons. Take it away and the society built on babies having babies cannot sustain itself.

Moreover, society will not long sustain such a system. Americans feel a civic obligation to help the unfortunate. There is no great protest when their tax dollars go for widows and orphans.

SUBSIDIZING IMMORALITY

But by what moral logic should a taxpayer be asked to give a part of his earnings to sustain a child fathered by a young man who disappears leaving mother and child as wards of the state?

Subsidizing tragedy is one thing. Subsidizing wantonness is quite another.

In October 1993, Sen. Daniel Patrick Moynihan held a finance committee hearing on "social behavior and health care costs." In his opening statement, he drew attention to the explosion of illegitimacy in the general population. It has now reached about 30 percent of all births, 5.5 times what it was 30 years ago. It is tragedy for the people involved, a calamity for society at large. "Now then," asked Moynihan, "what are we going to do?"

Try this. Don't reform welfare. Don't reinvent it. When it comes to illegitimacy, abolish it.

| "The current welfare system is actually producing more poverty, more dependency, and much more illegitimacy."

WELFARE ENCOURAGES TEENAGE PREGNANCY

Donald Lambro

In August 1996, President Bill Clinton signed a comprehensive welfare reform bill that, among other changes, gave states the option to deny benefits to unwed teenage parents. This measure was advocated by politicians and others who believe that the availability of welfare payments encourages teenagers to become pregnant and have babies. In the following viewpoint, which was written prior to the passage of the welfare bill, conservative columnist Donald Lambro expresses this view. He contends that the welfare system, which was originally created to reduce poverty, has instead contributed to various social problems, including poverty and teenage pregnancy.

As you read, consider the following questions:

1. According to Lambro, what is one problem with having seventy-seven different federal welfare programs in place?
2. What proportion of American children are currently being reared on welfare, according to the author?
3. In the overhaul of welfare proposed by Lambro, what would all recipients be required to do to qualify for assistance?

Donald Lambro, "Welfare Increases Poverty and Illegitimacy," *Conservative Chronicle*, June 28, 1995. Reprinted by permission of United Feature Syndicate, Inc.

If you still doubt that the welfare system needs to be reformed, then you need to read Robert Rector's compelling 1995 study, "America's Failed $5.4 trillion War on Poverty."

Rector, a senior analyst at the Heritage Foundation and a specialist on welfare policy, not only shows how costly the current system is, but how counterproductive and damaging it has become and what should be done to fix it.

The $5.4 trillion in his study's title is what welfare has cost taxpayers since Lyndon Johnson's War on Poverty began in 1965. That was the year that LBJ promised us that poverty would disappear if we just spent enough money on it. We did and it didn't.

A LOT OF MONEY

Not that $5.4 trillion isn't a lot of money: It would buy every factory, office building, airline and railroad, every trucking, telephone, television, radio, and power company in the country, along with every hotel, retail and wholesale store, and the nation's commercial maritime fleet to boot.

The price tag for LBJ's war on poverty, when adjusted for inflation, is 70 percent higher than the cost of defeating Nazi Germany and Japan in World War II.

Yet the costliest welfare system that money can buy could not alleviate the problems of poverty and dependency. Indeed, if we continue doing what we're doing now, federal, state and local governments will spend another $2.38 trillion on welfare between 1995 and 2000—"all to pay for a system that is not ending poverty, but instead is rapidly destroying the family structure of America's low-income neighborhoods."

AN INSIDIOUS CYCLE

Rector's findings are that, contrary to conventional wisdom about helping the poor, the current welfare system is actually producing more poverty, more dependency, and much more illegitimacy.

The feds run 77 major welfare programs for poor and low-income Americans that frequently overlap and duplicate one another. There are, for example, 11 food aid programs costing $36 billion, eight medical aid programs costing $155.8 billion, 15 housing aid programs costing $23.5 billion, 10 education aid programs costing $17.3 billion.

More than 94 percent of the money in these programs is "means-tested" and goes directly to individuals.

But for all of this assistance, the problems that Lyndon Johnson wanted to solve in the 1960s have only grown worse—much worse.

"In welfare, as in most other things, you get what you pay for—and for 30 years the welfare system has paid for non-work and non-marriage. Now we have massive increases in both, and an explosion of illegitimacy, which breeds all manner of social ills," he says.

"By undermining the work ethic and rewarding illegitimacy, the welfare system thus insidiously generates its own clientele," he says. The more that is spent, the more people in apparent need of aid who appear. The taxpayer is trapped in a cycle in which spending generates illegitimacy and dependency, which in turn generate demands for even greater spending."

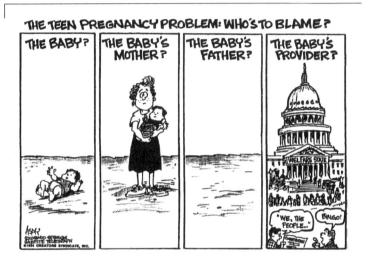

Reprinted by permission of Chuck Asay and Creators Syndicate.

The numbers then and now stunningly reveal the tragic consequences from this failed system on the breakdown of the family structure and sharply higher out-of-wedlock births.

One in every seven children is now being raised on welfare. When LBJ began his expansion of the welfare state, about one black child out of four was born out of wedlock, and overall one child out of 14 was born to an unwed mother.

Today two out of three black children are raised out of wedlock and the illegitimacy rate among low-income white high school dropouts has soared to 48 percent. Nearly one-third of America's children overall are born to unwed mothers.

This is why Rector thinks the No. 1 priority in any welfare reform must be to promote stable two-parent families and reduce illegitimacy. "Any reform that does not dramatically reduce the illegitimate birth rate will not save money and will fail to help America's children."

Any overhaul of the system must also include the requirement that welfare recipients work for their assistance from the beginning; costs must be controlled; and charities, churches and community self-help groups must be given a greater role in rebuilding moral behavior among children, including a school choice voucher program that includes religious schools.

Wisconsin State Rep. Polly Williams' inner-city school choice program will do more to lift its participants out of poverty than a dozen welfare programs ever could.

"Welfare bribes individuals into courses of behavior which in the long run are self-defeating to the individual, harmful to children and, increasingly, a threat to society," Rector wrote in a Heritage paper in 1994.

That is why any welfare reform bill that passes Congress must end cash payments to teen-age mothers and welfare recipients who continue to have children. We must stop subsidizing illegitimacy.

"[Teens] don't intend to become pregnant for any reason, much less [plan] to become pregnant so they can have a baby and go on welfare."

WELFARE DOES NOT ENCOURAGE TEENAGE PREGNANCY

Barbara Vobeja

Welfare reform legislation passed in August 1996 gave states the option to eliminate welfare benefits to unmarried teenage parents. This measure was supported by those who contend that the possibility of receiving welfare benefits encourages teenagers to have children. In the following viewpoint, which was written prior to the passage of the welfare bill, Barbara Vobeja disputes this argument. Vobeja, a staff writer for the *Washington Post*, interviews two teenage girls who say that neither their pregnancy nor their decision to keep their babies was motivated by the prospect of receiving welfare payments. Vobeja also cites social scientific studies that conclude that welfare does not play a major role in causing teenage pregnancy and childbearing.

As you read, consider the following questions:

1. According to Vobeja, why do so many teenage pregnancies seem "irresponsible" to many conservatives?
2. What percentage of unwed teenage mothers receives Aid to Families with Dependent Children within four years of giving birth, according to the author?
3. What evidence does Vobeja cite to support her argument that little correlation exists between high welfare benefits and illegitimacy rates?

Barbara Vobeja, "Welfare Check, Reality Check," *Washington Post National Weekly Edition*, March 13-19, 1995, ©1995, The Washington Post. Reprinted with permission.

Seventeen-year-old April Whetstone, a pale, weary-eyed mother of a month-old girl, has her own theories about why so many teenagers are having babies. "A lot of girls get pregnant so they can keep their boyfriends," she says. Others do it for attention. "I didn't intend for it to happen," she says, cradling her baby Natalie, on her shoulder. "I guess I was looking forward to have somebody love me back."

On one point, Whetstone is absolutely clear: She was not thinking about a welfare check when she became pregnant.

A BURDEN TO SOCIETY

The forces behind teenage childbearing are at the heart of the current national debate over welfare reform, with Congress arguing over a fundamental question: Can lawmakers bring down the high number of births to unwed teenage mothers by rewriting federal welfare regulations?

Whetstone is among more than 1 million American teenagers who become pregnant each year. About half will go on to give birth, and of those, 70 percent will be unmarried. They make up less than one-third of out-of-wedlock births, but for a variety of reasons, they present a disproportionate economic and social burden to society.

In his State of the Union address for 1995, President Clinton called teenage pregnancy "our most serious social problem."

Studies have shown that the costs to society are enormous: Children of teenage mothers are more likely to have behavioral problems, fail in school and become teenage parents themselves, some of which is related to poverty. Nearly half of the current caseload on Aid to Families with Dependent Children (AFDC), the nation's basic cash welfare program, began their families as teenagers.

Convinced that the availability of welfare has contributed to teenage births, a group of House Republicans is proposing that unwed mothers under age 18 be denied AFDC. [Legislation passed in August 1996 gives states the option to deny benefits to unwed teenage mothers.]

"It is irresponsible to give grants to somebody you would not let baby-sit your kids or your grandkids," says Republican Rep. E. Clay Shaw Jr. of Florida, chairman of the House subcommittee responsible for welfare reform.

Shaw and other conservatives argue that the nation's welfare system has underwritten the irresponsible behavior of teenagers and other unmarried couples who conceive and bear children when they are not able to support them.

The provision . . . also would allow states to use the savings to provide other services to young mothers—including education, training and group homes.

The proposal to cut off federal assistance has drawn sharp criticism from advocates for the poor, who say innocent children would suffer. And social scientists are skeptical that such a policy would make a significant difference in birthrates.

CHANGING BEHAVIOR

The challenge of changing behavior by tinkering with federal policy is underscored in a red-brick, white-trimmed group home outside Atlanta where Whetstone and a dozen other young mothers live with their babies. Their histories make clear the interplay between teenage parenthood and welfare is complex and the reasons young women become pregnant are difficult to tease apart and deal with.

Whetstone says she is not sure why she became pregnant. Her mother knew she was sexually active and warned her to use contraceptives, but Whetstone didn't believe it would happen to her. "I don't blame nobody," she says. "I should have known better. I was young and stupid. . . . I'm still young."

With adolescent bravado, Whetstone describes how her boyfriend and family pressured her to give up the baby for adoption. She considered it, but at the last minute she decided against it. She wasn't sure how she would take care of her daughter. "I quit school. I didn't have a car, I didn't have a job. I didn't have nothing. My mom didn't want me to live off her. . . . I agree. . . . You need to be responsible for your own actions."

At no point, Whetstone says, was her decision to have or keep her baby influenced by the availability of welfare. She says she doesn't want to apply for AFDC now because she fears the government would go after her boyfriend for child support. He gives her $100 every two weeks, she says.

Whetstone has moved into the Family Development Center—a complex of 14 efficiency apartments for young, unmarried mothers who are considered homeless—run by a nonprofit agency, Families First.

She hopes to get her high school equivalency diploma, take computer classes and get a part-time job. She finds it kind of exciting, she says, to be on her own, living in a dorm-like room furnished with a single bed, a chest of drawers and a crib.

Nationally, half of unwed teenage mothers go on AFDC rolls within four years of giving birth. And many of the women at the Family Development Center receive a monthly AFDC check for $235—the benefit allowed a mother and child in Georgia.

Quara Harbin, 19, the mother of a 2-month-old girl, says she too became pregnant unintentionally. "It happened," she says. She knew she couldn't stay with her mother, a single parent with seven children. So she moved into a maternity home, also run by Families First.

PLAIN LUNACY

We have become a society in which sex and the exploitation of it dominates American mores. Pre-marital and extra-marital sex are now commonplace. The stigma of bearing a baby without the convenience (or inconvenience) of marriage has virtually vanished. . . .

It is lunacy to believe that withdrawing a pittance of money to support teenagers and their babies will counteract all the sexual forces that are at work in America, causing young women to stop having sex—and babies—before marriage. Yes, lunacy. Plain, unadulterated lunacy.

Carl Rowan, *Liberal Opinion Week*, January 22, 1996.

When she was pregnant, she says, she worried about how she would care for her child, and considered abortion and giving up her baby for adoption. "I had my mind on other things," she says. "I wasn't thinking about AFDC."

But after she gave birth, Harbin applied for welfare. Now, she pays about $60 a month in rent and uses the rest of her check to cover formula, diapers and supplies for the baby. Losing that check, she says, "would hurt me. I'm struggling. The money is really not for us, it's our children. It's hard enough trying to depend on the baby's daddy. I really need the AFDC."

PREVENTING SEX?

At the same time, Harbin, like many other mothers here, complains about welfare abuse and says she has known of women who got pregnant to get on welfare. Still, most of the mothers say they do not believe that cutting welfare would keep very many teenagers from having sex.

Tanya Davis, 22, who gave birth to a baby girl, echoes the argument of some antiabortion groups and academics that such a policy won't keep young women from becoming pregnant, but it might keep them from having the baby.

In Washington, proponents of the policy . . . argue that even if it does little to hold down teenage birthrates, it will send the proper signal to the nation: that taxpayers will no longer subsidize irresponsible behavior.

Gary Bauer, president of the Family Research Council, suggests that benefits should be cut off for any out-of-wedlock births, not just for teenagers, and that a national campaign should discourage sexual activity outside marriage. "I may be unrealistic, but I think . . . sending that cultural message and ending the subsidies would influence behavior," he says.

Critics disagree.

RESEARCH RESULTS

Kristin Moore, executive director of Child Trends, a research organization in Washington, says research does not show that welfare benefits are a major factor in teenage births.

Social scientists cite as evidence of the minor role welfare plays in decisions to have a baby the fact that states with high benefit levels do not have higher out-of-wedlock birthrates than those with very low benefits.

Social scientists also note that as benefit levels nationally have fallen over the past 15 years, out-of-wedlock birthrates have risen rapidly. Moreover, teenage birthrates are much higher in the United States than they are in other industrialized countries, including those with much more generous welfare programs.

"Teens are not planners," Moore says. "They don't intend to become pregnant for any reason, much less planning to become pregnant so they can have a baby and go on welfare."

Frank Furstenberg Jr., a sociologist at the University of Pennsylvania, says there is "no prospect" that the policy of denying aid would lead teenagers to defer sexual activity or use contraception more carefully.

"What's likely to occur is probably more abortions and more children ill cared for and that much poorer." The policy, he says, is "an emotional response . . . based on a tremendous amount of misinformation."

THE POVERTY CONNECTION

Furstenberg and others call for longer-range strategies, including programs that help at-risk students stay in school and move from school to work. Critics of the welfare cutoff proposal do not, however, minimize the problems of youthful pregnancies, most obviously poverty.

A study by the Annie E. Casey Foundation, for example, found that nearly 80 percent of children born to unmarried teenagers without a high school diploma were living in poverty at ages 7 to 12, compared with 8 percent of children born to older, married mothers who finished high school.

The recurring nature of the problem is obvious at the Family Development Center, where many of the residents were themselves born to teenage mothers. A few months after giving birth, often before they have hit their twenties, these young women have crossed a great divide.

"I had to find out the hard way," says 17-year-old Netaya Chambers, whose daughter, Shaniya, is about 6 months old. Chambers applied for welfare, but does not know if she will qualify because she has been working, after school, as a waitress. Even so, she says welfare did not enter into her decision to keep her baby.

"Some girls act like they want a baby," she says. "They don't know how hard it is. Babies are cute, but they also cost money. It's hard. I have to go to school and she wakes up in the middle of the night. . . . For me, being so young, I had to grow up. I notice I can't get everything my way."

"*A 1992 Washington state study found that 62 percent of 535 teen mothers had been raped or molested before they became pregnant; the offenders' mean age was 27.4 years.*"

SEXUAL ABUSE IS A FACTOR IN TEENAGE PREGNANCY

Joe Klein

Joe Klein, a columnist on social issues for *Newsweek* magazine, focuses in the following viewpoint on the strong correlation between teenage pregnancy and sexual abuse. Klein argues that a large percentage of teenage girls who become pregnant are victims of seduction and rape by adult men. He criticizes both liberals and conservatives for failing to address this dimension of the teenage pregnancy problem.

As you read, consider the following questions:

1. According to Klein, why does the social work community's philosophy of keeping families together frequently produce disastrous results?
2. What desire or yearning in many young girls fuels the "predator problem," according to the author?
3. Why, according to the author, is it so hard to prosecute male predators under statutory rape laws?

S he wants to be called Charlette. She lives in a New York shelter for teenagers who've had babies. Her story is not unusual. The guy's name was Mickey. He was older, in his mid-20s. Charlette was going through a bad time: her stepfather had come home from prison, was beating her mother, was beating on her. "I lived in the streets for a while, starting when I was 14," she said. "I was young and vulnerable, I had problems. He was going to protect me, teach me things, discipline my mind. But when I told him I was pregnant, he was gone. I began to ask around. I asked his cousin. I found he had six other children, mostly with younger girls. I was naive, and he took advantage of me."

A FORM OF CHILD ABUSE

This is what we're learning about teen pregnancy: it is, too often, a form of child abuse. An Alan Guttmacher Institute study in the summer of 1995 found that 66 percent of all teen mothers had children by men who were 20 or older. In many cases, the age spread isn't extreme—three or four years. But a 1990 California survey seemed to indicate that the younger the girl, the older the guy (among mothers aged 11–12, the father was an average 10 years older). And a 1992 Washington state study found that 62 percent of 535 teen mothers had been raped or molested before they became pregnant; the offenders' mean age was 27.4 years. "This is a situation that no one really wants to talk about," says Aurora Zapata of Homes for the Homeless in New York, "but everyone knows it's true."

No one wants to talk about the situation because it is inconsistent with the prevailing mythologies about teen pregnancy, both liberal and conservative. No one wants to talk about it because it exposes the criminal stupidity of the national debate over welfare reform. Conservatives are uncomfortable because it posits another victim class: girls who become pregnant aren't just amoral, premature tarts—they are prey. Who could support cutting off these children's benefits, as some Republicans have proposed? But liberals are also uncomfortable because the data are further proof that an intense social pathology—a culture of poverty—has overwhelmed the slums. Certainly, these studies raise huge new questions about the social work community's disastrous ideology of "family preservation." The "families" preserved too often house a sexual predator: a stepfather, mom's boyfriend, an "uncle." In any case, single parents—usually former teenage mothers themselves—seem quite unable, and sometimes unwilling, to stop the abuse. "They do not want to admit it's their men who are doing this," says Zapata. "In many cases they're not unhappy their daughter is having a baby. It brings more [welfare] money into the household."

POWERLESS AND FATHERLESS

The psychology at work is deep and discouraging. For the men, hitting on young girls may be a consequence of powerlessness—though one wonders what sort of man is empowered by the rape of an 11-year-old—compounded by the absence of all ethical moorings and by a welfare system ready to bankroll irresponsibility. As for the girls, who are inevitably fatherless, Charlette's yearning for protection—for a *father*—seems entirely comprehensible. (No doubt many young girls also expect that a new baby would bring fulfillment and status in an otherwise bleak world.) "The most depressing thing is, these behavior patterns are tacitly condoned," says Kathleen Sylvester of the Progressive Policy Institute. "Not enough mothers say, 'You're too young to be with a man' or 'That guy's too old for you.'"

NOT "STRANGER DANGER"

A 1992 report by the American Medical Association estimates that 61% of all U.S. victims of sexual assault are under the age of 18. That is, according to the AMA, most of the sexual violence that occurs in this country is directed against children. U.S. Bureau of Justice figures for the same year revealed that one of every six rape victims is under 12. And in spite of a few highly publicized incidents and many urgent warnings about "stranger danger," 80% of all sexual assaults against children are committed by family members, friends, and acquaintances. . . .

Unfortunately, as reported in a 1987 American Bar Association study, offenders known to the victim—the vast majority—are far less likely to be prosecuted and incarcerated than those who victimize strangers. When sentences are handed down for child sexual abuse, they are generally shorter than sentences for adult-adult sex crimes—in spite of the long-term consequences of child assault.

Bronwyn Mayden, *Children's Voice*, Winter 1996.

What to do? Enforcement of statutory rape laws, especially for serial progenitors like Charlette's partner, would seem a good idea. "Child abuse is a crime," says Sylvester. "A lot of these guys should be in jail. But it's very hard to get the girls to testify—they're ashamed, they're frightened and in many cases they still have an emotional attachment." What to do? The nostrum that pregnant teenagers must live at home in order to receive welfare money seems exactly the wrong thing. "The only way to break the cycle," says Aurora Zapata, "is to get them out of those homes."

A Return to Orphanages

Kathleen Sylvester has proposed a system of government funded, privately run "second-chance homes" where pregnant teens could be protected from predators, given something like the structure and support of a permanent home, taught motherhood and morality. In other words: orphanages. But liberals, enthralled by social work ideologues and "family preservation" fantasists, tend to blanch at both the word and the concept; most conservatives simply don't want to spend the money. Still, there was surprising support for a $150 million "second-chance home" pilot project—especially among conservatives, who see it as an alternative to cash payments—in the Welfare Reform Act vetoed by the president.

But . . . a stray "second-chance home" here or there isn't going to put much of a dent in this disgraceful situation, nor will it provide much evidence about the effectiveness of removing these children from dysfunctional families. Someone—some small state or big city—has to propose an intensive experiment with the idea, perhaps even a mandatory program for pregnant children under the age of 15: if you want government support, you can only get it at a "second-chance home." "I'd like to see it given a try," says Charles Murray, the sociologist who first proposed cutting teenagers off the dole. "At the very least, it might have a deterrent effect. Of course, I'd also like to see some city try a complete suspension of benefits, so we could compare the results." That's probably a bridge too far, even for most conservatives. But I wonder: Breathes there a Republican governor with the courage to request a federal waiver for a real "second-chance" project in one of his cities? Breathes there a New Democrat president with the courage to grant it?

"Until we are ready to take a hard look
at the real causes of teen pregnancy—
in large part, the sexual exploitation of
teenage women by much older
men—the hysteria will remain and
the problem will go unsolved."

ADULT MEN ARE LARGELY RESPONSIBLE FOR TEENAGE PREGNANCY

Linda Villarosa

In the following viewpoint, Linda Villarosa argues that most teenage pregnancies are the result of sexual exploitation of teenage girls by adult men. Because they fail to account for this, she insists, both liberal and conservative solutions for teenage pregnancy are ineffective. She maintains that neither reforming welfare nor increasing sex education programs will solve the problem. Instead, she contends, men must be held accountable for their sexual behavior. Villarosa is the coauthor of *Finding Our Way: The Teen Girls' Survival Guide*, and the editor of *Body & Soul: A Black Woman's Guide to Health*.

As you read, consider the following questions:

1. According to the author, why would cutting welfare benefits make a bad situation worse?
2. Why, according to Villarosa, are sex education approaches to preventing teenage pregnancy ineffective?
3. What does Villarosa say is the most important component of the effort to reduce teenage pregnancy?

Linda Villarosa, "Who's Really Makin' Babies?" *Third Force*, March/April 1996. Reprinted by permission of the Center for Third World Organizing.

The subject of teenage pregnancy draws a great deal of hysterical political attention. Politicians have used the 370,000 babies born each year to teenage mothers to justify their own agendas for everything from establishing national morality to dismantling or saving the welfare safety net. Driven by political motives, they have offered up a number of solutions.

THE ROLE OF OLDER MEN

Pregnancy and childbearing can be devastating to teenage girls. Adolescent mothers are less likely than older mothers to be employed and to find work with adequate wages. They are far more likely than their peers to drop out of school. But none of the solutions—from the shortsighted and narrow-minded ("close your legs, pull down your skirt") to the misguided and cruel ("cut off welfare benefits to unmarried women who have children and require unwed teen mothers to live at home") to the well-meaning and progressive ("provide birth control and sex education in schools")—make any real sense on their own. Virtually all the current solutions designed to attack teen pregnancy individualize the problem, telling teenage women to avoid or manage pregnancy by making them take action on their own. Until we are ready to take a hard look at the real causes of teen pregnancy—in large part, the sexual exploitation of teenage women by much older men—the hysteria will remain and the problem will go unsolved.

Two recent studies shed new light on the subject of teen pregnancy. A survey by the National Center for Health Statistics notes that 67 percent of teenage mothers are impregnated by men who are over 20 years old. In other words, approximately 700,000 teenage pregnancies every year involve men who are 20 to 50 years old. Whether coerced or voluntary, couplings between teenage girls and adult males are many times more likely to result in pregnancy than teen-teen sex. In fact, the younger the girl, the older the man. Several other studies are equally shocking: researchers Debra Boyer and David Fine note that two-thirds of young women who become pregnant during adolescence have previously been sexually abused or raped, nearly always by fathers, stepfathers, other relatives or guardians.

The Alan Guttmacher Institute (AGI) reports that 74 percent of girls under age 14 who have had sex are victims of rape. A study by the American Association of University Women finds that one in five girls in grades 8 to 11 is sexually harassed by teachers or staff.

Conservative proposals have merged the reshaping of American morality with racist political expediency. Cutting off welfare benefits to unwed teens not only won't help but could send a young family spiraling rapidly downward. AGI reports that 83 percent of teenagers giving birth are from poor or low-income families. Their initial economic disadvantage explains their poverty after childbirth. In the majority of cases, having a child only worsens the already existing problem. Child Trends, a non-profit research organization, has found that childbirth is not tied to welfare payments and that states with higher benefits don't necessarily have higher birth rates. The ridiculous proposal to force young mothers to live at home puts them back in the hands of the male relatives who may have sexually abused them in the first place.

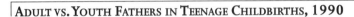

ADULT VS. YOUTH FATHERS IN TEENAGE CHILDBIRTHS, 1990

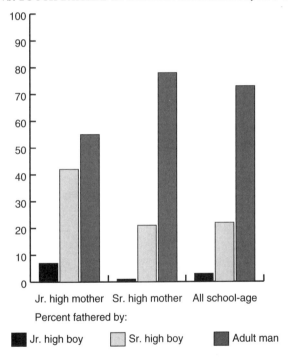

Source: Mike Males, EXTRA!, March/April 1994.

The same organizations putting forth these proposals have rabidly dismantled sex education in schools in an attempt to "return" power and control to parents, especially fathers. Emphasizing an abstract notion of family values and demanding abstinence—as groups such at the Traditional Values Coalition and the American Enterprise Institute insist must be done—is a waste of time and resources. But self-righteously scapegoating and bullying young women is easier for conservative groups than taking a hard look at the sexual exploitation and incest that is going on within families and schools.

POWER RELATIONS

It is tempting to simply discredit traditional right-wing approaches to deterring teen pregnancy, but solutions on the other end of the political spectrum are almost as ineffective. Merely offering sex education and even distributing birth control in school ignores the fact that many teens are impregnated by rape and, worse, exploited by some of the very educators who would be teaching their sex-education classes. Even more to the point, school sex education fails to reach the older men who have either graduated or dropped out of school and who are fathering most of the babies born to teen girls. Such solutions, motivated in part by the urge to protect sexual liberty and choice, still do not address the fundamental power relations between men and women, and between adults and children, that lie at the heart of this issue.

DEMANDING RESPONSIBILITY

Given all the information available, it is time for parents, politicians, educators, health advocates and community organizations to take bold and thoughtful action. The first and most difficult step is to eradicate the poverty that is directly linked to so many social problems, including adolescent pregnancy. This project requires us to include a structural economic analysis as we intervene in this issue. Second, we must stop turning a blind eye on the sexual exploitation of teenage girls—both inside and outside the family. It's time to quit pretending that these young women become pregnant from space aliens or through immaculate conception and demand that men, especially older men, take responsibility for their actions. We have to be prepared to fight that fight aggressively in all the institutions through which men learn to own women's sexuality and women learn to give it up. Those institutions include churches, the media and schools, as well as the family. Teachers and parents, supported by their organizations, must also begin to speak to young women and men honestly about dealing with sexual abuse, having or postponing sex, contraception, safer sex and personal responsibility.

Most important of all, young women must learn to fight together for the kinds of deep-reaching programs that will help them to learn physical and verbal self-defense, protect their right to set sexual boundaries and give them space to develop self-esteem that extends far beyond their sexual value to men. Girls who are strong—who have something going on in their lives and who care about themselves, their bodies and their communities—are better able to fend off sexual exploitation and avoid unwanted pregnancy.

| "*A girl growing up with a close father internalizes a sense of love, which sends up warning signals when a boy on the prowl begins to strut near her.*"

LACK OF PARENTAL INFLUENCE IS A FACTOR IN TEENAGE PREGNANCY

Kay S. Hymowitz

Much of the current debate about the causes of teenage pregnancy has focused on the topics of welfare benefits and sex education. Kay S. Hymowitz argues that parental influence, or lack thereof, is the most significant variable in the teenage pregnancy equation. Through interviews with many pregnant teenagers, Hymowitz has concluded that the absence of a father is the primary factor that leads many teenage girls to become pregnant and to have children. Hymowitz is a journalist writing for *City Journal*, published by the Manhattan Institute, a nonpartisan public policy research organization.

As you read, consider the following questions:

1. According to Hymowitz, what do many teenage girls believe is the best evidence of their maturity?
2. What two social changes of the late 1960s have promoted extended adolescence and increased teenage pregnancy, according to the author?
3. In the author's view, how does the experience of Asian-Americans tend to validate her theory about parental influence?

From Kay S. Hymowitz, "The Teen Mommy Track," *City Journal*, Autumn 1994. Reprinted by permission of the Manhattan Institute for Policy Research.

Fourteen-year-old Taisha Brown is thinking of having a baby. She doesn't say so directly, and it doesn't seem about to happen tomorrow, but she smiles coyly at the question. Around her way—a housing project in the South Bronx—lots of girls have babies. Her 16-year-old cousin just gave birth a few months ago, and she enjoys helping with the infant. "I love babies," the braided, long-legged youngster says sweetly. "They're so cute. My mother already told me, 'If you get pregnant, you won't have an abortion. You'll have the baby, and your grandmother and I will help out.'" What about school or making sure the baby has a father? "I want to be a lawyer . . . or maybe a teacher. Why do I need to worry about a father? My mother raised me and my sister just fine without one."

ACTUAL EXPERIENCES OF TEENAGERS

Taisha Brown seems likely to become one of the nearly half-million teenagers who give birth each year in the United States, a number that gives the nation the dubious honor of the highest teen birth rate in the developed world. About two-thirds of those girls are unmarried; many are poor. Americans debating welfare reform and the state of the family have no shortage of opinions about the cause of the problem: welfare dependency, low self-esteem, economic decline, ignorance about birth control—the list could go on and on. All these theories fail to explain the actual experiences of teenagers, because they ignore the psychology of adolescence, the differences between underclass and mainstream cultural norms, and the pivotal role of family structure in shaping young people's values and expectations.

To get a clearer focus on the teen pregnancy problem, I spoke with some thirty new or expectant young mothers and sometimes with their boyfriends, nurses, teachers, and social workers. (To protect their privacy, I've identified the teenagers with fictitious names.) I asked about their lives, their expectations, and their babies. The girls' stories vary widely: from a 15-year-old, forced to live in seven different foster homes over the last five years, whose sunken eyes hint of Blakean misery, to a 17-year-old college student who describes herself as "old-fashioned" and has been cheerfully dating the same boy for five years.

It gradually became clear that, however separated they may be by degrees of poverty and family disorder, these girls all live in a similar world: a culture—or subculture to be precise—with its own values, beliefs, sexual mores, and, to a certain extent, its own economy. It is, by and large, a culture created and ruled by children, a never-never land almost completely abandoned by fathers and, in some sad cases, by mothers as well. But if such a culture is made possible by adult negligence, it is also enabled by mixed messages coming from parents, teachers, social workers, and the media—from mainstream society itself.

Sociologists sometimes use the term "life script" to refer to the sense individuals have of the timing and progression of the major events in their lives. At an early age, we internalize our life script as it is modeled for us by our family and community. The typical middle-class American script is familiar to most readers: childhood, a protracted period of adolescence and young adulthood required for training in a complex society, beginning of work, and, only then, marriage and childbearing. The assumption is not merely that young adults should be financially self-supporting before they have children. It is also that they must achieve a degree of maturity by putting the storms of adolescence well behind them before taking on the demanding responsibility of molding their own children's identity.

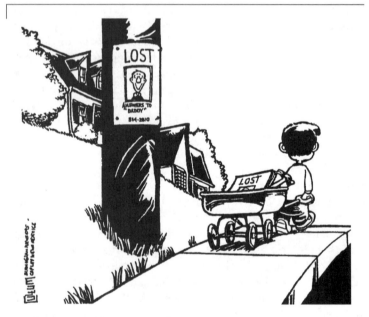

Cullum. Reprinted by permission of Copley News Service.

But for the minority teens I spoke with, isolated as they are from mainstream mores, this script is unrecognizable. With little adult involvement in young people's daily activities and decisions, their adolescence takes on a different form. It is less a stormy but necessary continuation of childhood—a time of emotional, social, and intellectual development—than a quasi-adulthood. The mainstream rites of maturity—college, first apartment, first serious job—hold little emotional meaning for these youngsters. Many of the girls I spoke with say they aspire to a career, but these ambitions do not appear to arise out of any deep need to place themselves in the world. Few dream of living on their own. And all view marriage as irrelevant, vestigial.

To these girls and young women, the only thing that symbolizes maturity is a baby. A pregnant 14-year-old may refer to herself as a "woman" and her boyfriend as her "husband." Someone who waits until 30 or even 25 to have her first child seems a little weird, like the spinster aunt of yesteryear. "I don't want to wait to have a baby until I'm old," one 17-year-old Latino boy told me. "At 30, I run around with him, I have a heart attack."

The teen mommy track has the tacit support of elders like Taisha's mother, many of whom themselves gave birth as teenagers. Even if they felt otherwise, the fact is that single mothers in the inner city don't expect to have much control over their kids, especially their sons, after age 13—on any matter. And, with few exceptions, the fathers of the kids I spoke with were at best a ghostly presence in their lives. . . .

NEVER-NEVER LAND

The failure to understand the power of cultural norms over youngsters, especially norms that coincide so neatly with biological urges, has created a policy world that parallels but never quite touches the never-never land of underclass teenagers. Dwellers in the policy world seem unable to make the leap of sympathetic imagination needed to understand the mindset of the underclass adolescent. Instead, they assume that everyone is born internally programmed to follow the middle-class life script. If you don't follow the mainstream script, it's not because you don't have it there inside you, but because something has gotten in your way and derailed you—poverty, say, or low self-esteem, or lack of instruction in some technique such as birth control.

According to this view, to say that teen pregnancy perpetuates poverty has it backwards. Instead, writes Katha Pollit in the *Nation*, "It would be closer to the truth to say that poverty causes early and unplanned childbearing. . . . Girls with bright futures—college, jobs, travel—have abortions. It's the girls who have nothing to postpone who become mothers." But evidence contradicts the notion that early childbearing is an automatic response to poverty and dim futures. After all, birth rates of women aged 15 to 19 reached their lowest point this century during the hard times of the Depression. And in the past forty years, while the U.S. economy has risen and fallen, out-of-wedlock teen births have only gone in one direction—up, and steeply. Meanwhile, in rural states like Maine, Montana, and Idaho, the out-of-wedlock birth rate among African-Americans is low, not because there is less poverty but because traditional, mainstream norms hold sway.

A related but also flawed theory is that a lack of self-esteem caused by poverty and neglect is at the root of early pregnancy. But the responses of the girls I spoke with were characterized more by a naive adolescent optimism than by a sad humility, depression, or hopelessness. Indeed, a study commissioned by the American Association of University Women found that the group with the highest self-esteem is African-American boys, followed closely by African-American girls.

POOR SELF-ESTEEM?

Self-esteem has a different foundation in a subculture that, unlike elite culture, values motherhood over career achievement. To listen to some policymakers, one might think that wanting to become a lawyer or anchorwoman—and possessing the requisite orderliness, discipline, foresight, and bourgeois willingness to delay gratification—are natural instincts rather than traits developed over time through adults' prodding and example. With little sympathetic understanding of the underclass teen heart, David Ellwood, an assistant secretary of Health and Human Services, has written: "The overwhelming proportion of teenagers do not want children, and those who do simply cannot realize what they are in for. It is not rational to get pregnant at 17, no matter what the alternatives appear to be."

Ellwood's notion of rationality presupposes that a teenager is following the middle-class life script. This failure to understand the underclass teen's world view leads him to embrace another deep-seated but mistaken theory: that unwed teen childbearing is the result of inadequate sex education. "Teenage pregnancy is a matter of information, contraception, and sexual activity, all of which might plausibly be changed," he writes. Most sex education curriculums, including those that "stress abstinence," rely on the same belief in a fundamentally rational teenager. They set out to train students in "decision making skills," "planning skills," or something mysteriously called "life skills." Explain the facts, detail the process, the bulb will go on, and the kids will get their condoms ready or just say no. . . .

Governor Mario Cuomo took the fallacy of the underclass teenager with a bourgeois soul to its logical extreme when he remarked recently: "If you took a 15-year-old with a child, but put her in a clean apartment, got her a diploma, gave her the hope of a job . . . that would change everything." But it takes more than a governor's decree to transform an underclass 15-year-old into a middle-class adult. Many programs for teen mothers find it necessary to teach them not only how to interview for a job, but also how to shop for food, how to budget money, how to plan a menu, even how to brush their teeth. Programs like these point to the devilishly tricky problem of resolving the tension between the mainstream and underclass life scripts.

Moreover, instead of discouraging unwed teen pregnancy, such programs often end up smoothing it into an alternative lifestyle. If Taisha Brown does become pregnant, she will be able to leave her dull, impersonal school for a homey, nurturing middle school for pregnant girls like herself. Later, she will very likely find a high school with a nursery where she can stop by between classes and visit with her baby, attend parenting classes, receive advice about public assistance, and share experiences with other teen mothers in counseling groups. Kathleen Sylvester of the Progressive Policy Institute, who has visited such a school in Baltimore, says it is far nicer than ordinary public schools. "It's cheerful, warm; you get hugs and lots of attention." These programs have been introduced with the best of intentions—to ensure that teen mothers will continue their education. But because of them, it will seem to Taisha that the world around her fully endorses early motherhood.

THE ROLE OF WELFARE

Conservatives, most notably Charles Murray, see the roots of this normalization in Aid to Families with Dependent Children and other welfare subsidies that provide an economic incentive for illegitimacy. But even if welfare ignited the initial explosion of out-of-wedlock births in the 1960s, its role in shaping social norms today seems less vital. The Census Bureau reports that the number of children living with a never-married parent soared by more than 70 percent between 1983 and 1993. The birth rate among single women in professional and managerial jobs tripled during the same period. Increasingly America seems a land in which, as Mort Sahl has joked, the only people who want to get married are a few Catholic priests, and the only people who want to have babies are lawyers nearing menopause—and impoverished children. In a world so out of whack, welfare seems only a bit player.

All of the prevailing analyses of teen childbearing, both liberal and conservative, neglect a troubling truth apparent throughout most of human history: nothing could be more natural than a 16-year-old having a baby. But in complex societies such as our own, which require not just more schooling but what the great German sociologist Norbert Elias calls a longer "civilizing process," the 16-year-old, though physically mature, is considered an adolescent, a late-stage child, unready for parenthood. This quasi-childhood constitutes a fragile limbo between physical maturation and social or technical competence, between puberty and childbearing, one that requires careful ordering of insistent, awakening sexual urges. This century's gallery of juvenile delinquents, gangs, hippies, and teen parents should remind us of the difficulty of this project. Even now, social workers report seeing 14- and 15-year-old wives from immigrant Albanian and Yugoslavian families coming to pregnancy clinics. The truth is that adolescent childbearing was commonplace even in the staid 1950s, when a quarter of all American women had babies before the age of twenty, though of course almost always within wedlock.

Social Changes of the 1960s

But two related social changes occurred in the late 1960s: early marriage came under suspicion, and the sexual revolution caught fire. This meant that the strategies societies generally use to control the hormonal riot of adolescence—prohibiting sex entirely and encouraging marriage within a few years of puberty—both became less workable. The "shotgun wedding" became a thing of the past. As a result, American adolescence became longer, looser, more hazardous.

Adolescents at the bottom of the socioeconomic ladder were most harshly affected by these changes. Middle-class kids have more adult eyes watching over them during this precarious period. They also have numerous opportunities for sublimation—a useful Freudian term unfortunately banished along with its coiner from current intellectual fashion—of their urges: sports teams, church or temple groups, vacations, and camp, not to mention decent schools. Their poorer counterparts don't get that attention. It's much less likely that someone watches to see whom they're hanging out with or whether they've done their homework. Their teachers and counselors often don't even know their names. And "solutions" like contraceptive giveaways, decision-making-skill classes, and even abstinence training only ratify their precocious independence.

Far better would be programs that recognized and channeled the emotional demands of adolescence—intensive sports teams or drama groups, for instance, which simultaneously engage kids' affections and offer constructive, supervised outlets for their energies. According to some teachers who work closely with pregnant teens, births go up nine months after summer and Christmas vacation—further evidence of adolescents' profound need for structure and direction.

KEEPING THE GENIE IN THE BOTTLE

Given that unwed teen childbearing has become the norm for a significant subset of American society, the salient question is not why so many girls are having babies, but what prevents some of their peers from following this path? I explored that question with a group of five young black and Latino women in their twenties, all of whom had grown up in neighborhoods where the teen mommy track was common. All were college students or graduates acting as peer AIDS counselors for teens in poor areas of the city. None had children. All but one grew up with both parents; the other was the product of a strict Catholic education in Aruba. If the meeting hadn't been arranged by the New York City Department of Health, I might have suspected a family values agenda at work.

All of these young women said their parents, in addition to loving them, watched and prodded them. "My father used to come out on the street and call me inside," Jocelyn recalls, laughing. "It was so embarrassing, I just learned to get in their before he came out." Intact families seem to provide the emotional weight needed to ballast the increasingly compelling peer group. Clearly, two parents are vastly better than one at keeping the genie of adolescent pregnancy inside the bottle.

These experiences jibe with both common sense and research. Asians, who have strong families and the lowest divorce rate of any ethnic group (3 percent), also have the lowest teen pregnancy rate (6 percent). In a longitudinal study that may be the only one of its kind, sociologist Frank Furstenberg of the University of Pennsylvania periodically followed the children of teen mothers from birth in the 1960s to as old as 21 in 1987. His findings couldn't be more dramatic: kids with close relationships with a *residential* father or long-term stepfather simply did not follow the teenage mommy track. One out of four of the 253 mostly black Baltimoreans in the study had a baby before age 19. But *not one* who had a good relationship with a live-in father had a baby. A close relationship with a father not living at home did not help; indeed, those children were more likely to have a child before 19 than those with little or no contact with their fathers.

Some social critics, most forcefully Senator Daniel Patrick Moynihan, have insisted on the profound importance of fathers in the lives of adolescent boys. But for girls a father is just as central. Inez, one of the peer AIDS counselors, says she always bristled on hearing boys boast of their female acquaintances, "I can do her anytime," or, "I had her." Any woman who had grown up in a home with an affectionate and devoted father would be similarly disapproving. Having had a first-hand education of the heart, a girl is far less likely to be swayed by the first boy who attempts to snow her with the compliments she may never have heard from a man: "Baby, you look so good," or, "You know I love you."

Warning Signals

The ways of love, it seems, must be learned, not from decision-making or abstinence classes, not from watching soap operas or, heaven forbid, from listening to rap music, but through the lived experience of loving and being loved. Judith S. Musick, a developmental psychologist with the Ounce of Prevention Fund, explains that through her relationship with her father, a girl "acquires her attitudes about men and, most importantly, about herself in relation to them." In other words, a girl growing up with a close father internalizes a sense of love, which sends up warning signals when a boy on the prowl begins to strut near her.

Further, a girl hesitates before replacing the attachment she has to her own father with a new love. I recently watched a girl of about 12 walking down the street with her parents. As she skipped along next to them, busily chattering, she held her father's hand and occasionally rested her head against his arm. The introduction of a serious boyfriend into this family romance is unlikely to come soon. Marian Wright Edelman's aphorism has received wide currency: "The best contraceptive is a real future." It would be more accurate to say, "The best contraceptive is a real father and mother."

If it is true that fatherless girls are far more likely to begin sex early, to fall under the sway of swaggering, unreliable men, to become teen parents, and quite simply to accept single parenthood as a norm, then we are faced with a gloomy prophecy: the teen mommy track is likely to become more crowded. Nationwide, 57 percent of black children are living with a never-married mother. In many inner-city schools, like those in Central Harlem where the rate of out-of-wedlock births is 85 percent, kids with two parents are oddballs, a status youngsters don't take kindly to. When Taisha Brown has her baby, that child may eventually repeat Taisha's question: "Why do I need to worry about a father? My mother raised me just fine without one." Indeed, it seems inevitable, without a transformation of the culture that gave birth to the teen mommy track.

PERIODICAL BIBLIOGRAPHY

The following articles have been selected to supplement the diverse views presented in this chapter. Addresses are provided for periodicals not indexed in the *Readers' Guide to Periodical Literature*, the *Alternative Press Index*, the *Social Sciences Index*, or the *Index to Legal Periodicals and Books*.

Jonathan Alter	"The Name of the Game Is Shame," *Newsweek*, December 12, 1994.
Michael A. Carrera	"Preventing Adolescent Pregnancy: In Hot Pursuit," *SIECUS Report*, August/September 1995. Available from 130 W. 42nd St., Suite 2500, New York, NY 10036.
Ralph deTolando	"Teenage Mothers—Lots of Talk, Little Action," *Conservative Chronicle*, August 28, 1996. Available from PO Box 11297, Des Moines, IA 50340-1297.
Don Feder	"Keeping 'Em Barefoot and Pregnant with Title X," *Conservative Chronicle*, August 23, 1995.
Maggie Gallagher	"The Abolition of Marriage," *Common Sense*, Summer 1996.
D.H. Klepinger, S. Lundberg, and R.D. Plotnick	"Adolescent Fertility and the Educational Attainment of Young Women," *Family Planning Perspectives*, January/February 1995. Available from the Alan Guttmacher Institute, 120 Wall St., 21st Fl., New York, NY 10005.
Robert Lerman and Theodora Ooms	"Unwed Fathers," *American Enterprise*, September/October 1993.
Anthony Lewis	"Condom Classes," *Family in America* (New Research), December 1995. Available from 934 N. Main St., Rockford, IL 61103.
Shelley Lundberg and Robert Plotnick	"Adolescent Premarital Childbearing: Do Economic Incentives Matter?" *Journal of Labor Economics*, April 1995.
Bronwyn Mayden	"Child Sexual Abuse: Teen Pregnancy's Silent Partner," *Children's Voice*, Winter 1996. Available from 440 First St. NW, Suite 300, Washington, DC 20001.
J.P. Shapiro	"Sins of the Fathers," *U.S. News & World Report*, August 14, 1995.

CHAPTER 3

HOW CAN TEENAGE PREGNANCY BE PREVENTED?

CHAPTER PREFACE

Since 1975, when the federal government first recognized teenage pregnancy as a pressing social problem, the two most discussed approaches to preventing pregnancy among teens have been the creation of sex education programs in schools and the distribution of contraceptives to teenagers. These efforts are based on the belief that because a significant number of teenagers are sexually active, the best way to help them avoid the risk of pregnancy and sexually transmitted diseases is to provide them with information and protection.

Opponents of sex education programs in schools contend that the rise in teenage pregnancy rates in recent years proves that such programs are ineffective. They argue that providing contraceptives to teenagers promotes sexual activity among teens because it sends the message that such behavior is acceptable and expected. Furthermore, according to critics, because contraceptives are not 100 percent effective and are often misused (especially by teenagers), they do not eliminate the risks associated with sexual activity and therefore fail to protect young people from pregnancy and sexually transmitted diseases. For these critics, sex education and the provision of contraceptives actually increase rather than reduce the risk of teenage pregnancy. The most responsible means of preventing teenage pregnancy, sex education opponents maintain, is to adopt education programs that stress abstinence from sex.

Defenders of sex education insist that such programs, when properly instituted, can help teenagers avoid pregnancy. They contend that too many sex education programs still consist of a few perfunctory lectures and slides. Comprehensive sex education—which involves ongoing instruction on sexuality and reproduction beginning in the early primary grades—is in place in only a few school districts nationwide, proponents argue, so it is too soon to judge the effectiveness of these programs. Moreover, defenders of sex education note, the pregnancy rate measured as a proportion of teenagers who are sexually active has declined significantly in recent years, suggesting that existing programs may have had some success at preventing pregnancy.

The effectiveness of sex education is among the issues debated in the following chapter on measures to prevent teenage pregnancy.

| "It is simplistic, and mistaken, to claim that the efforts of the past two decades to help teens [prevent pregnancy] have been either ineffective or counterproductive."

SEX EDUCATION CAN PREVENT TEENAGE PREGNANCY

Jane Mauldon and Kristin Luker

In the following viewpoint, Jane Mauldon and Kristin Luker respond to the most frequent conservative objections to sex education, including the arguments that sex education promotes sexual activity and is ineffective in reducing teenage pregnancy. Stating that the pregnancy rate among sexually active teenagers has declined, the authors reject the idea that there is an epidemic of teenage pregnancy and argue that sex education programs have been generally successful. Mauldon is assistant professor at the Graduate School of Public Policy at the University of California, Berkeley. Luker, a professor of sociology and law at the University of California, Berkeley, is author of *Dubious Conceptions: The Politics of Teenage Pregnancy*.

As you read, consider the following questions:

1. Why is the overall teen pregnancy rate higher now than in the past, according to the authors?
2. How do the authors refute the idea that providing contraceptives increases sexual activity?
3. According to Mauldon and Luker, which students are most positively affected by sex education programs?

Jane Mauldon and Kristin Luker, "Does Liberalism Cause Sex?" Reprinted with permission from the *American Prospect*, Winter 1996, ©1996 The American Prospect, Inc.

The drumbeat of criticism that eventually drove Joycelyn Elders out of office as Surgeon General may be only a fading memory, but the controversies over sex education and contraception that dogged her tenure linger on. To conservatives, nothing symbolizes the illusions of liberalism better than the failure of permissive sexual policies. In the years since contraceptives became widely available and schools began offering sex education, haven't kids become more promiscuous? Aren't births to unmarried teenage mothers soaring? Therefore, conservatives say, the government ought to practice some abstinence of its own and stop sex education in our schools and programs that promote contraception.

But, like so many conservative arguments that appeal to a general sense of social decline, this one ignores some well-established facts. More teenagers use contraception, they use it sooner after starting sex, and they are becoming more sophisticated about its use. Pregnancy rates among sexually active teenagers have dropped, decreasing by 20 percent between 1970 and 1990. Recent evidence also suggests that sex and AIDS education programs in the public schools have encouraged youth to delay sex, limit the number of partners, and use condoms.

But, conservatives say, increased access to contraceptives and sex education has stimulated more sexual activity among teenagers. These fears were cogently voiced in 1978 by Archbishop (now Cardinal) Bernardin, who doubted, he said, whether "more and better contraceptive information and services will make major inroads in the number of teenage pregnancies—it will motivate them to precocious sexual activity but by no means to the practice of contraception. In which case the solution will merely have made the problem worse."

Was the Archbishop right? For if he was, Americans might have reason to shut down the great enterprise of sexual enlightenment that America launched thirty years ago. . . .

TEENAGE PREGNANCY RATE

Although ready access to contraceptives is now part of the fabric of American life, conservatives hold it partly responsible for what they see as deepening moral decline. Among the sources of misperception about the consequences of liberalized contraceptive access is a series of misunderstandings about teenage pregnancy and the use of birth control. Constant references to "an epidemic of teenage pregnancy" suggest that the pregnancy rate for teens is dramatically higher than in the past and different from pregnancy rates among older women. In fact, the overall teenage pregnancy rate rose modestly between the early 1970s and the late 1980s, from 95 to 107 pregnancies annually per 1,000 women aged 15 to 19; it rose a little more rapidly from 1987 to 1991, and then fell in 1992 and 1993 (the last year for which we have data). Changes in the rate for teenagers closely track the somewhat higher pregnancy rates among women aged 20 to 29.

It is natural to assume that a higher teen pregnancy rate means that sexually active young women are more likely to conceive than they used to be, but this assumption is false. For most of the last two decades the pregnancy rate rose because more teenagers were sexually active, not because more sexually active teens were becoming pregnant. As more teens started to have sex while unmarried, they also became much more likely to use condoms, the pill, and other forms of birth control. . . .

In 1964 only one-third of sexually active 15- to 19-year-olds used protection during their first sexual experiences, while 40 percent did nothing to prevent pregnancy for at least a year after their first sexual intercourse. But by 1988, 56 percent of sexually active teens used contraception from the start, and fewer than 16 percent were delaying contraception by more than a year. The unsurprising result is that a smaller fraction of the sexually active teens became pregnant with every year that passed between 1972 and 1990.

Encouraging Sexual Activity?

But what about Archbishop Bernardin's thesis that offering contraception to teenagers increases the odds that they will become sexually active and, more precisely, that they will be sexually active without using contraception? Based on the historical record in the United States and other developed nations, no one has yet been able to show that liberalized contraceptive policies increase teenage sexual activity in general or unprotected sex in particular.

Looking overseas first, we find that almost all European nations report increases similar to ours in sexual activity among teens, although they have followed widely divergent policies on access to birth control. Some have long offered publicly funded birth control to women of all ages as part of their national health care systems. Others make it difficult for even adult women to acquire contraception. These varied national strategies make up a kind of natural experiment. The evidence shows that sexual activity among teenagers is independent of any changes in the public provision of contraceptives.

In the United States the policy changes of the 1960s and

1970s responded to social changes already under way. Young people were delaying marriage but not forgoing sex. In the early 1950s American women had a one-in-two chance of being married by the age of twenty. After 1960 the median age at marriage rose four years, lengthening by about 50 percent the time that sexually mature young women (and men) are single. Norms about sex and marriage changed, and the rate of sex outside of marriage increased accordingly. The proportion of American adolescents who were sexually active and unmarried was growing steadily before any public subsidy for birth control. Not only was teen sex already on the increase, but sexual activity leveled off as funding became relatively generous in the 1970s.

Thus the first part of Archbishop Bernardin's hypothesis—providing contraception increases sexual activity—is unsupported by the available data. His second claim, that as more teens become sexually active more of them engage in unprotected sex, was somewhat true during the 1970s but not during the 1980s (when our data end). . . .

In short, as more young unmarried women have become sexually involved, they have also become more likely to use contraception. And while unmarried virgins are less numerous among teens than they used to be, they still remain in the majority. It is married teens who have almost vanished from the landscape.

These data, however, cut two ways. While public funding of contraception has not caused more teens to have sex, neither is there any clear correlation between public funds and teenage use of contraceptives. When federal funds were cut in the 1980s, overall teenage contraceptive use did not decline too, although these broad national data may not pick up the difference public funding makes in low-income and minority communities. Clearly, other factors affect the use of contraceptives: the determination of many teens to avoid pregnancy; increased commercial access to contraceptives in large anonymous drugstores and supermarkets, and the dissemination of knowledge about birth control—including sex education programs in schools and throughout the community that conservatives have also attacked.

THE SUCCESS OF SEX EDUCATION
Critics claim that sex education has failed primarily on the basis of research that has shown no appreciable difference in behavior between students who have taken sex education courses and those who have not. But only in recent years have most schools offered education about birth control to young teens, timed to occur before most of them are sexually active.

For many young people, sex education has come from a partner, not from a class. In the 1988 National Survey of Family Growth—the most recent, large-scale survey available—almost half of all young women (44 percent) born between 1963 and 1965 had sex education about contraception after they had become sexually active. But as schools became willing to teach sex education in lower grades, this pattern began to change. Of teens born between 1966 and 1968, 38 percent had sex before sex education, but of those born between 1971 and 1972, only 19 percent had been sexually active prior to any instruction about contraception.

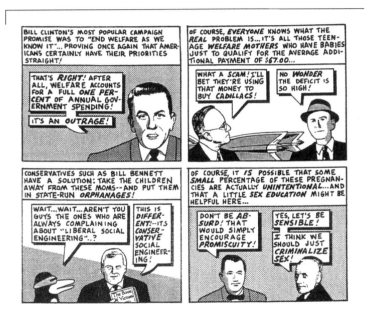

Tom Tomorrow, ©1994. Reprinted by permission.

Most types of sex education offered after sexual initiation have little effect on behavior. Yet the popular view that sex education does not work was based on early studies that did not distinguish youngsters who received sex education from those who sat through the instruction when they were already having sex. Any beneficial effects of sex education on the students who were still virgins were likely masked by the absence of effects among the sexually active.

Our own analyses of the 1988 survey data show a strong relationship between prior sex education and contraceptive use by teens. We found a difference of about 10 percentage points in the likelihood of contraceptive use. By 1988 young women who had had sex education were only half as likely as those who had not to delay contraception for a year or more.

The impact of sex education stems from small changes among many students. It can hasten their use of birth control, encourage more effective methods, and (though this is not our theme here) help students to resist premature or unwanted sexual activities. In short, it will nudge some students—not all—in the direction of safer behavior.

Some, of course, do not need to be nudged in school. Half of sexually active teens in the 1980s used some type of contraception at first sex even without formal sex education. Others cannot be reached even through a good program. About 3 percent of students who had had sex education had never used contraceptives even though they had been sexually active for more than a year. But between these extremes lie half of sexually active youth, whose behavior can be shaped by the information, skills, peer expectations, and adult counsel that constitute an effective sex education curriculum.

DESIGNING EFFECTIVE PROGRAMS

While our research suggests that sex education can work, aggregate data tell us nothing about what goes into an effective program. Fortunately, thanks to a panel of 14 national experts convened at the request of the Centers for Disease Control (CDC) and a recent analysis for the Office of Technology Assessment (OTA), we know more than ever before on this question. Under the leadership of Douglas Kirby of ETR Associates, the panel carefully reviewed the evaluations of 16 school-based programs and 7 studies using national data with an eye to establishing what works. Kirby subsequently reviewed an additional 33 studies for the OTA.

Both reviews first address the Bernardin hypothesis that sex education increases sexual activity among teens. None of the evaluated curricula hastened sexual intercourse or increased its frequency among participating students. Kirby and colleagues are unequivocal: "These data strongly support the conclusion that sexuality and AIDS education curriculums that include discussions of contraception in combination with other topics—such as resistance [to sexual pressure] skills—do not hasten the onset of intercourse." In fact, even those sex education programs associated with school-based clinics, which provide birth control to students, did not find that rates of sexual initiation went up.

Indeed, the news is that sometimes sex education can postpone sexual initiation if the program is based on carefully evaluated strategies and is offered to groups of students who are mostly still virgins. Kirby and colleagues note that "two curriculums that specified delaying the onset of intercourse as a clear goal . . . successfully reduced the proportion of sexually inexperienced students who initiated sex during the following 12 to 18 months. Notably, both groups also received instruction on contraception." This result may not have been found in earlier research into sex education because until recently, most curricula did not explicitly seek to discourage students from initiating sex at young ages.

Other programs that successfully influenced student behavior were focused on increasing contraceptive use or, more specifically, increasing condom use, among participating students. These programs had several features in common. They had clear goals and a relatively narrow focus, whether on postponing sexual involvement or on reducing risks of pregnancy or sexually transmitted diseases. They acknowledged the importance of peer group behavior in student learning. They offered accurate information through experiential exercises designed to let students personalize the information. And they let students practice skills in sexual communication, negotiation, and refusal.

In part because of their controversial character, the early sex education curricula that addressed contraception were often forced to adopt a tone of value neutrality, focusing on clinical information to the exclusion of the social, emotional, and moral aspects of sex. The research by Kirby and his colleagues suggests that this strategy was a mistake. In many respects, the most successful sex education programs are liberal in the breadth of their discussion but conservative in their directive message.

A MIDDLE GROUND

The Europeans reached this conclusion first. They have carved out a middle ground between absolute prohibition of adolescent sexuality and the total abdication of any adult responsibilities for guiding it. The new sex education programs in the United States are trying to create an analogous middle ground. Feminists and conservatives alike can find something to admire in programs that encourage young women (and men) to resist peer pressure and take responsibility when and if they feel truly ready for sexual intimacy. While the far right will still insist on a policy of "just say no" and sexual libertarians will resent any attempt to tell adolescents what to do, the emerging consensus of the middle has much to recommend it.

The CDC's team of reviewers emphasizes that we are just beginning to understand which factors contribute most to the overall success of the programs. Their main message is that some programs do work and that the next generation of programs should take advantage of the lessons that varied approaches teach.

A Long Way to Go

American youngsters in the 1990s face a different world from the one that confronted their parents. More young people are sexually active, and more report that some sexual activity is coerced. Sexually transmitted diseases that threaten health and fertility (gonorrhea and chlamydia) or life itself (AIDS) afflict many young as well as older people. Helping teens handle these challenges isn't easy. Their needs change rapidly as they mature: A youngster may need encouragement to postpone sexual involvement when she or he is fifteen, easy access to contraceptives when he or she is eighteen, and, throughout, increasingly sophisticated help in sexual negotiation and refusal.

America has a long way to go before our teenagers are as effective in preventing pregnancy as are most of their European counterparts. While we understand the desire of many people to turn the clock back to a simpler age, the crucial task now is to continue studying open-mindedly what works for adolescents, and for whom it works. It is simplistic, and mistaken, to claim that the efforts of the past two decades to help teens have been either ineffective or counterproductive. Young people from across the social spectrum have taken advantage of public policies to help them take care of themselves. Legally imposed barriers that once imperiled their well-being have been lowered or removed. That these new policies and programs have made only slow and partial progress is evidence for strengthening them and designing them more intelligently. To abandon the effort now would be a kind of collective, parental irresponsibility.

> "Sex education has little effect on
> teenagers' decisions to engage in or
> postpone sex. Nor . . . do knowledge-
> based sex-education programs
> significantly reduce teenage
> pregnancy."

MOST SEX EDUCATION PROGRAMS FAIL TO PREVENT TEENAGE PREGNANCY

Barbara Dafoe Whitehead

Comprehensive sex education programs provide students, beginning in kindergarten, with extensive ongoing instruction in sexuality, reproduction, and contraception. In the following viewpoint, Barbara Dafoe Whitehead argues that although these programs are helpful in purveying basic knowledge about sexuality to America's youth, they fail to reduce sexual activity and teenage pregnancy. To support this conclusion, the author focuses on the long-established comprehensive sex education program in New Jersey, a state that has seen a steady increase in unwed teenage childbearing. Whitehead holds a doctorate in social history and lives in Massachusetts.

As you read, consider the following questions:

1. What does the author mean when she calls comprehensive sex education a "technocratic approach" to teenage sexuality?
2. According to Whitehead, what is the problem with teaching "noncoital" sex?
3. What predictable social consequences await the teenage unwed mother, according to Whitehead?

Barbara Dafoe Whitehead, "The Failure of Sex Education," *Atlantic Monthly*, October 1994. Reprinted by permission of the author.

A mid rising concern about the hazards of teenage sex, health and school leaders are calling for an expanded effort to teach sex education in the schools. At the moment the favored approach is called comprehensive sex education. . . .

Sex education in the schools is not new, of course, but never before has it attempted to expose children to so much so soon. Comprehensive sex education includes much more than a movie about menstruation and a class or two in human reproduction. It begins in kindergarten and continues into high school. It sweeps across disciplines, taking up the biology of reproduction, the psychology of relationships, the sociology of the family, and the sexology of masturbation and massage. It seeks not simply to reduce health risks to teenagers but also to build self-esteem, prevent sexual abuse, promote respect for all kinds of families, and make little boys more nurturant and little girls more assertive. . . .

Comprehensive sex education has provoked vigorous opposition, both at the grass roots and especially in the organized ranks of the religious right. Its critics argue that when it comes to teaching children about sex, the public schools should convey one message only: abstinence. In response, sex educators point to the statistics. Face facts, they say. A growing number of teenagers are engaging in sex and suffering its harmful consequences. It is foolish, if not irresponsible, to deny that reality. If more teenagers are sexually active, why deprive them of the information they need to avoid early pregnancy and disease? What's more, why insist on a standard of conduct for teenagers that adults themselves no longer honor or obey? . . .

THE NEW JERSEY MODEL

Few states have worked harder or longer than New Jersey to bring sexual enlightenment to schoolchildren. In 1980 the state adopted one of the nation's first mandates for comprehensive sex education—or family-life education, as it is called there—and it was the very first state to require sex education for children in the primary grades. Its pioneering efforts have earned New Jersey the equivalent of a five-star rating from the Sex Information and Education Council of the U.S. (SIECUS), a national advocacy organization that promotes comprehensive sex education.

Virtually every public school student in New Jersey receives sex education (the average is twenty-four hours a year), and some schoolchildren, like those in the Irvington public schools, have an early and full immersion. Overall, teachers are trained and experienced, averaging close to ten years of teaching a family-life curriculum. . . .

In New Jersey two closely allied organizations advance the sex-education cause. Rutgers, the state university, administers grants and provides office space to the advocacy campaign. It is, though, the small but ubiquitous New Jersey Network for Family Life Education that conducts the daily business of winning support for sex education across the state.

Susan Wilson runs the Network from her handsome gated home in Princeton. (The Network is officially headquartered at Rutgers.) Wilson, who has been an indefatigable crusader for comprehensive sex education for more than a decade, helped to write and pass the state mandate in the late 1970s, while she was a member of the State Board of Education. A few years later she took over as the head of the Network. With a budget of about $200,000, mostly from foundations and the state government, Wilson and her small staff publish a newsletter, testify at hearings, train teachers, develop sex-education materials, fight efforts to overturn the mandate, and perform the scores of other duties required in their advocacy work. But Wilson's single most important task, which she clearly enjoys, is traveling up and down the state making the case for comprehensive sex education.

THE EARLIER THE BETTER

Because the case that she makes represents today's comprehensive-sex-education orthodoxy, it deserves close attention. It has several tenets. First, children are "sexual from birth." Like many sex educators, Wilson rejects the classic notion that a latency period occurs between the ages of about six and twelve, when children are sexually quiescent. "Ever since I've gotten into this field, the opponents have used that argument to frighten policymakers," she says. "But there is a body of developmental knowledge that says this is not true." And, according to Wilson, it is not simply that children are born sexual or that their sexuality is constantly unfolding. It is also that sexuality is much broader than most imagine: "You are not just being sexual by having intercourse. You are being sexual when you throw your arms around your grandpa and give him a hug."

Second, children are sexually miseducated. Unlike Europeans, who learn about sex as matter-of-factly as they learn about brushing their teeth, American children grow up sexually absurd—caught between opposing but equally distorted views of sex. One kind of distortion comes from parents. Instead of affirming the child's sexuality, parents convey the message that sex is harmful, shameful, or sinful. Or, out of a misguided protectiveness, they cling to the notion of childhood innocence and fail to provide timely or accurate information about sex. The second kind of distortion comes from those who would make sex into a commodity. While parents withhold information, the media and the marketplace spew sexual misinformation. It is this peculiar American combination of repressiveness and permissiveness that leads to sexual wrong thinking and poor sexual decision-making, and thus to high rates of teenage pregnancy and STDs [sexually transmitted diseases].

EXPECTING THE WORST

Abstinence programs mean believing in young people, while contraceptive programs mean expecting the worst from them. Abstinence programs require an investment of time and energy, while contraceptives promise a quick technological fix.

Gary Bauer, *National Review*, August 15, 1994.

Third, if miseducation is the problem, then sex education is the solution. Since parents are failing miserably at the task, it is time to turn the job over to the schools. Schools occupy a safe middle ground between Mom and MTV. They are places where "trusted adults" can teach children how to protect themselves against the hazards of sex and sexual abuse.

Moreover, unlike homes, schools do not burden children with moral strictures. As Wilson explains, schools can resolve the "conflict between morality and reality" by offering unbiased statements of fact. Here, for example, is how a teacher might handle the subject of masturbation in a factually accurate way: "Some people think it is okay to masturbate and some people think it is not okay to masturbate, but most people think that no harm comes to you if you masturbate." Consequently, when it comes to sex, schools rather than homes offer a haven in the heartless world.

A fourth and defining tenet is that sex education must begin in the earliest grades. Like math or reading, comprehensive sex education takes a "building blocks" approach that moves from basic facts to more sophisticated concepts, from simple skills to more complex competencies. Just as it would be unthinkable to withhold math education until the sixth grade, so, too, is it unwise to delay the introduction of sex education until the eighth grade.

In the beginning, before there is sex, there is sex literacy. Just as boys and girls learn their number facts in the first grade, they acquire the basic sex vocabulary, starting with the proper names for genitalia and progressing toward an understanding of masturbation, intercourse, and contraception. As they gain fluency and ease in talking about sexual matters, students become more comfortable with their own sexuality and more skillful in communicating their feelings and desires. Boys and girls can chat with one another about sex, and children can confide in adults without embarrassment.

Early sex education readies grade school children for the onslaught of puberty. By the time they reach adolescence, they are cognitively as well as biologically primed for sex. Moreover, with early sex training, teenagers are much more likely to engage in what Wilson and her colleagues consider responsible sexual conduct: abstinence, noncoital sex, or coitus with a condom. Since abstinence will not lead to pregnancy or STDs, and noncoital and protected sex are not likely to do so, comprehensive sex education will help to reduce the incidence of these problems among teenagers. This is the philosophy of comprehensive sex education. . . .

SEX WITHOUT RISK?

Sex-education advocates agree that abstaining from sex is the best way to avoid STDs and early pregnancy. But they reject an approach that is limited to teaching abstinence. First, they say, abstinence-based teaching ignores the growing number of adolescents who are already sexually active at age twelve or thirteen. One Trenton schoolteacher said to me, "How can I teach abstinence when there are three pregnant girls sitting in my eighth-grade class?" Second, abstinence overlooks the fact that, as Susan Wilson explains, "it is developmentally appropriate for teenagers to learn to give and receive pleasure."

Consequently, the New Jersey sex-education advocates call for teaching middle-schoolers about condoms, abortion, and the advantages of "protected" sex. But given the risks to teenagers, they are not crazy about sexual intercourse either. Indeed, Wilson says, Americans are fixated on "this narrow little thing called intercourse." The alternative is a broad thing called noncoital sex or, in the argot of advocates, "sexual expression without risk."

Noncoital sex includes a range of behaviors, from deep kissing to masturbation to mutual masturbation to full body massage. Since none of these involves intercourse, sex educators see them as ways for teenagers to explore their sexuality without harm or penalty. . . .

A TECHNOCRATIC APPROACH

There is something radically new about comprehensive sex education. As both a philosophy and a pedagogy, it is rooted in a deeply technocratic understanding of teenage sexuality. It assumes that once teenagers acquire a formal body of sex knowledge and skills, along with the proper contraceptive technology, they will be able to govern their own sexual behavior responsibly. In brief, what comprehensive sex education envisions is a regime of teenage sexual self-rule.

The sex educators offer their technocratic approach as an alternative to what they see as a failed effort to regulate teenage sexuality through social norms and religious values. Face facts. In a climate of sexual freedom the old standard of sexual conduct for teenagers—a standard separate from adult sexual standards—is breaking down. Increasingly teenagers are playing by the same sexual rules as adults. Therefore, why withhold from adolescents the information and technologies that are available to adults?

To be sure, sex educators have a point. Traditional sexual morality, along with the old codes of social conduct, is demonstrably less effective today than it once was in governing teenage sexual conduct. But although moral standards can exist even in the midst of a breakdown of morality, a technocratic view cannot be sustained if the techniques fizzle. Thus comprehensive sex education stands or falls on the proven effectiveness of its techniques.

For a variety of reasons the body of research on sex-education programs is not as rich and robust as we might wish. However, the available evidence suggests that we must be skeptical of the technocratic approach. First, comprehensive sex education places its faith in the power of knowledge to change behavior. Yet the evidence overwhelmingly suggests that sexual knowledge is only weakly related to teenage sexual behavior. The researcher Douglas Kirby, of ETR Associates, a nonprofit health-education firm in Santa Cruz, California, has been studying sex-education programs for more than a decade. . . . His research shows that students who take sex education do know more about such matters as menstruation, intercourse, contraception, pregnancy, and sexually transmitted diseases than students who do not. (Thanks to federal funding for AIDS education in the schools, students tend to be very knowledgeable about the sources and prevention of HIV infection.)

But more accurate knowledge does not have a measurable impact on sexual behavior. As it is typically taught, sex education has little effect on teenagers' decisions to engage in or postpone sex. Nor, according to Kirby, do knowledge-based sex-education programs significantly reduce teenage pregnancy. And although teenagers who learn about contraception may be more likely to use it, their contraceptive practices tend to be irregular and therefore ultimately unreliable. . . .

EDUCATIONAL MALPRACTICE

Unsurprisingly, there is not a shred of evidence to support the claim that noncoital sex, with or without communication, will reduce the likelihood of coitus. William Firestone, of Rutgers, who wrote the study for the Network for Family Life Education, concedes that his enthusiasm is empirically unfounded. In fact, several studies show just the opposite. Outercourse is a precursor of intercourse. But do we need studies to tell us this? Is it not graven in our memory that getting to third base vastly increases the chances of scoring a run? In fact, it could be argued that teaching noncoital sex techniques as a way of reducing the risks of coitus comes close to educational malpractice.

And what about empowering students to make their own sexual decisions? Douglas Kirby's work shows that teaching decision-making skills is not effective, either, in influencing teenage sexual behavior. Similarly, there is little empirical support for the claim made by comprehensive sex education's advocates that responsible sexual behavior depends on long years of sexual schooling. In fact, the evidence points in the opposite direction. Math and reading do require instruction over a period of time, but sex education may be most effective at a key developmental moment. This is not in grade school but in middle school, when pre-teens are hormonally gearing up for sex but are still mainly uninitiated.

In pursuit of a more effective sex pedagogy, researchers have turned away from technocratic approaches and dusted off that old chestnut, norms. According to Kirby's research review, several new and promising sex-education programs focus on sending clear messages about what is desirable behavior. When middle-schoolers ask "What is the best time to begin having sex?" teachers in these programs have an answer. It is "Not yet. You are not ready for sex."

Evidently, too, sex education works best when it combines clear messages about behavior with strong moral and logistical support for the behavior sought. One of the most carefully designed and evaluated sex-education courses available is Postponing Sexual Involvement, a program developed by researchers at

Grady Memorial Hospital, in Atlanta, Georgia, and originally targeted at minority eighth-graders who are at high risk for unwed motherhood and sexually transmitted diseases. Its goal is to help boys and girls resist pressures to engage in sex.

PRACTICE IN SAYING NO

The Grady Hospital program offers more than a "Just say no" message. It reinforces the message by having young people practice the desired behavior. The classes are led by popular older teenagers who teach middle-schoolers how to reject sexual advances and refuse sexual intercourse. The eighth-graders perform skits in which they practice refusals. Some of them take the part of "angel on my shoulder," intervening with advice and support if the sexually beleaguered student runs out of ideas. Boys practice resisting pressure from other boys. According to the program evaluator, Marion Howard, a professor of gynecology and obstetrics at Emory University, the skits are not like conventional "role plays," in which students are allowed to come up with their own endings. All skits must end with a successful rebuff.

The program is short: five class periods. It is not comprehensive but is focused on a single goal. It is not therapeutic but normative. It establishes and reinforces a socially desirable behavior. And it has had encouraging results. By the end of ninth grade only 24 percent in the program group had had sexual intercourse, as compared with 39 percent in the nonprogram group. Studies of similar programs show similar results: abstinence messages can help students put off sex. It is noteworthy that although the purpose of the Grady Hospital program was to help students postpone sex, it also had an impact on the behavior of students who later engaged in sexual intercourse. Among those who had sex, half used contraception, whereas only a third did in a control group that had not taken the course.

Postponing Sexual Involvement and similarly designed sex-education programs offer this useful insight: formal sex education is perhaps most successful when it reinforces the behavior of abstinence among young adolescents who are practicing that behavior. Its effectiveness diminishes significantly when the goal is to influence the behavior of teenagers who are already engaging in sex. Thus teaching sexually active middle-school students to engage in protected intercourse is likely to be more difficult and less successful than teaching abstinent students to continue refraining from sex. This seems to hold for older teens as well. In a 1991 study Kirby points to one curriculum for tenth-graders,

Reducing the Risk, which has been successful in increasing the likelihood that abstinent students will continue to postpone sex over the eighteen months following the course. However, although the program emphasizes contraception as well as sexual postponement, it does not increase the likelihood that already sexually active tenth-graders will engage in protected sex. "Once patterns of sexual intercourse and contraceptive use are established," Kirby writes, "they may be difficult to change." For that reason the Grady Hospital researchers have developed a program for sixth-graders, since 44 percent of the boys taking their course in the eighth grade were already sexually experienced (this was true of just nine percent of the girls). . . .

None of the technocratic assumptions of comprehensive sex education hold up under scrutiny. Research does not support the idea that early sex education will lead to more-responsible sexual behavior in adolescence. Nor is there reason to believe that franker communication will reduce the risks of early-teenage sex. Nor does instruction about feelings or decision-making seem to have any measurable impact on sexual conduct. Teaching teenagers to explore their sexuality through noncoital techniques has perverse effects, since it is likely to lead to coitus. Finally, although teenagers may be sexually miseducated, there is no reason to believe that miseducation is the principal source of sexual misbehavior. The most important influences on teenage sexual behavior lie elsewhere.

Moreover, if comprehensive sex education has had a significant impact on teenage sexual behavior in New Jersey, there is little evidence to show it. The advocates cannot point to any evaluative studies of comprehensive sex education in the state. Absent such specific measures, one can only fall back on gross measures like the glum statistics on unwed teenage childbearing in the state. In 1980, 67.6 percent of teenage births were to unmarried mothers; eleven years later the figure had increased to 84 percent. Arguably, the percentage might be even higher if comprehensive sex education did not exist. Nevertheless, it is hard for advocates to claim that the state with the nation's fourth highest percentage of unwed teenage births is a showcase for their approach.

> "*Although their contraceptive use is often less than perfect, a large majority of these young people [who use contraception] succeed in avoiding unintended pregnancy.*"

CONTRACEPTIVES HELP PREVENT TEENAGE PREGNANCY

The Alan Guttmacher Institute

The Alan Guttmacher Institute promotes family planning and sex education through research, educational projects, and policy analysis. In the following viewpoint, writers for the institute argue that while more teenagers are sexually active now than in the past, the majority of those who are active use contraception to prevent unintended pregnancy and the transmission of sexually transmitted diseases (STDs). The authors concede that the ineffective use of contraceptives by teenagers sometimes results in pregnancy or infection, but they insist that the failure rate among teenagers is comparable to that of adults.

As you read, consider the following questions:

1. According to the authors, what traditional markers of adulthood are occurring at later ages now than in past generations?
2. What are the two predominant ways teenagers deal with pregnancy, according to the authors?
3. Why, in the view of the authors, is there more teenage pregnancy in the United States than elsewhere in the industrialized world?

Over the last century, the transition from childhood to adulthood has been radically, and probably irrevocably, altered. Many of the traditional markers of adulthood, such as full-time employment, economic independence, marriage and childbearing, now generally occur at later ages than in past generations. At the same time, young people initiate sexual intercourse much earlier than in the past, and long before they marry. Most adolescents today begin to have intercourse in their middle to late teens. More than half of women and almost three-quarters of men have had intercourse before their 18th birthday; in the mid-1950s, by contrast, just over a quarter of women were sexually experienced by age 18. As sex has become more common at younger ages, differences in sexual activity between gender, racial, socioeconomic and religious groups have narrowed considerably.

SEXUAL INITIATION

Despite these trends, teenagers generally do not initiate sexual intercourse as early as most adults believe. Nor do all teenagers have sex. Although the likelihood of having intercourse increases steadily with age, nearly 20% of adolescents do not have intercourse at all during their teenage years. Moreover, many of the youngest teenagers who have had intercourse report that they were forced to do so.

BETTER THAN ADULTS

Most adolescents who are sexually experienced try to protect themselves and their partners from the negative consequences of sex—namely, sexually transmitted diseases (STDs) and unintended pregnancy—even the first time they have intercourse. Two-thirds of adolescents use some method of contraception—usually the male condom—the first time they have sex, and between 72% and 84% of teenage women use a method of contraception on an ongoing basis. Although their contraceptive use is often less than perfect, a large majority of these young people succeed in avoiding unintended pregnancy. In fact, teenagers use contraceptives as effectively as or even better than adults; adolescents have lower rates of unintended pregnancy, for example, than unmarried method users in their early 20s.

For adolescents who are not effective contraceptive users or who do not use a method, the consequences can be serious, especially for young women. Every year, 3 million teenagers acquire an STD, which can imperil their ability to have children or lead to serious health problems, such as cancer and infection with the AIDS virus. In addition, 1 million teenage women become pregnant every year, the vast majority unintentionally. Pregnancy rates among sexually experienced teenagers have declined substantially over the last two decades, but because the proportion of teenagers who have had intercourse has grown, the overall teenage pregnancy rate has increased. Older teenagers and adolescents who are poor or black are more likely to get pregnant than are their younger, more advantaged and white counterparts.

THE NEEDS OF THE MAJORITY

By the age of 19, 82% of adolescents in the U.S. have had intercourse. The interval between the onset of puberty and the average age of first marriage has increased dramatically so that young people today begin having intercourse an average of eight years prior to marriage. Thus, although abstinence is the only 100% effective way to avoid pregnancy and STDs [sexually transmitted diseases], parents, schools and communities must address the needs of the majority of adolescents for pregnancy and STD prevention.

Leslie M. Kantor, Priorities, vol. 6, no. 4, 1994.

Teenagers who become pregnant almost always have an abortion or give birth and raise the child themselves; placing a child for adoption is rare. About half of adolescent pregnancies end in birth, slightly over a third in abortion and the rest in miscarriage. The way in which adolescent women resolve their pregnancies is determined largely by their socioeconomic status. Young women who come from advantaged families generally have abortions. Childbearing, on the other hand, is concentrated among teenagers who are poor and low-income; in fact, more than 80% of young women who give birth fall into one of these income categories.

TEENAGE DISADVANTAGES

Young mothers tend not only to be disadvantaged economically, educationally and socially at the time of their child's birth, but also to be at risk of falling further behind their more advantaged peers who postponed childbearing to obtain more education and to advance their careers. Teenage mothers, for example, obtain less education and have lower future family incomes than young women who delay their first birth. Many are poor later in life, and while it is clear that their initial disadvantaged background is a major reason for their subsequent poverty, it is also clear that early childbearing has a lasting impact on the lives and future opportunities of young mothers and of their children.

Current trends in sexual behavior among U.S. teenagers are similar to trends both among U.S. adults and among teenage and adult women and men in other countries. For example, the proportion of births to U.S. women in their 20s that were out of wedlock has increased fourfold in the last 20 years. In fact, adult women, not teenagers, account for large majorities of the unintended pregnancies, abortions and out-of-wedlock births that occur each year. Furthermore, even though nearly 70% of births to adolescents occur outside of marriage, teenagers account for a smaller proportion of out-of-wedlock births today than they did in 1970.

INTERVENTIONS NEEDED

If adults are going to help teenagers avoid the outcomes of sex that are clearly negative—STDs, unintended pregnancies, abortions and out-of-wedlock births—they must accept the reality of adolescent sexual activity and deal with it directly and honestly. Certain interventions are needed by all teenagers. All adolescents, for example, need sex education that teaches them communication skills that will help them postpone sex until they are ready and that provides information about specific methods to prevent pregnancy and STDs. All young people also need clear and frequent reminders from their parents, the media and other sources about the importance of behaving responsibly when they initiate sexual intercourse. Sexually experienced teenagers need accessible contraceptive services, STD screening and treatment, and prenatal and abortion services, regardless of their income status.

As important as these interventions are, they do not address the entrenched poverty that is a major cause of early childbearing among disadvantaged teenage women. Only when their poverty is alleviated, and these young women—and their partners—have access to good schools and jobs and come to believe that their futures can be brighter, is real change in their sexual behavior and its outcomes likely to occur.

LEARNING FROM SUCCESS

Other industrialized countries are also dealing with issues related to adolescent sexual activity, but teenage pregnancy, abortion and childbearing are bigger problems in this country, for several reasons: Elsewhere in the industrialized world, there is a greater openness about sexual relationships; the media reinforce the importance of using contraceptives to avoid pregnancy and STDs; and contraceptives are generally more accessible to teenagers because reproductive health care is better integrated into general health services. We can learn from the successes of other countries, as well as from programs in this country that have had a positive impact on teenagers' initiation of sexual intercourse and contraceptive use, to better help young people avoid being adversely and needlessly affected by sexual behavior.

| "The bottom-line is that condoms are not effective in preventing pregnancy or the transmission of HIV."

CONTRACEPTIVES FAIL TO PREVENT TEENAGE PREGNANCY

Charmaine Crouse Yoest

Supporters of contraceptive use for teenagers concede that all contraceptives have the potential to fail, but they insist that some form of contraception is better than none at all. One critic of this view is Charmaine Crouse Yoest, who argues that the current emphasis on condoms as a contraceptive is actually unhealthy for teenagers. Yoest contends that condoms promote a false sense of safety concerning the transmission of HIV and the prevention of pregnancy. Yoest is a public policy consultant and a Bradley Fellow at the University of Virginia.

As you read, consider the following questions:

1. On what evidence does Yoest base her assertion that condoms have a "very high failure rate"?
2. Why does Yoest argue that better education about the use of condoms will not make a difference in the failure rate?
3. In the author's opinion, what negative view of sexuality is reinforced by the distribution of condoms to teenagers?

Charmaine Crouse Yoest, "Should Condoms Be Distributed in Schools? No." Priorities, vol. 6, no. 4, 1994. Reprinted with permission from Priorities, a publication of the American Council on Science and Health, 1995 Broadway, 2nd Floor, New York, NY 10023-5860.

How safe is "safe"? Or "safer"? In any discussion of condom distribution in schools, this fundamental question must be kept clearly in focus. The bottom-line is that condoms are not effective in preventing pregnancy or the transmission of HIV. Presenting condoms to immature teenagers—particularly in a school setting—as safe, or "safer," is irresponsible public policy.

As a contraceptive, condoms have a very high failure rate. Planned Parenthood's research shows that condoms have a failure rate of 15.7% at preventing pregnancy over the course of a year. This is a standardized rate; for specific age and demographic groups, the rates soar to 36 and 44 percent.

Despite this unpromising performance, Planned Parenthood, SIECUS [Sex Information and Education Council of the U.S.] and others remain vocal advocates of distributing condoms in schools. They argue that more education would cut down on the user failure factor that contributes to these fluctuating failure rates.

Would it? Research from the Alan Guttmacher Institute, an organization with close ties to Planned Parenthood, found that of women ages 15–44, women 20–24 had the highest failure rates. Surprisingly, women 15–19 and women 25–34 had very similar failure rates. The women in each age range were grouped into "high" and "low" rankings, reflecting the low and high rates of pregnancy among groups of women who have higher rates of user-failure—*only among women over 35 were all of the women in an age range able to achieve failure rates of less than 19%.* Even this last group of women—presumably more mature, in more stable relationships, better educated, and with overall lower fertility rates—report failure rates as high as 5%.

This gives us a rough idea of how well "more education" might work: Age, which generally correlates with more education and greater maturity, does make a difference. But not enough. When we switch to evaluating condoms for HIV prevention, the stakes are a lot higher: Failure is no longer measured by unwanted pregnancies. Failure is measured by death.

A DANGEROUS LIE

Nevertheless, despite its poor showing as a contraceptive, the condom has been reincarnated as a disease-preventing device. We now see dancing condoms in federally-funded television commercials, and hear from the Centers for Disease Control and Prevention and the Surgeon General that using a condom is the way to prevent the spread of HIV. This is simply not true. It is, in fact, a dangerous lie.

In a study published in *Social Science & Medicine*, Dr. Susan Weller, Associate Professor of Preventive Medicine and Community Health at the University of Texas, Medical Branch at Galveston, found that condoms had higher rates of failure in preventing HIV transmission than in preventing pregnancy. "Since some contraceptive research indicates condoms are about 90 percent effective in preventing pregnancy, many people, even physicians, assume condoms prevent HIV transmission with the same degree of effectiveness," said Dr. Weller. "However, HIV transmission studies do not show that to be true. Effectiveness may be as low as 48 percent or as high as 82 percent."

MEN AND CONTRACEPTIVES

Men don't help matters. Their aversion to condoms is well-known. Seventy-five percent of 20- to 39-year-old men interviewed by researchers at Battelle Human Affairs Research Center in Seattle, for example, said that condoms reduced sensation. But some disadvantaged men don't want their girlfriends to use contraception either. Kay Armstrong, research director of the Southeastern Pennsylvania Family Planning Association, studied women in drug treatment programs; she found that many of the women were afraid to use birth control because it "implies something negative about the relationship," in the words of one client.

According to many women in Armstrong's study, birth control is often equated with prostitutes and trading sex for drugs. "Some women preferred to hide their use of contraceptives and avoid their partners' wrath. . . . One woman's partner cut up the condoms and sponges she had received from the family planning counselor," Armstrong notes.

For men who have had few successes in life, getting a girlfriend pregnant can be a way of showing masculine prowess like "so many notches on one's belt," according to Elijah Anderson, a University of Pennsylvania sociologist who studied disadvantaged black teens in a Philadelphia neighborhood. Patricia Stern, a graduate student at Penn, found that control was also a central theme in the sexual relations of white inner-city youths. "Boys 'get girls pregnant' to keep them from 'being with' other guys," she says.

Douglas J. Besharov, *Washington Post National Weekly Edition*, March 20–26, 1995.

Weller's conclusions are based on a meta-analysis of 11 studies of HIV transmission which involved a total of 593 partners of infected people. "Exposed condom users will be about a third as likely to become infected as exposed individuals practicing 'unprotected' sex," concluded Dr. Weller. "Thus, condom effectiveness or the risk reduction due to condom use can be estimated at 69%." Should our teenagers be told that a risk reduction method that fails 31% of the time is "safe"? Statistically, both teens and adults alike who are sexually active outside a monogamous marital relationship are protected far more by another factor: The relatively low risk that their partner is HIV-positive. Dr. Robert Redfield, one of our nation's top AIDS researchers at Walter Reed Army Medical Center, has stated publicly that condoms "protect" only if both partners are HIV-negative. "Condoms may possibly be less dangerous," says Redfield, "but I would never call it 'safe sex' or even 'safer sex.' If one partner is HIV-positive, it is not safe. Period."

The underpinning of the universal condom use philosophy is the idea that *everyone* is at risk. Everyone. As a result, a negative view of sexuality is creeping—subtly and unacknowledged—into our public sex education. By distributing condoms to school children, and publicly urging everyone to use a condom every time they have intercourse, we are teaching our children—as well as adults—to distrust the people with whom they are having sex. *Why are we accepting, even promoting, the idea that one would sleep with someone one does not trust?*

NEGATIVE MESSAGES

Most people do not behave that way. This is perhaps the most unrealistic element of the universal condom use policy: Most people (particularly teens) have convinced themselves that there is at least a minimum level, usually more, of trust involved before they decide to have sex with someone. The condom philosophy says just the opposite. Passing out condoms in schools is a fear-based approach to sexuality.

It communicates other negative messages to our teens. Is it possible that a teen can receive a condom from a teacher and then honestly think that teacher believes he or she has the strength of character to say, "no"? Do we want our teenagers to live up to this kind of expectation?

Imagine the scenario: A young man is trying to convince his date to have sex. She knows he has in his pocket a condom he received in school. Planned Parenthood's research shows that peer pressure and "thinking that everyone else is doing it" are the top two reasons teens have sex. What kind of added pressure is she feeling *now*? Even her school thinks everyone else is doing it.

These two teens go on to have sex, using that condom with

fear, inexperience and fumbling. How realistic is it to think it was used correctly? Even if it was, how sad. The young girl probably didn't get HIV, but the condom didn't protect her from other sexually transmitted diseases, like chlamydia, that could impair her fertility later in life. And it certainly didn't protect her self-esteem.

The alternative scenario of two teens who use the condom flawlessly isn't a much prettier picture. That takes experience. Is that what we want for our teens? This isn't just a debate about pregnancy and HIV prevention. It's about teaching teens to be healthy in all areas of their lives. The research is quite clear: Teens who get involved in sexual activity have multiple partners, high rates of sexually transmitted diseases, lower grades and higher rates of suicide. Condoms don't provide protection for any of those consequences. Our teens deserve better advice. They deserve the truth about the power of abstinence.

"If young people are having sex—with or without a condom— they still are placing themselves at significant risk for unwanted pregnancies, disease and economic and educational poverty."

TEACHING ABSTINENCE CAN PREVENT TEENAGE PREGNANCY

Patricia Funderburk

Formerly director of the adolescent pregnancy program for the George Bush administration, Patricia Funderburk is director of educational services at Americans for a Sound AIDS/HIV Policy. In the following viewpoint, Funderburk argues against the current government strategy of promoting condom use for the prevention of HIV infection and teenage pregnancy. In place of the condom-centered approach, the author advocates abstinence-based sex education programs. For Funderburk, abstinence is the solution to the problems of increasing teenage pregnancy and HIV transmission.

As you read, consider the following questions:

1. What values besides abstinence are taught in abstinence-based programs, according to the author?
2. According to Funderburk, what is wrong with the comprehensive sex education approach to sexuality?
3. Funderburk argues that programs that promote abstinence but also promote condom use have no effect in what specific areas?

From Patricia Funderburk, "None, Not Safer, Is the Real Answer," Insight, May 9, 1994. Reprinted with permission from Insight. Copyright 1996, News World Communications. All rights reserved.

It is inarguable that the Public Health Service's (PHS) charge is to provide the very best medical information to the American public to prevent or stop disease, save lives and limit suffering. Since there are risks of HIV infection with all sexual activity, the message of abstinence is the best the Centers for Disease Control and Prevention (CDC), a part of PHS, can offer.

Then why is the government spending the vast majority of its time, money and effort promoting the use of condoms? The PHS's own literature admits that there are better alternatives: abstinence until establishing a lifelong monogamous relationship with an uninfected partner; knowing your HIV status and that of your partner; and limiting the number of sexual partners. . . .

NOT RELIGION OR FEAR

The entire concept of abstinence as perpetuated in abstinence-based sex-education curricula frequently has been misrepresented. To teach abstinence in the schools is not to teach religion or fear. An effective abstinence-based curriculum focuses on universal values and activities such as discipline, self-control, delaying self-gratification, respect for oneself and others, developing and maintaining meaningful relationships, developing future goals and understanding and respecting the potential joys and dangers of sexual involvement. It helps teens understand why it is important to delay sex; teaches them the skills to resist peer pressure; provides support from peers, teachers, parents and the community in general that will help them to follow through on their decision to delay; and finds something positive to which young people can say "yes" as they are saying "no" to sex.

In July 1993, Central State University in Wilberforce, Ohio, sponsored a conference titled "Abstinence and the African-American Youth." In his opening remarks at the event, University President Arthur Thomas explained why the conference was necessary: "To save our children . . . to teach them about marriage and parenting; how to date and not date rape; to delay gratification; and to develop a meaningful relationship."

Thomas and the diverse group of attendees clearly saw sexual abstinence for adolescents as a realistic goal that also has a significant impact on other societal problems such as drug abuse, violence and school dropout rates. It is extremely irresponsible to imply to young people that they can control their passions in the area of violence and other abuses but cannot control their sexual urges. If young people are having sex—with or without a condom—they still are placing themselves at significant risk for unwanted pregnancies, disease and economic and educational poverty (a breeding ground for violence, substance abuse and welfare dependence).

Project Sister, an abstinence-based program developed and administered by the University of California at San Diego, reports that not only are girls in the program waiting longer to have sex, but they also are less inclined to cut class and use drugs than are girls in the control group and report being more satisfied with themselves.

Best Friends in Washington reports only one pregnancy out of the nearly 400 inner-city elementary through senior high school girls in its abstinence-based program over a seven-year period.

Charles Ballard, president of the Cleveland-headquartered National Institute for Responsible Fatherhood and Family Development, is quick to share the impressive outcomes of his 12-year-old program, which boasts of not distributing condoms or endorsing sex outside of marriage. Of the nearly 2,000 young men, most of whom already were unwed fathers, 75 percent have not caused an additional pregnancy since participating in the program.

Ester Alexanian, director of the Kenosha County, Wisconsin, Health Department's abstinence-based program, reports that a significant number of previously sexually active students in the program made the decision to return to abstinence.

Kimi Gray, chairwoman of Kenilworth Parkside Resident Management Corp. in Washington talks about how setting guidelines and boundaries and teaching adolescents to say no to sex and drugs changed their lives: "TV and music need to change, but the most important thing is how adults in the child's life behave and the messages they give them. Instead of watching our young people go off to jail, a drug rehab center or the welfare office like we used to do, we are now sending them to college," she said.

JUST SAYING NO

When Emory University asked nearly 2,000 sexually active girls what they would most like to learn in an effort to reduce teen pregnancy, over 85 percent answered, "How to say no without hurting the other person's feelings." Students—boys and girls—in Emory University's Postponing Sexual Involvement, an abstinence-based program, were five times less likely to become sexually active than those not enrolled in the program.

ABC correspondent Diane Sawyer noted that she made a sad discovery in the course of her report on Norplant, the long-term contraceptive made available at schools in Baltimore: "Every single one of these sexually active girls confided to us they wish they'd said no [to sex]." When pressed to say how long they would wait to have sex, each girl replied that they'd wait until they got married. The sad part is that abstinence until marriage probably was not seriously presented as a viable option for these girls. Someone made a judgment that it was unrealistic— an unacceptable concept for them—perhaps because most were black, poor and in the inner city.

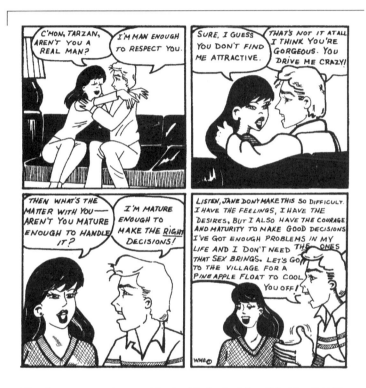

Taken from *Sex Respect: The Option of True Sexual Freedom* by Coleen Kelly Mast, ©1990, Respect Inc., PO Box 349, Bradley, IL 60915. Used by permission.

One of the significant differences in abstinence-based and comprehensive sex-education programs is emphasis. If waiting to have sex until a lifelong, mutually faithful relationship is attained is the best message we can give our young people, why is this approach dealt with so briefly in most sex-ed curricula—almost in passing, or as an equal option among other sexual behaviors? Where are the public service announcements, curricula, brochures and videos funded by the government to promote this message?

The Title XX Family Life Act of the Department of Health and Human Services is the only federal government entity that provides funding for abstinence-based programs. Although the office had approximately $7.8 million awarded annually to support demonstration programs throughout the country, only about $2.5 million could be used for abstinence-based programs. Contrast this with an estimated $50 million used for contraceptive services and counseling for adolescents in the Title X Family Planning Program. (A portion of Title XX money also was used for family-planning services for adolescents.)

Most advocates of comprehensive sex-ed believe it is very important to help adolescents explore ways of experiencing sexual intimacy and pleasure. Indeed, in the fall 1992 issue of *Family Life Matters*, published by Rutgers University in New Jersey, Joan Saltzer, a teacher in the Cherry Hill, New Jersey, school district, described her method (endorsed by the paper) of teaching sexual pleasure to high school students: "I teach that the key to good sex is lubrication. . . . I talk about sexual positions. . . . We talk about the taste of different people, how kissing tastes. . . . The topic leads to discussion of masturbation, how it feels to touch our genitals."

In the age of AIDS, to encourage adolescents (who are notoriously poor contraception and condom users) to be involved in sexual activity for pleasure or any other reason is incomprehensible. Unfortunately, today we are reaping the consequences of our abdication of responsibilities to instill values in this generation of young people. It is also unfortunate that we, in many cases, still have not made the connection between our behavior as adults, the messages we send to these kids and their behavior. We've left child rearing to the TV executives and video producers. We've abandoned sound and proven psychological studies that tell us young people need and want boundaries, clear guidance and direction. Instead, we now affirm their right to certain behaviors—many with the potential for devastating consequences—simply because "it's their decision."

Abstinence-based programs do talk about condoms and contraceptives. But these devices are discussed in a realistic manner only after significant effort is made to encourage and support a youth's decision to delay sexual involvement. Accurate facts are given about their use and effectiveness, but they do not become the highlight of the presentation. Settings such as family-planning clinics are very appropriate for more detailed information about condoms and contraceptives.

The abstinence-based approach also recognizes that parental

guidance is essential and irreplaceable. In more nondirective sex-ed programs, the emphasis often is not on empowering parents to share their values with their children, but on supporting whatever choices the children have made.

A recent proliferation of media coverage has featured the "new" focus on chastity programs. Maryland's Campaign for Our Children, which focuses on abstinence and responsibility with no specific mention of contraception, has been distributing materials for seven years and now sends out publications to all 50 states. Health departments, including the Baltimore City Department of Health, began sponsoring abstinence conferences in 1994. Programs such as True Love Waits, a nationwide movement by teenagers to promote waiting for sex, and Athletes for Abstinence, an organization headed by Phoenix Suns player A.C. Green, are cropping up.

Perhaps they've heard that San Francisco has the lowest teen pregnancy rate of any major metropolitan area in the country (significantly lower than the next closest city). Experts attribute that phenomenon to the large Asian-American population in the public schools there. What's different about Asian-Americans? They generally promote strong family ties and delaying sex until marriage.

Maybe the recent attention on chastity programs relates to the fact that data show that even programs such as the highly touted Reducing the Risk, which significantly encourages abstinence but also strongly promotes condom use, lowered by 24 percent the odds that participating students would begin having sexual relations. However, the program had little effect on contraceptive use by sexually active teens or reducing the pregnancy rate of program participants.

We should applaud the CDC for its efforts to stem the spread of the deadly AIDS epidemic. However, those who proclaim themselves experts in the area of preventing the spread of a disease that already is on its way to decimating large numbers in many American communities should be held accountable for their actions. The policies they promote, the services they provide and the advice they advocate should all be weighed against time-honored medical strategies and good old common sense. Each American citizen should, without hesitation, encourage PHS to vigorously seek input from those who have been successful in promoting an HIV-prevention approach for school-age children that also positively impacts other debilitating social ills confronting us as a nation. That approach is unquestionably the abstinence-based sex education and HIV prevention model.

"*Vows of abstinence break more often than condoms do—especially in today's atmosphere of growing peer pressure and sexual hype in the media.*"

TEACHING ABSTINENCE IS NOT A REALISTIC APPROACH

Planned Parenthood Federation of America

The Planned Parenthood Federation is a national organization that provides reproductive services, including counseling, contraception, and sterilization. In the following viewpoint, Planned Parenthood contends that although abstinence is a healthy option for teenagers, sex education programs must account for the fact that many teenagers are sexually active. Educators have a responsibility to provide these teens with information on how to avoid pregnancy and sexually transmitted diseases, according to Planned Parenthood.

As you read, consider the following questions:

1. Why is abstinence-only sex education unrealistic, according to Planned Parenthood?
2. According to Planned Parenthood, how can abstinence-only sex education damage the self-esteem of teenagers?
3. Why is it not contradictory to teach both abstinence and contraception to teenagers, according to Planned Parenthood?

From the Planned Parenthood Federation of America publication "Sexuality Education: Issues and Answers for Parents, Educators, and Policy Makers." ©1993 by Planned Parenthood Federation of America, Inc. Reprinted with permission.

What's wrong with teaching kids to abstain? Nothing, as long as it isn't the only message. The bottom line is that the "Just Say No" message doesn't work. That message has been around for many years, in many cultures—and it has failed. Vows of abstinence break more often than condoms do—especially in today's atmosphere of growing peer pressure and sexual hype in the media. Millions of teens each year continue to make the choice to engage in sexual intercourse. Withholding information that can preserve their health and save their lives is cruel, counterproductive, and immoral.

While abstaining from intercourse is the most effective way to avoid pregnancy and disease, both teenagers and adults know that fewer than 50% of teens are abstinent. Curricula that ignore this reality, in the face of all evidence, only serve to undermine the credibility of adults, teachers, and other authority figures in teens' eyes. When abstinence is presented as the only choice, students who have already rejected that choice are made to feel condemned, guilty, and sick. This stigmatization not only harms them emotionally—it makes them tune out to other educational messages. They become isolated, marginalized, and unreachable by adults who could help them.

Teaching young people that there is only one acceptable choice does not help them develop critical thinking skills, clarify their own values, and achieve empowerment. Good education isn't just for today—it's for life. Very, very few human beings will choose life-long sexual abstinence. Young people need to acquire the information and decision-making skills that will guide them throughout their lives.

REALITY-BASED EDUCATION

What *should* teens be taught about abstinence? Reality-based education teaches that abstinence is the only 100% effective way to protect against unintended pregnancy and sexually transmitted diseases, including AIDS. It also encourages young people to view abstinence as a healthy choice that people may make at different times in their lives. Every Planned Parenthood program or curriculum includes abstinence as a healthy option; one of Planned Parenthood's most popular pamphlets is "Teensex? It's OK to Say No Way"—hundreds of thousands of copies have been distributed to young people over the past several years.

However, reality-based education recognizes that by age 15, one-fourth of all girls and one-third of all boys have had intercourse; by age 20, 77% of females and 86% of males have had intercourse. For the sake of their health and lives, these young people need and deserve straightforward information on sexuality—including (but not limited to) facts on how to reduce the risks that can accompany sexual activity. Even for teens who choose to postpone sex, abstinence is not likely to be their lifelong choice. And while many parents hope their teens will abstain now, most also hope their children will have a satisfying sexual relationship later in life. Without appropriate knowledge and skills, young people cannot be expected to become sexually responsible and healthy adults.

ABSTINENCE-ONLY PROGRAMS ARE INEFFECTIVE

Only three studies of school-based abstinence-only programs have been published in the professional literature. These studies did not find any impact of such programs on adolescents' initiation of intercourse.

Sexuality education programs that teach only abstinence have not proven effective. The research that exists on these programs tends to have serious methodological flaws, such as not asking students about their sexual behavior before and after their participation in the program.

No available evidence supports the effectiveness of having young people sign pledges that they will not engage in intercourse until marriage.

Nearly two-thirds of teenagers think teaching "Just Say No" is an ineffective deterrent to teenage sexual activity.

Leslie Kantor, *SIECUS Report*, August/September 1994.

Isn't it hypocritical to teach kids to abstain, then teach them about contraception? No. Teaching facts is not the same as telling kids what to do, and teens know the difference. Teaching both the benefits of abstinence and the facts about contraception is not a mixed message—it's a balanced message, which teenagers are perfectly capable of understanding. They grow up learning many such messages, for example: "Drive safely so you can avoid accidents; and wear your seat belt just in case." "Candy tastes good, but eating a lot of it isn't good for you." "It's best to avoid too much sun exposure; but if you're going to be in the sun a lot, wear a sunscreen." In all the above examples, there are two halves to the message—and censoring the second half would be both cruel and unwise.

But isn't it just like telling kids not to use drugs, then telling them where to get them? Or telling them not to rob banks, then supplying them with a getaway car? (The latter analogy is used in the fear- and shame-based "Teen Aid" curriculum.) Sexual urges are healthy and normal for teens, and they need to learn how to handle those feelings in ways that are responsible and caring. Healthy sexual behavior should *never* be compared with substance abuse or criminal behavior. Such comparisons only further stigmatize sexually active teenagers, making them harder to reach with messages about responsibility and safety. Sexual intercourse is a behavior that most human beings practice at some time in their lives. When it is respectful, responsible and healthy, it can be a positive, life-enhancing experience. That is not the case with substance abuse or crime.

ENCOURAGING SEXUAL ACTIVITY?

Won't teaching about contraception and making condoms available encourage kids to have sex? No. Teaching young people to use condoms properly can only protect their health and lives. Research indicates that educated, correct use increases the effectiveness of condoms in preventing pregnancy and sexually transmitted disease. Condoms and foam have been available to teenagers in pharmacies, supermarkets, and convenience stores for years. The National Research Council, in its 1986 report on teen pregnancy, found that "there is no available evidence to indicate that availability and access to contraceptive services influences adolescents' decisions to become sexually active, while it does significantly affect their capacity to avoid pregnancy if they are engaging in intercourse."

In a three-year study of school-based clinics that dispense contraception, the Center for Population Options concluded that making birth control available in schools "neither hastened the onset of sexual activity nor increased its frequency." In a 1992 national Gallup poll, 68% of American adults supported the availability of condoms in public schools. As Jeannie Rosoff, president of the Alan Guttmacher Institute, has said, "Fire engines are present at the site of fires, but they do not cause them. They only limit their destructiveness to property and their harm to human beings. The causes of fires must be sought elsewhere."

PERIODICAL BIBLIOGRAPHY

The following articles have been selected to supplement the diverse views presented in this chapter. Addresses are provided for periodicals not indexed in the *Readers' Guide to Periodical Literature*, the *Alternative Press Index*, the *Social Sciences Index*, or the *Index to Legal Periodicals and Books*.

Mary Abowd	"What Are Your Kids Learning About Sex?" *U.S. Catholic*, April 1996.
Douglas Besharov	"The Contraceptive Gap," *Washington Post*, March 20–26, 1995. Available from Reprints, 1150 15th St. NW, Washington, DC 20071.
Robert Coles	"On Sex Education for the Young," *New Oxford Review*, March 1995. Available from 1069 Kains Ave., Berkeley, CA 94706.
Jennifer J. Frost and Jacqueline Darroch Forrest	"Understanding the Impact of Effective Teenage Pregnancy Prevention Programs," *Family Planning Perspectives*, September/October 1995. Available from the Alan Guttmacher Institute, 120 Wall St., 21st Fl., New York, NY 10005.
Michael E. Gress	"Sex Education in Schools: In Praise of Mystery," *Conservative Review*, December 1992. Available from 1307 Dolley Madison Blvd., Rm. 203, McLean, VA 22101.
Jessica Gress-Wright	"The Contraception Paradox," *Public Interest*, Fall 1993.
Leslie M. Kantor	"Should Condoms Be Distributed in Schools?" *Priorities*, Winter 1994. Available from ACSH, 1995 Broadway, 2nd Fl., New York, NY 10023.
Leslie M. Kantor and Debra W. Haffner	"Adolescents and Abstinence," *SIECUS Report*, August/September 1994. Available from 130 W. 42nd St., Suite 2500, New York, NY 10036.
Douglas Kirby	"School-Based Programs to Reduce Sexual Risk Behaviors: A Review of Effectiveness," *Public Health Reports*, May/June 1994.
Donna Schaper	"Condoms, Carelessness, and Caring," *Christian Social Action*, February 1994.

CHAPTER 4

WHAT NEW INITIATIVES WOULD REDUCE TEEN PREGNANCY?

CHAPTER PREFACE

In August 1996, President Bill Clinton signed a major welfare reform bill, the Federal Responsibility and Work Opportunity Reconciliation Act. This law gives states the option of denying benefits to unwed teenage mothers. It also stipulates that federal funds cannot be used to aid unmarried parents younger than eighteen unless they live with an adult and attend school.

During the months prior to the passage of the welfare bill, a great deal of debate took place as numerous welfare reform proposals were offered and rejected by both liberals and conservatives. Several of the viewpoints in the following chapter were written during this time and are directed at specific pieces of legislation. Although the final outcome of this welfare reform debate has been decided, many of the crucial issues concerning teenage pregnancy either remain undecided or are now being debated at the state level.

The following viewpoints present cogent arguments for and against cutting benefits for and imposing restrictions on teenage mothers who receive welfare. Many critics maintain that teenage girls find welfare benefits an inducement to become pregnant because, in the words of James M. Talent, a Republican congressman from Missouri, those benefits provide "status, independence, and some money every month." Cutting off or reducing welfare benefits would deter teenagers from becoming pregnant, Talent and others argue.

However, other commentators question the correlation between out-of-wedlock childbearing and welfare benefits. Mike Males, the author of *The Scapegoat Generation: America's War on Adolescents*, points out that the states with the lowest welfare payments have the highest illegitimacy rates and the states with the highest benefit levels have the lowest illegitimacy rates. If the availability of welfare benefits had a significant influence on pregnancy, Males contends, the opposite should be true. Males and others insist that cutting welfare benefits will only intensify the poverty faced by many young mothers.

The authors in this chapter also raise new initiatives for consideration. For example, some experts favor requiring unwed teenage mothers to live in maternity homes as a condition of receiving benefits. Others advocate vigorously enforcing statutory rape laws in order to deter adult males from preying on teenage girls. These and other issues are debated in the following chapter on the most effective ways to reduce teenage pregnancy.

| "New legislation . . . should end payments of cash and cash-related benefits to young, unwed parents."

ENDING WELFARE BENEFITS WILL REDUCE TEENAGE PREGNANCY

James M. Talent and Mona Charen

Many social commentators have endorsed the idea of cutting off all welfare benefits for unwed teenage mothers as a strategy for reducing teenage pregnancy. In the following two-part viewpoint, James M. Talent and Mona Charen advocate this approach. Talent, the author of Part I, and Charen, the author of Part II, argue that eliminating benefits for teenage mothers would remove a major incentive for teenagers to become pregnant. Talent is a Republican representative from Missouri. Charen is a conservative columnist who writes on social issues.

As you read, consider the following questions:

1. What will be achieved through an emphasis on adoption and group homes, according to Talent?
2. Why does Charen believe that requiring work in place of welfare will not work?
3. What does Charen mean by the "ruthless application of social stigma"?

Part I: James M. Talent, "Should Congress Halt Welfare Benefits for Unwed Mothers?" *American Legion Magazine*, May 1995. Reprinted by permission, the *American Legion Magazine*, ©1995. Part II: Mona Charen, "Withholding Welfare Is a First Step," *Conservative Chronicle*, August 23, 1995. Reprinted by permission of Mona Charen and Creators Syndicate.

I

It is time to end welfare as we know it. That is the consensus of the American people.

At the outset of the War on Poverty 30 years ago, the out-of-wedlock birthrate in the United States was roughly 7 percent. Since then, the government has spent $5 trillion on programs to end poverty. Yet today, one third of the babies in the United States are born out of wedlock. In many low-income urban communities, nearly eight out of 10 are born into a culture where fatherhood does not exist. These children are three times as likely to fail in school; twice as likely to commit crimes and end up in jail; and almost twice as likely to bear children out of wedlock themselves.

The current welfare system subsidizes out-of-wedlock births, rewards young men for being irresponsible, lures young women into a course of action that often destroys them and their children, and undermines the stability of American society.

WORK AND MARRIAGE

The two most effective anti-poverty programs are work and marriage. Yet the welfare system offers even teenage girls benefits up to $15,000 a year, provided they have a child, do not work and do not marry an employed male.

In my parents' generation, people understood that they simply could not afford children until they had a work skill and had married someone who was committed to help raise a family. Great Society programs changed this reality. We need to provide assistance in a way that tells young people the truth: Having a child means responsibility.

The key feature of new legislation to achieve this should end payments of cash and cash-related benefits to young, unwed parents and offer primary options that emphasize adoption and group homes. The immediate impact of such legislation would be a reduction of the out-of-wedlock birthrate, because pregnancy would no longer mean status, independence and some money every month. It would mean giving the child up for adoption or moving into a group home with regimented schedules and the real expectation of assuming the responsibilities of life.

The states need freedom to experiment with assistance of this kind. There is no reason the welfare system should continue offering quicksand instead of a safety net to single teenage mothers.

II

Sen. Phil Gramm's (R-TX) 1995 welfare reform bill would for-bid states from giving benefits to unwed teen-age mothers, to women who have additional babies while on welfare and to im-migrants before they obtain citizenship.

The debate has been interesting. Sen. Pat Moynihan (D-N.Y.), who has made a career of sounding the alarm about family breakdown in America, has once again allied himself with the status quo. In the greatest disconnect between means and ends since the Polish army tried to fend off the Wehrmacht with cav-alry, Sen. Moynihan warns that our very civilization is in peril unless we are able to reduce the rate of illegitimate births (now at 32 percent)—and then proposes that we stick with (essen-tially) current policy!

The Uses of Shame

Shame doesn't mean someone calling your baby a bastard. It means being forced to live with your parents instead of using welfare to get your own apartment. Instead of the young mother getting to leave school after getting pregnant, she should have to go to *more* school.

Jonathan Alter, *Newsweek*, December 12, 1994.

Sen. Bob Dole, never a conservative ideologue, seems to have been drawn to the block-grant approach because it frees him from having to commit to specific reforms. By adopting a block-grant strategy, he gets some conservative points for devolution while side-stepping the distasteful matter of illegitimacy.

The Work Requirement

But central to the Dole approach, and not widely noticed by conservatives, is the work requirement. There is a great deal of doubt that requiring welfare mothers, especially mothers of children under the age of 2, to work is a conservative approach.

In the first place, very young children are almost always bet-ter off with their mothers than with the kindest of strangers. Abundant psychological research demonstrates that in order to become well-adjusted adults, children need to form a primary attachment to their care givers during this crucial period in in-fancy. (There is a subset of mothers who are so incompetent or emotionally dead that their children would be better off with-out them, but even among the welfare population, this amounts to a small minority.) Almost all babies are better off with the mothers who love them than in group day care, even good day care. And the quality of day care available to the very poor is unlikely to be very good.

Additionally, as Karl Zinsmeister has noted in his review of the literature in *American Enterprise* magazine, workfare has been tried in many ways and in many guises and has consistently failed. People who have gotten themselves on welfare—specifically the long-term population that gets there by having an illegitimate child—are often without the discipline or work habits necessary to hold even the simplest job.

APPLYING SOCIAL STIGMA

The answer to the welfare problem is not to force women to drop their babies and go to work but to prevent women from getting on welfare in the first place.

Ah, but we don't know how to mold behavior by fiddling with incentives, comes the reply. This has become the mantra of the shrug-your-shoulders, Moynihanesque crowd. We just don't know what to do.

I think that's false. Other societies—Japan comes to mind—suppress illegitimate child bearing through the ruthless application of social stigma. Our own society did so as recently as 30 years ago. Loose mores, more than financial incentives, have given rise to this crisis. And we won't truly solve it until we recover a sense of shame about bringing children into the world without fathers.

But in the meantime, while we are adjusting our culture, we can at least stop subsidizing the behavior we all recognize as so destructive. The AFDC [Aid to Families with Dependent Children] check has been the enabler for disastrous conduct. Withholding it from people who behave badly will not eliminate the behavior—human conduct is too complex—but it is a necessary first step.

"Most Democrats and Republicans share the core belief that welfare provokes and rewards illegitimacy—especially among teens. . . . But that assumption . . . is just plain wrong."

ENDING WELFARE BENEFITS WILL DEVASTATE TEENAGE MOTHERS

Mike Males

In the following viewpoint, Mike Males argues that, contrary to popular belief, no causal link exists between welfare benefits and a recent increase in teenage pregnancy. Males cites a number of statistical studies demonstrating that the increase in teenage pregnancy is unrelated to the availability of welfare. Hence, the author believes, the reduction or elimination of welfare benefits will do nothing but punish teenage mothers unfairly. Males is a reporter on youth issues for In These Times magazine and author of The Scapegoat Generation: America's War on Adolescents.

As you read, consider the following questions:

1. According to Males, states with the highest welfare payments have what kind of unwed birthrates?
2. What racial prejudice lurks behind the term "teenage," according to the author?
3. Instead of welfare benefits, where should Congress look to make budget cuts, in Males's view?

From Mike Males, "Poor Logic," In These Times, January 9, 1995. Reprinted by permission of the publisher.

In early 1994 sociologist Charles Murray made a startling admission. Writing in the spring 1994 issue of *Public Interest*, Murray retracted his claim that federal welfare policy has been a key culprit in the rising number of America's out-of-wedlock births—a central tenet of his enormously influential 1984 book, *Losing Ground*. "It seems likely," Murray conceded, "that welfare will be found to cause some portion of illegitimacy, but not a lot."

FLAWED ASSUMPTIONS

Although Murray's retraction undermines a central belief of both Republican and Democratic welfare reformers—that government handouts are feeding an illegitimacy crisis—it has received virtually no notice in the press. Even today, as Congress prepares to radically revise the nation's welfare system, that flawed assumption—and dozens of equally wrongheaded notions—is driving the debate in Washington.

In order to unravel the myths of the congressional debate, one must examine the complex trends being cited—including illegitimacy rates, welfare payments and child poverty rates. By tracking those statistics over the last 50 years one can learn what is really wrong with welfare, and what can be done to fix it.

In Washington today, welfare reformers from both parties are arguing that overly generous welfare benefits are responsible for the current welfare crisis. In fact, the value of the average benefit for recipients of Aid to Families with Dependent Children (AFDC) has declined nearly 50 percent over the last two decades. In inflation-adjusted dollars that's a loss of roughly $400 per family per month.

Not surprisingly, that drop in income has been accompanied by sharply rising poverty rates. Though these figures suggest that what welfare recipients need are more benefits, not less, both parties are considering reforms that would substantially cut government assistance for poor people. . . .

TEENAGE MOTHERS ARE THE TARGET

Unfortunately for unwed teenage mothers, they are the primary target of Republican reformers. "The federal government has made it possible through welfare for unwed women to have babies without having to suffer," says Steve Boriss, press secretary for Rep. James M. Talent (R-MO). . . . "These women do not have to have kids.". . .

Most Democrats and Republicans share the core belief that welfare provokes and rewards illegitimacy—especially among teens—and that lowering or eliminating benefits is an essential tool to enforce reform. But that assumption—as Murray was forced to admit—is just plain wrong.

No Clear Welfare Link

Across the nation today, the states with the highest welfare payments to poor families have the lowest rates of unwed births, especially among teenagers. Conversely, the states with the lowest welfare payments have the highest rates of illegitimacy.

Historically, it has proved extraordinarily difficult to link supposedly generous welfare payments to illegitimacy.

• The real value (adjusted for inflation) of poor-family welfare benefits increased slowly from 1940 to 1960, rose rapidly from 1960 to 1970 during the War on Poverty, leveled off in the Nixon years and then decreased rapidly from 1975 to 1993.

• From 1940 to 1990, unwed birthrates rose steadily, sharply and identically (sixfold) among both teenage mothers and adult mothers. But it's important to note that unwed birthrates increased at roughly the same rates during the '40s and '50s—the "family values" decades—as they did during the counterculture '60s. The most marked increase in unwed birthrates took place after 1975—when the value of welfare benefits began falling sharply.

• The percentage of children living below federal poverty guidelines stood at over 30 percent during the '40s and '50s, plummeted to 14 percent by 1973, then rocketed upward to 23 percent by 1993. Contrary to what congressional reformers imply, there is no relationship between unwed mothers having babies and higher levels of child poverty, simultaneously or delayed, over the past 30 years.

Poverty and Childbearing

It is clear, however, that female children who grow up in poverty are more likely to become teenage mothers. Over the last three decades, the rate of poverty among children almost perfectly correlates with the birthrates among teenage mothers a decade later. That is, child poverty seems to lead to teenage childbearing, not the other way around. . . .

But today's shrunken public aid no longer provides a boost out of poverty, only a marginal subsistence that cements long-term dependence. Any "reform" Congress produces is likely only to deepen the cuts that quietly added 5 million children and adolescents to poverty rolls since 1973.

Today, government officials are more likely to blame victims than to seek the true causes for their condition. Health and Human Services Secretary Donna Shalala takes aim at the misbehavior of unwed teen mothers while remaining silent on their backgrounds of poverty and socially imposed racial obstacles. Three-quarters of unwed teen mothers on welfare are black, Latina or other non-white, and 85 percent were poor or near-poor before giving birth, a 1994 study by the Alan Guttmacher Institute found. But Shalala simply declares that unwed teen mothers who drop out of school are eight times more likely to be on welfare than mothers who are married, over 20 and high school graduates, period—without emphasizing the social or economic context.

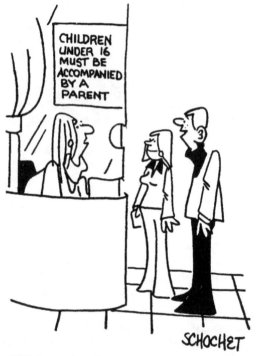

"We're under sixteen, but we're parents."

From the *Wall Street Journal*—Permission, Cartoon Features Syndicate.

"Teenage" has become a Democratic euphemism for "non-white" and "low income." Thus, Democrats tacitly accede to Murray's *Bell Curve* wisdom, which claims that blacks (in particular) are inherently more disposed to illegitimacy and poverty. This acceptance of Murrayesque assumptions leaves them unable to mount arguments against his absolutist, punishment-oriented cures.

President Clinton's proposal that unwed teen mothers should simply return home is a classic New Democrat sham. A June 1994 study released by the Center for Law and Social Policy in Washington shows that only a small minority (perhaps 14,000 out of 350,000) of teen mothers under age 18 live on their own. The study, noting that many of them had faced sexual or physical abuse at home, had "valid reasons" for leaving. Consistent research has found that large majorities of teenage mothers, both white and non-white, were the victims of physical and sexual abuse while growing up—mostly inflicted by adult male family members averaging well over 21 years old.

THE AGE GAP

Contrary to New Democratic biology popularized by Shalala, school-age girls do not "become pregnant" all by themselves or "contemplate motherhood" in monastic solitude. More than half the so-called "sexually active" girls under age 15 reported having been raped by "substantially older" men, the two-year Guttmacher study found.

California's near-complete records of 40,000 births among school-age girls in 1993 show that 71 percent were fathered by adult men averaging over 22 years of age, not by schoolboy peers. The age gaps between 3,000 California junior-high mothers and the adult men who fathered their babies averaged 6.5 years in 1993. National figures are similar.

Poverty, rape, sexual abuse, family violence, much-older adult "partners," racial disadvantage: these are matters that New Democratic "values" and "character" crusaders do not address. The administration's ongoing "national mobilization against teen pregnancy" included a "Democratic family values" campaign featuring shamings of pregnant girls and excessive victim-blaming rhetoric. The effect was to shift the welfare debate further to the right, allowing Republicans to offer more drastic schemes and making their harsh rhetoric sound almost reasonable.

In this atmosphere, one confronts the following conventional wisdom on the adult male impregnation of school-age girls: "That is a serious problem, we agree," says GOP Rep. Talent's press secretary Boriss. "But if the man isn't a fit father, the girl has to make a decision not to get pregnant."

Like the assumptions that underlie teen-mom bashing, the mathematics of welfare reform are little short of lunacy. The "budget-busting" welfare programs targeted by both parties—AFDC, food stamps, nutrition programs and housing subsidies—account for less than 4 percent of the total federal spending. Another target that has recently come on the table is Supplemental Security Income, a program that delivers roughly $25 billion per year to the disabled and elderly poor.

BENEFITS TO NON-POOR ADULTS

By contrast, over $1 trillion in government subsidies, special tax breaks and other benefits flowed to thousands of corporations and 180 million individuals in 1993, according to federal budget figures. A bipartisan commission led by Sens. Bob Kerrey (D-NE) and William Danforth (R-MO) was supposed to find ways to reduce those outlays, but the commission concluded its work in December 1994 after failing to agree on a single cut. Congress finds it far easier to focus its attention on the benefits of the nation's politically powerless.

As former Nixon Commerce Secretary Peter Peterson exhaustively detailed in his 1993 book *Facing Up*, it is the exploding benefits for non-poor adults that are the true cause of the nation's erupting deficit and entitlement crisis. "In 1991, about half of all federal entitlements went to households with incomes over $30,000," Peterson wrote. Unlike Europe, whose social insurance programs serve as income "equalizers," U.S. welfare "has nothing to do with economic equality."

The elderly receive three times more in local, state, and federal benefits than do children, even when schooling is added. Yet welfare to the old is so maldistributed—$75 billion in Social Security goes to seniors whose cash incomes exceed $50,000 per year—that the United States still has by far the highest elder (and child) poverty rates of any industrial nation. Scheduled Social Security cost-of-living increases for just the next year will cost more than the entire combined budgets for Head Start and school lunch programs. . . .

The Progressive Policy Institute has listed $225 billion in annual corporate subsidies that could be redirected to ameliorating poverty and income disparities. But Democrats are not championing such reforms at either an individual or a corporate level.

Given the inability of lawmakers to honestly confront these facts, it is likely that any welfare reform that does make it through Congress will produce a consensus like that forged on the crime bill: emphasizing punitive measures while throttling social spending. As a result, teenage mothers and their babies, like tens of thousands of now-homeless veterans and mentally ill before them, are at risk of being cut off completely, with few choices except life on the street and survival in a grim shadow economy.

"The group maternity home would provide much less encouragement than the current welfare system for out-of-wedlock births."

MATERNITY HOMES WOULD DETER TEENAGE PREGNANCY

George W. Liebmann

In the following viewpoint, George W. Liebmann advocates a welfare reform proposal that would end cash benefits and require unwed teenage mothers to live in maternity homes, where they would receive supervision and education in parenting. According to Liebmann, the maternity home environment would benefit unmarried teenage mothers and their children, and eliminating cash incentives would deter additional young women from becoming pregnant. An attorney from Baltimore, Maryland, Liebmann is a former counsel to the Maryland State Department of Social Services and a former executive assistant to the governor of Maryland.

As you read, consider the following questions:

1. How would maternity homes discourage teenagers from becoming pregnant, according to Liebmann?
2. According to the author, what is the main objection to maternity homes?
3. What physical facilities does Liebmann believe could be adapted into maternity homes?

From George W. Liebmann, "Addressing Illegitimacy: The Root of Real Welfare Reform," *Backgrounder*, April 6, 1995, ©1995 by The Heritage Foundation. Reprinted with permission.

It is clear that illegitimacy must be deterred by moving back to the structure of disincentives favored by the original generation of social workers: no cash aid as a matter of right, the active fostering of adoptions, and the moral education and reformation of mothers in maternity homes run by the voluntary sector. . . .

The Faircloth-Talent bill, first proposed in 1994, takes the first clear step in reversing the sixty-year-old mistaken policy of federal cash subsidies to women who bear children out of wedlock. The bill intends to remove or diminish many of the current welfare incentives which promote illegitimacy. The legislation provides that one year after enactment, women age 21 and under who prospectively bear children out of wedlock will no longer be eligible for direct cash, food, or housing aid from the federal government. Eligibility for direct federal aid will be restored only if the mother subsequently marries or if the child is adopted.

The bill focuses initially on limiting direct welfare to young unmarried women precisely because the consequences of illegitimacy are most severe among members of that age group. . . .

NOT COLD TURKEY

However, the Faircloth-Talent bill does not propose simply to go "cold turkey" by denying aid with no alternative. Under the bill, all aid which ordinarily would have gone directly to the unmarried mother is given instead to the state government for a special grant. The grant may be used for two purposes: 1) to prevent out-of-wedlock pregnancies and 2) to support those children who are born out of wedlock through alternative means that do not involve conventional welfare payments to the mother. The bill encourages use of these funds for pregnancy prevention, adoption, and closely supervised group homes for unmarried mothers and their children.

Under the type of group maternity home envisioned in the Faircloth-Talent bill, the behavior of the mothers would be closely monitored. They would receive no cash for drugs, cigarettes, alcohol, and non-working boyfriends. Instead, constructive behavior would be required. For example, mothers in the group home could be required to take parenting classes, to do their homework, and to complete high school. Thus, while the group maternity home would provide much less encouragement than the current welfare system for out-of-wedlock births, it would also provide a higher quality of environment for children born out of wedlock. . . .

The concept of maternity homes for unmarried mothers is gaining support from both sides of the political spectrum. For example, use of maternity homes was advocated by the liberal Progressive Policy Institute, a research organization closely linked to the Democratic Leadership Council, in a 1994 report on teen pregnancy. Criticism of supervised group homes is largely restricted to the charge that they will be far more costly than the current system of direct cash, food, and housing aid to unmarried mothers. Several points can be made in response to this charge. First, the Faircloth-Talent legislation and similar bills do not call for a direct one-for-one exchange in which all young unmarried mothers who otherwise would have enrolled in AFDC [Aid to Families with Dependent Children] will be placed in maternity homes. Instead, the backers of the bill predict a sharp redirection in the number of out-of-wedlock births as well as an increase in the number of young mothers supported by family and friends rather than welfare. Thus, the number of young mothers who would enter group homes would be only a fraction of those who would enroll in AFDC under the current welfare system.

EASIER TO INFLUENCE

Our welfare system should separate pregnant girls who are not yet 16 years old. It should remove them from wherever they are staying—with boyfriends, sisters, parents, or in the streets. Our system should have a residential base where these girls can stay, be protected, and grow up. Why not have supervised group housing? Why not provide counselors during the pregnancy and, in those cases where the mother decides to keep the baby, for the first eight months of the infant's life? Why not require school attendance and nightly check-ins? Why not create a haven where a girl can learn about her new responsibility?

Girls in group homes are easier to reach with services and easier to influence than girls living on their own. . . .

Why shouldn't our welfare system send the message before teens risk pregnancy that they cannot escape the responsibilities of parenthood?

Lynn Martin, *Responsive Community*, Spring 1994.

Second, mothers on AFDC currently must be housed somewhere. The simple fact is that congregate housing, in which bath and kitchen facilities are shared, costs less than providing a separate housing unit for each mother. The extra cost, if any, involved in a maternity home will come from the additional supervision provided. But welfare systems already provide a large array of fragmented social services to mothers on AFDC, often designed to deal with crises after the fact. These services could be provided better by maternity home supervisors on site.

Most states currently assign portions of their bureaucracies to fitful and inadequate efforts to ensure that young mothers attend school, secure required immunizations, keep prenatal medical appointments, and refrain from physical abuse of their children. All these functions are performed more appropriately by a resident supervisor. Even the most rudimentary regime of residential supervision by a trained adult in control of the purse strings should suffice to reduce inner-city rates of infant mortality that are now of Third-World proportions. The states pay for the absence of this supervision in the emergency room and pediatric hospital components of their Medicaid programs, in their special education programs and institutions for the retarded, and ultimately in their juvenile justice and prison systems.

Third, there are a number of ways to keep the costs of maternity homes low. The cities in which the AFDC caseload is greatest are, by no particular coincidence, those that also are depopulating most rapidly. Characteristically, they possess a number of recently closed hospitals or wings of hospitals. In consequence of the deinstitutionalization of the mentally ill, many state governments also possess hospitals or wings of hospitals which are susceptible of adaptive use. Finding physical facilities for maternity homes would not seem to present a large problem. The use of wings of operating hospitals also would greatly facilitate the rendition of medical services necessary in the first few months of life and now gravely neglected by this population. Corridors of public housing complexes also could be sealed off from the rest of the housing units and converted into supervised group quarters.

Estimates that maternity homes will cost as much as $7,000 to $30,000 per mother per year to operate are grossly inflated. Such estimates are based on facilities where the staff-to-client ratio is as high as 1 to 2. Clearly, homes can be operated at much lower expense, as is demonstrated by many small church-related homes sponsored by organizations like Loving and Caring, Inc., of Lancaster, Pennsylvania.

SUPERVISION, NOT INDEPENDENCE

Unwed motherhood should no longer create entitlement to public cash aid or be perceived by teenage girls as a path to economic independence. Rather, as the timid 1988 Family Support Act began to suggest, young unwed mothers should receive their principal assistance from their own families where possible

148

and from private group homes subsidized with government funds, and supervised living arrangements sponsored by them, where family support is unavailable.

It will not work to provide maternity homes merely as an add-on to the current welfare system. Governments simultaneously must stop providing recipients with other more convenient and attractive types of aid. Maternity homes, with the requirements they place on their residents, will be widely used only if the alternative of responsibility-free cash payments is no longer provided to women who bear children they cannot support.

Decades of experience have demonstrated that the policy of defining cash benefits as "rights" of teenage mothers has failed. The effect of the policy has been not to assist such mothers in becoming part of society, but to isolate them at a time when their greatest need is for education, supervision, and direction. Those who claim that reversing the policy will generate abandoned children, a new class of homeless, or teenage prostitution ignore the existence of responsible alternatives to it. Government should provide support for maternity homes and social assistance. It also should give the institutions and social workers with whom young mothers become affiliated the means to provide limited supervised assistance where it is needed. But if illegitimacy and dependency are to be reduced, unsupervised cash aid must be brought to an end, and teenagers must be told in unmistakable terms that supervision—and not a fraudulent form of independence—is the consequence of irresponsibility.

> "Second-chance homes aren't really about protecting waifs and reviving Ophelias—who come, as feminists know, from all economic levels. They're about cutting welfare."

MATERNITY HOMES WOULD UNFAIRLY PUNISH PREGNANT TEENAGERS

Katha Pollitt

Some commentators have advocated maternity homes as part of welfare reform. Maternity homes, also called second chance homes, would be group homes where unmarried teenage mothers would live and receive instruction and guidance in parenting. In the following viewpoint, Katha Pollitt, a feminist and columnist for the *Nation* magazine, contends that such homes would be excessively punitive and moralistic. She points out that many teenagers become pregnant as a result of sexual victimization, while many others consent to sex. In either case, according to Pollitt, confinement and moral education would be an inappropriate solution.

As you read, consider the following questions:

1. How do the statistics on rape and sexual coercion undercut the rationale for maternity homes, according to the author?
2. Second chance homes would be run by private institutions rather than the government. What is Pollitt's objection to this arrangement?
3. According to Pollitt, why is it inaccurate to assume that all families receiving welfare must be dysfunctional families?

Katha Pollitt, "Motherhood and Morality," *Nation*, May 27, 1996. Reprinted with permission of the *Nation* magazine; © The Nation Company, L.P.

For years feminists have argued that there is a great deal of sexual coercion and violence against girls and women and that most of it goes unreported. For their pains, they have been labeled victimologists, paranoids, man-haters, hysterics, prudes, New Victorians and falsifiers of research data, even as study after study confirms the basic outlines of this unflattering portrait of American life. (See, for example, Nina Bernstein's excellent May 5–6, 1996, *New York Times* series on campus crime, which exposes the many clever ways colleges keep gang rapes and acquaintance rapes out of their official crime statistics—exactly as rape counselors charged, to widespread skepticism, when Katie Roiphe cited official campus rape figures to "prove" date rape was hyped.)

For years, too, feminists have pointed out that sexual coercion and violence against girls and women are causally bound up with a wide variety of social ills, from unwanted pregnancy to mental illness to homelessness. In May 1996, for example, NOW [National Organization for Women] announced the results of a Taylor Institute study suggesting that up to 80 percent of current welfare recipients are or have been victims of physical domestic abuse. This analysis has not, to put it mildly, made much of a dent in the family-values cheerleading that dominates the policy hot-air-waves.

THE "SECRET TRUTH"

Enter *Newsweek*'s Joe Klein, scourge of black men and single mothers, twin carriers of the dreaded "culture of poverty." In his April 29, 1996, column Klein reveals what he calls the "secret truth" about pregnant teens, which is that many of them are victims of sexual abuse and have been impregnated by predatory older men. Stop the presses! Isn't this exactly what feminists have been saying since forever? The research Klein cites—an Alan Guttmacher Institute study that found that two-thirds of teen mothers were impregnated by men over 20; a Washington State study that found 62 percent of pregnant teens had been raped or molested before becoming pregnant—along with other studies showing high rates of coercive sex generally and by older men particularly, has been widely cited by feminists and others concerned with young girls, including me (!) many times (!) right here (!). The clinical psychologist Mary Pipher's *Reviving Ophelia: Saving the Selves of Adolescent Girls*, which gives much the same picture of attention-starved and insecure girls from troubled families who are easily exploited by lupine boys and men, has been on the *New York Times* best-seller list for more than a year with half a million copies in print. Some secret!

What's made Joe Klein suddenly so interested in the victimization of teenage girls by older men is an idea being pushed by the Progressive Policy Institute: privately run "second-chance homes" for teenage welfare mothers instead of A.F.D.C. [Aid to Families with Dependent Children]. It's easy to see why Klein would go for this idea and even urge states to make it mandatory: He gets to send a whole lot of black men off to jail for statutory rape and establish welfare receipt as proof positive of family dysfunction. True, the plan does require expressing some sympathy for inner-city Magdalenes—not Klein's favorite charity—but at least it allows for their confinement and instruction in "motherhood and morality." The hostility Klein feels toward welfare mothers is simply pushed back a generation—from today's teen moms to their moms, whom he portrays as helpless or even complicitous in their daughters' plight.

THE PROSPECT OF GROUP HOMES

Have [conservative Republicans] ever had any candid conversations with teenagers about sex?

Do they really believe the prospect of living in group homes with other unwed mothers will counteract the influence of peer pressure, which is pushing kids into sexual activity at younger and younger ages? Have any of them ever watched "Beverly Hills 90210," "My So-Called Life," or any of the shows aimed at adolescents in which sexual activity among the young is neither shameful nor surprising?

Cynthia Tucker, *Liberal Opinion Week*, January 30, 1995.

Certainly there are plenty of teen mothers in desperate straits: girls trapped in abusive families and exploitative relationships, runaways and throwaways. It would be nice if society provided them with kindly, safe living alternatives—on a voluntary basis. As the P.P.I.'s Kathleen Sylvester described various second-chance homes to me, they sounded pleasanter than the genteel reform schools envisioned by Klein. ("Motherhood and morality are his words," she said pointedly.) It speaks volumes about how vengeful and cruel and loaded with woman-blame the welfare reform debate has become that I wanted to like this proposal, which at least acknowledges that teenagers are valuable people who can be good mothers and who have a claim on society. President Clinton's recent decision requiring states to force teen welfare moms to live at home, by contrast, comes from a much more punitive vision.

The problem, though, is that second-chance homes aren't really about protecting waifs and reviving Ophelias—who come, as feminists know, from all economic levels. They're about cutting welfare. (The reliance on volunteers—churches, Rotary Clubs, the Junior League—is a tipoff. If the girls are in such trouble they need to be in an institution, don't they need more help than the local bourgeoisie can give?) Like Klein, the P.P.I. makes welfare receipt a proxy for dysfunctional family, and teen motherhood a proxy for sexual victimization and bad parenting by a girl's own mother. But none of this is so simple: Most teenage mothers don't go on welfare; many welfare mothers are good parents; many middle-class and upper-class homes are spectacularly dysfunctional; many teenage girls from stable, intact families have sex with older men. Construing teen sex as all victimization seems more compassionate than construing it, like Newt Gingrich, as all sluttishness. But do we really want to say that a 15-year-old girl is always and invariably incapable of giving consent to sex with her 18-year-old boyfriend?

The truth is, second-chance homes are like those "lavishly funded" orphanages Charles Murray proposes for welfare babies: a mental conscience-salve for those who can't quite stomach the ongoing war against the poor. Once the homes got beyond the demonstration-project phase, they'd be like the other institutions, public and private, to which we confine the poor— the daycare centers, public schools and clinics, foster care systems and group homes. An America willing to give poor teen mothers and their babies a true second-chance home wouldn't need to. It would have made sure they had a first chance.

> "Men who have sexual relations with girls below the legal age of consent are committing the crime of statutory rape, a crime for which they can go to jail."

ENFORCING STATUTORY RAPE LAWS WOULD REDUCE TEENAGE PREGNANCY

Arnold Beichman

Because such a high percentage of teenage pregnancies are caused by adult men, sometimes through rape or sexual coercion, some politicians and social commentators are calling for increased enforcement of statutory rape laws, which currently are rarely enforced. In this viewpoint, Arnold Beichman contends that serious enforcement of statutory rape laws could deter adult males from having sex with teenage girls, and thus reduce teenage pregnancy. Beichman is a research fellow at the Hoover Institution and a columnist for the *Washington Times*.

As you read, consider the following questions:

1. According to Beichman, what is the definition of "statutory rape" and how does it differ from state to state?
2. What approaches to reducing teenage pregnancy will receive less emphasis in California's new approach, according to Beichman?

Arnold Beichman, "Statutory Rape Laws Must Be Enforced," *Insight*, May 13, 1996. Reprinted by permission of the *Washington Times*.

One of Supreme Court Justice Oliver Wendell Holmes' wisest maxims is that it's sometimes more important to emphasize the obvious than to elucidate the obscure.

The obvious is the fact that men who have sexual relations with girls below the legal age of consent are committing the crime of statutory rape, a crime for which they can go to jail. Rarely is there such a prosecution. Perhaps it is regarded as politically incorrect to try the male responsible for adolescent pregnancy for what is defined as a crime in state penal codes.

Republican Gov. Pete Wilson of California has undertaken to emphasize the obvious. In 1995 he proposed a teenage pregnancy–prevention program with a $12 million price tag. In 1996 he proposed to increase the 1996–1997 cost to $16 million. What is unusual about the program is that it is going to deal with a legal violation long ignored by state and local governments.

One-fifth of the governor's 1995–1996 $12 million appropriation—$2.4 million—was budgeted for the prosecution of men who engage in sex with girls under 18, the California age of consent. For the fiscal year, Wilson increased the prosecution fund by $6 million for a total of $8.4 million. The objective is to strengthen enforcement of statutory-rape laws throughout the state. Every state has a statutory-rape law that prohibits adult males from having sexual intercourse with girls under the age of consent. States have different age limits ranging from 16 to 18.

A NEW APPROACH

The Wilson policy represents a major change in the approach to teenage pregnancy. Instead of pressuring teenage mothers with threats of welfare-benefit cutbacks or distributing condoms in the classroom or telling pubescent and adolescent girls to "just say no," the governor proposes to go after the adult fathers—with the threat of prosecution and jail sentences for statutory rape. The assumption here is that a 13- or 14-year-old girl no more can give meaningful consent to sexual activity than she could consent to work nights as a stripper.

California is facing a dramatic statewide increase in out-of-wedlock pregnancies. Whereas in the sixties in California 10 percent of births were to unmarried women, today births to unmarried women of all ages account for more than 30 percent of all live births. In 1994, nearly one-fourth of all births to unmarried women in California were to teens.

According to the Guttmacher Institute, the majority of births nationally to adolescent women (70 percent in 1992) occur out of wedlock. At least half of the babies born to teenage girls are fathered by adults. These adults are violating a law that for too long has been more honored in the breach than the observance.

The Maximum Penalty

In the case of teen-age pregnancies, all that is needed is thorough and systematic enforcement of laws pertaining to statutory rape. A girl of 16 and under has by law been raped, whether she consented to or even initiated the sex act. She should be required to name and testify against the male, of any age, who should be prosecuted for rape and given the maximum penalty. Once upon a time, this was done routinely, but the liberal bleeding hearts have tied the hands of police, prosecutors and the government agencies that handle and subsidize these pregnancies.

If these predatory males knew for certain that they would face prison and fines for every casual roll in the hay, you would see a tremendous decline in the teen-age pregnancies that result.

Ralph de Toledano, *Conservative Chronicle*, August 28, 1996.

Statutory rape used to be penalized. That's why a long time ago the coarse alliterative expression for girls under the age of consent was "Quentin Quail." This was a reference to the then–San Quentin prison where a convicted defendant in a rape case might do time.

The Guttmacher Institute's findings are based on 1989–1991 survey data from the National Maternal and Infant Health Survey of the National Center for Health Statistics. A full report of the survey is to be found in the August 1995 edition of the journal *Family Planning Perspectives*.

Older Fathers

Between 1989 and 1991, interviews were conducted of 10,000 underage mothers. The survey found that half of the fathers of babies born to mothers between ages 15 and 17 were 20 years of age or older. Twenty percent of the fathers were six or more years older than the teenage mothers. The survey found a significant correlation in age between the sex partners: The younger a mother was, the greater the age difference between the girl and her partner.

The question of sexual abuse arises from a finding that about 18 percent of women 17 or younger who have had intercourse were, they say, forced at least once to do so. In such cases, the adult male could be tried for aggravated sexual assault.

In California, a survey showed that of 47,000 births to teen-age mothers in 1993, as many as two-thirds were fathered by men who were of post-high-school age. With high-school girls, fathers averaged 4.2 years older than their partners. With junior high-school mothers, the fathers were, on average, 6.7 years older.

The survey showed that among California mothers between the ages of 11 and 15, 51 percent of the fathers were adults, 40 percent were high-school boys and 9 percent junior high-school boys. Another survey in the state of Washington showed that of 535 mothers ages 12 to 17, the average age of the father was 24. More than two-thirds of these teenage mothers said they had been sexually abused.

It is possible that a few jail sentences for statutory rape—and why not prosecutions for pedophilia as well?—may influence adult males to leave children alone. Go to it, Wilson.

| "Preventing teen pregnancy requires more than implementing tough sexual predator laws and enforcing them."

ENFORCING STATUTORY RAPE LAWS IS ONLY A PARTIAL SOLUTION

Regina T. Montoya

In the following viewpoint, Regina T. Montoya agrees that enforcement of statutory rape laws may help deter older men from preying on young girls, thus lowering the teenage pregnancy rate. Enforcement of these laws would temporarily remove predatory males from society, Montoya contends, but this step alone would not solve the problem of teenage pregnancy. She argues that young girls will remain vulnerable unless they are better able to understand and control their own sexuality. Montoya is on the national board of directors of Girls, Inc., a youth organization for girls.

As you read, consider the following questions:

1. What do oversize sweatshirts on teenage girls indicate, according to Montoya?
2. In the author's view, what provides a more lasting solution to the problem of teenage pregnancy than prosecuting the fathers?

Regina T. Montoya, "We Need Tough Laws, Consistent Messages," *Los Angeles Times*, February 4, 1996. Reprinted by permission of the author.

At dinner recently, my mother, a high school teacher for more than 25 years, told me she was disappointed because one of her star students, a bright and energetic 15-year-old girl, had worn a sweatshirt that day and the day before.

When I asked my mother why wearing a sweatshirt two days in a row was so tragic, she looked at me, as if I were from another planet. "Mi hijita," she said, "that's how you know the young girls are pregnant." She said the girls hide their conditions for as long as possible and once they start to show, they wear oversized sweatshirts.

My mother's disappointment was palpable. She knew that it would be more difficult for her star pupil to finish high school and, given the time and financial demands of providing for another human being, to attain the career and family goals she had told my mother about.

THE THREAT OF JAIL

The girl's experience is not unique. Each year, 1 million teenagers become pregnant, statistics that prompted President Clinton to begin a national campaign against teen pregnancy. California has the highest teen pregnancy rate in the country; Gov. Pete Wilson has targeted the prosecution of adult men who engage in sex with girls under 18. This pilot program is important in light of the study by the Alan Guttmacher Institute in 1995, which found that the younger the mother was, the greater the usual age difference between her and the baby's father. According to the study, in 20% of cases, the father is six or more years older than the mother; fully half of the fathers of babies born to girls between 15 and 17 were 20 or older.

Adult men who prey on young girls should be punished and vilified. Perhaps the threat of incarceration will deter some of them from impregnating young girls. For those who still choose to break the law, at least they will not be able to target other young girls once they are prosecuted and incarcerated.

Yet one must contrast this with a recent case in Texas in which three adult male students, one of them 19, had sex with a 13-year-old girl during school hours. The girl provided each with a condom. Under Texas law, the male students committed aggravated sexual assault on a child, a felony punishable by life in prison. The first time the case went before a Dallas grand jury, the jury declined to indict the three students. The case went back to the grand jury and this time the three were indicted on charges of public lewdness, a misdemeanor that carries a maximum sentence of a year in jail. One cannot say for sure why the only charges were misdemeanors, but I suspect that because the girl provided condoms, the jurors decided that she had consented to have sex with the young men. But the fact remains that she was 13.

Punishing the adult male is important and cannot be discounted. But if a grand jury applies the law as it is written and the father of the child is actually jailed, what of the girl and her baby? Presumably the welfare system will provide the safety net. We all know that welfare is a shrinking net that may not be available. The answer is to educate underage girls. Some may know about contraception, as did the 13-year-old in Texas. But she was not mature enough to understand the consequences of her actions. Would it not have been better for her to have been educated about life's choices?

NOT MATURE ENOUGH

An alliance of progressives and conservatives has turned its attention to men and agreed that it is time to dust off the old statutory rape laws. In 1996, California Gov. Pete Wilson warned men who had sex with minors, "That's not just wrong, not just a shame. It's a crime, a crime called statutory rape."

But in Orange County, California, there are some judges and social workers trying to solve the concerns of unwed motherhood and statutory rape by marrying the two together. That is, by allowing the pregnant girl to marry the statutory rapist. . . .

Statutory rape laws are based on the notion that a girl below a certain age isn't mature enough to legally consent to sex. How then, is she old enough to consent to marriage?

Ellen Goodman, (San Diego) North County Times, September 13, 1996.

Research by Girls Inc., a youth organization that provides direct services and advocates for girls, shows that age-appropriate sexuality education that enhances girls' knowledge, skills and resources is effective in enabling them to delay sexual activity and pregnancy. Girls Inc. has learned that sexuality education must start by age 9 and continue through age 18, as a girl takes increasing responsibility for her well-being. Girls need to learn the skills to resist early sexual activity and to practice these skills.

Preventing teen pregnancy requires more than implementing tough sexual predator laws and enforcing them. A young girl who lacks self-esteem, parental involvement or basic information must receive consistent messages and reliable adult support at home, in school and in the community.

> "There is . . . a less drastic way to make welfare more inconvenient for unwed mothers: impose an unequivocal requirement to finish high school and then to work."

REQUIRING WELFARE RECIPIENTS TO WORK WOULD REDUCE TEENAGE PREGNANCY

Douglas J. Besharov

Like many social commentators, both liberal and conservative, Douglas J. Besharov believes that pregnancy and welfare have become attractive options for teenagers because other fulfilling opportunities seem closed off to them. Besharov would remedy this situation by making welfare inconvenient; he would require welfare recipients to participate in job training and work. Those who currently rely on the welfare system would be forced to acquire job skills and would gain in self-confidence and employability, according to Besharov. In addition, he contends, these strict requirements would discourage prospective teenage mothers from becoming pregnant. Besharov is a resident scholar at the American Enterprise Institute and a visiting professor at the University of Maryland School of Public Affairs.

As you read, consider the following questions:

1. Why, according to Besharov, do current job training programs fail?
2. What are the best contraceptives, according to the author?
3. In Besharov's view, what associated social problems can be avoided by requiring young welfare mothers to work?

Abridged from Douglas J. Besharov, "Making Illegitimacy Inconvenient," *Crisis*, March 1994. Reprinted with permission.

O fficial Washington is now in the midst of yet another effort to reform the nation's welfare system. But this time something is different: After 30 years of denial, almost everyone now agrees that real reform requires doing something about out-of-wedlock births, especially among teenagers. So far, though, most welfare planners are trying to use job training and public service jobs to make poorly educated unwed mothers self-sufficient, which won't work. Instead, training and work mandates should be used as tools to discourage out-of-wedlock births in the first place.

Attention is finally being focused on illegitimacy because the problem has simply grown too large to ignore. In 1991, about 30 percent of American children were born out of wedlock, reflecting a steady increase from 1960, when the figure was only 5 percent. More than one million children were born out of wedlock in 1990; over a third were to teenagers, often after they had dropped out of school.

Illegitimacy is not just a problem among black Americans. Although out-of-wedlock birth rates are much higher for blacks than for whites, they are rising faster among whites. In fact, since 1980, 776,000 more white babies than black have been born out of wedlock.

"The majority of teen mothers end up on welfare, and taxpayers paid about $29 billion in 1991 to assist families begun by a teenager," reports President Clinton's Working Group on Welfare Reform. The bulk of long-term welfare recipients are young, unmarried mothers, most of whom had their first baby as teenagers.

Unwed mothers now head half the families on welfare, double the proportion in 1970, further swelling the already-large number of long-term welfare dependents. According to the House Ways and Means Committee, unwed mothers average almost ten years on welfare, twice as long as divorced mothers. (The differences are actually greater because many unwed mothers later marry, although often for a short time, so they get counted in the divorced group.)

THE FAILURE OF JOB TRAINING

As these facts become better-known, agreement grows that reducing long-term dependency requires doing something constructive about the young unwed mothers who go on welfare in such large numbers—and stay there. But what?

President Clinton would start with up to two years of job training and education for all recipients. Unfortunately, even the best job training programs have had little success in helping these young unwed mothers to become economically self-sufficient. Five percent reductions in welfare rolls are considered major accomplishments—not nearly enough to "end welfare as we know it," Bill Clinton's much-repeated campaign pledge. . . .

Job training programs fail because they cannot overcome the financial mathematics of welfare dependency. A young girl who drops out of high school and then has two children (as do most long-term recipients) is all but trapped on welfare by the limits of her earning capacity compared to the size of contemporary welfare benefits. Even if she gets a job, she quickly realizes that she did just about as well on welfare as at work—with much less effort.

This is why Clinton also proposes a time-limit on welfare benefits. If, after two years, a welfare mother does not get a job, he says that she should be placed in a public service job. The job is supposed to give her work experience and to serve as an incentive to get off welfare, since she will have to work anyway.

WORTH TRYING

What might be done is to listen to some of the people who say we should try to change things, even over the objections of the sociologists and other experts whose advice is that doing nothing is always better than doing something.

Refusing welfare for more illegitimate children might be worth trying. Work programs instead of welfare might be worth trying. Requiring that fathers be named before new welfare checks are paid might be tried.

Leonard Larsen, *Washington Times*, February 25, 1995.

The evidence, however, suggests that work requirements do not reduce caseloads, at least not immediately. An initial evaluation of Ohio's workfare program found an impressive 34 percent reduction in caseloads for two-parent welfare households but only a modest 11 percent reduction among female-headed households. Even these results, however, have been called into question by subsequent analysis.

Worse, in September 1993, the Manpower Demonstration Research Corporation (MDRC) reviewed the impacts of the mandatory work programs in West Virginia; Cook County, Illinois; and in two sites in San Diego, California. In none of the sites were welfare payments reduced because of work requirements.

It should not be surprising that most single mothers stay on welfare, even after they are forced to work for their benefits. Their "welfare job" may be better than anything they can get in the real world of work, it is probably less demanding than an actual job, and there will be little chance of being laid off or fired. Moreover, especially in areas of high unemployment, there may be no other jobs available for poorly educated women with little work experience.

Recognizing these realities, and to save money, the president's welfare reform working group is now suggesting that Clinton's proposed public service requirement be watered down. This would be a mistake. In fact, work requirements should be strengthened—by applying them much earlier in the welfare careers of young, unwed mothers.

MAKING WELFARE INCONVENIENT

Former Surgeon General Joycelyn Elders often cites a 1988 survey in which 87 percent of unwed teen mothers said that their babies' births were "intended." But this includes 63 percent who said that the birth was "mistimed." And, when clinicians ask the more telling question, whether having a baby would disrupt their lives, that is, whether it would be inconvenient, few say "Yes." For example, in 1990, Laurie Zabin of the Johns Hopkins School of Public Health and Hygiene surveyed pregnant, inner-city black teens; only 31 percent said that they "believed a baby would present a problem." Making illegitimacy more inconvenient, what economists would call raising its opportunity cost, is the key to welfare reform.

Increasing the life prospects of disadvantaged teens is, of course, the best way to raise the opportunity costs of having a baby out of wedlock. Because those young people who have the most to look forward to are the most responsible about their sexual practices, it is not too much of an exaggeration to say that a good education and real job opportunities are the best contraceptives.

Nevertheless, welfare policies also can raise the opportunity costs of illegitimacy. The ultimate "inconvenience," of course, would be to deny welfare benefits altogether. But, although this position is gaining adherents, it is still unacceptable to most people. There is, however, a less drastic way to make welfare more inconvenient for unwed mothers: impose an unequivocal requirement to finish high school and then to work.

From almost the first day that a young, unwed mother goes on welfare, she should be engaged in mandatory skill-building activities. The first priority should be that she finish high school, or at least demonstrate basic proficiency in math and reading. After that, if she is unable to find work, she should be assigned to a public service job, as the president promised. However, the political pressure from unions will be for these public service positions to be "real jobs" at "decent wages." But, this would raise costs to prohibitive levels and make recipients even less likely to leave the rolls.

THE BENEFITS OF WORKING

Instead, the focus should be on activities that are appropriate for inexperienced young women, that is, on tasks that offer the discipline of job attendance and the boost to self-esteem that come with work. Examples of such activities were described by MDRC's Thomas Brock, who studied the four mandatory work programs mentioned above as well as six others. The activities "did not teach new skills, but neither were they 'make work.' Most were entry-level clerical positions or janitorial/maintenance jobs," such as office aides and receptionists for community nonprofit agencies, mail clerks for city agencies, assistants in day care programs for children or handicapped adults, helpers in public works department sweeping and repairing streets, and gardening in city parks. And, although the work requirement did not immediately reduce caseloads, in three of the four sites, the value of the services rendered together with other savings exceeded the program's cost to taxpayers.

Such activities probably also raise the self-discipline, social contacts, and skills of participants, and, therefore, their employability. This is all positive. However, it would be quite enough if the mandated work merely raised the inconvenience level of being on welfare by requiring these young women to be someplace—doing something constructive—every day. The object would be to discourage their younger sisters and friends from thinking that a life on welfare is an attractive option. (Strengthened child support enforcement would also increase the inconvenience level for their boyfriends who got them pregnant, but describing how to achieve that end is a complicated subject for another day.)

These requirements should not be considered punitive or vindictive, nor should they be implemented in a way that makes them so. Inactivity is bad for everyone. For young mothers on welfare, it can be even more dispiriting, spiraling some toward immobilizing depression. Child abuse, drug abuse, and a host of social problems are associated with long-term welfare dependency. A work requirement will help to reduce social isolation.

In addition, the welfare mother's parental responsibilities should be respected. A key argument in the debate about requiring welfare mothers to work is that, since so many middle-class mothers are now working, there is nothing wrong with expecting welfare mothers to work. And, in keeping with the careless way that the statistics are often used, the assumption is that welfare mothers should work full time. But most middle-class mothers are not working full time, with the exception of divorced mothers, who are often forced to do so because of failings in the alimony and child support systems. Also, divorced mothers and their children tend to be older than the average unwed welfare mother and her children. Therefore, training and work requirements for young welfare mothers should vary depending on the age (and any special needs) of their children.

MORE PRODUCTIVE LIVES

It will take some time before new expectations take root and behaviors begin to change. Hence, it is important to adopt a five- or even ten-year perspective on the effort. Moreover, the mandate would have to be universal. Half measures will not do. Since the community as a whole tends to establish and enforce behavioral norms, to achieve a change in expectations (and, hence, in behavior), all young women would have to feel that, if they went on welfare, they would be subject to school and work requirements.

Despite the real value of the services provided, such a program could be very expensive. But because of its prophylactic purpose, it could be imposed prospectively, that is, applied to new applicants only. This would result in a long phase-in period that would sharply lower initial costs—and allow modifications in program rules and administration based on what is learned during the first stages of implementation.

A decade-long commitment to making welfare "inconvenient" could change the reproductive behavior of disadvantaged teens—as the implications of the new regime begin to sink in. But even if disadvantaged young people didn't stop having so many babies out of wedlock, at least those on welfare might be helped to lead more productive lives. That would be reason enough to reform the system.

VIEWPOINT

"The high rate of early childbearing
is a measure of how bleak life is for
young people who are living in poor
communities and who have no
obvious arenas for success."

INCREASED EDUCATION AND ECONOMIC OPPORTUNITY WOULD REDUCE TEENAGE PREGNANCY

Kristin Luker

In the following viewpoint, Kristin Luker argues that poverty and diminished work opportunities for the poorest segment of society are the primary stimulants of early childbearing. Consequently, according to Luker, expanded sex education and increased job opportunities in poor communities are the best strategies for reducing teenage pregnancy. Luker is professor of sociology and law at the University of California, Berkeley, and the author of Dubious Conceptions: The Politics of Teenage Pregnancy, from which this viewpoint is excerpted.

As you read, consider the following questions:

1. Why does Luker consider conservative efforts to cut funding for contraceptive programs to be paradoxical and self-defeating?
2. When job markets are open to young women, what happens to teenage pregnancy rates, according to the author?
3. Why does Luker argue that cutting or ending welfare benefits to pregnant teenagers will have a negligible effect on teenage pregnancy rates?

Reprinted by permission of the publisher from Dubious Conceptions: The Politics of Teenage Pregnancy by Kristin Luker (Cambridge, MA: Harvard University Press, 1996). Copyright ©1996 by the Presidents and Fellows of Harvard College.

According to new research, effective sex education programs can change adolescents' behavior. Such programs typically begin before students have become sexually active and they are usually strongly prescriptive in nature. Effective programs focus clearly on goals and carefully evaluate what works. Not only do some programs delay the onset of sexual activity, but others lead to greater use of contraception. In comparison to people who have had no sex education, those who have attended a good sex-ed program are more likely to use contraception the first time they have sex, to obtain effective contraception sooner, and to use contraception more reliably in general.

SELF-DEFEATING INITIATIVES

Thus, in view of all the evidence that public policies have done a reasonably good job of containing early pregnancy despite a vast increase in sexual activity among teens, the current conservative initiatives seem paradoxical at best and self-defeating at worst. There are powerful pressures to cut public funding for contraceptive programs, even as these programs are becoming recognized for the success story they are. Similarly, people who oppose abortions, much like people in the nineteenth century who opposed contraception, have been stymied in their attempts to make abortion either illegal or unpopular for the affluent. They have instead contented themselves with policies that make abortion more difficult for young people and poor people to obtain. Finally, just as we have begun to sort out which sex education techniques work and which ones don't, the very notion of sex education is more contested than it has ever been. In the face of accumulating evidence which suggests that more students than ever are receiving sex education and that well-designed programs can indeed modify adolescents' risk-taking behavior, politically mobilized activists all over the United States are pushing for hasty adoption of abstinence-based programs before rigorous evaluation has been able to show whether they are capable of doing anything other than making adults feel better.

To put this in the bluntest terms, society seems to have become committed to *increasing* the rates of pregnancy among teens, especially among those who are poor and those who are most at risk. Affluent and successful young women see real costs to early pregnancy and thus have strong incentives to avoid it, but poor young women face greater obstacles, both internal and external. Cutting funding for public contraceptive clinics, imposing parental-consent requirements, and limiting access to abortion all increase the likelihood that a young woman will get pregnant and have a baby. Conversely, providing widespread contraceptive services (perhaps even making the Pill available over the counter), extending clinic hours, and affording greater access to abortion will give at least some poor young women an alternative to early childbearing.

BLEAK PROSPECTS

The news is even grimmer when it comes to preventing or postponing childbearing among teenagers who are not highly motivated in the first place. Even as we amass evidence showing that early childbearing is not a root cause of poverty in the United States, we are also realizing more clearly that the high rate of early childbearing is a measure of how bleak life is for young people who are living in poor communities and who have no obvious arenas for success. Here, too, just as we are developing a better sense of what it would take to offer these young women and men more choice in life, the political temper of the times makes even modest investments in young people seem like utopian dreams. Far from making lives easier for actual and potential teenage parents, society seems committed to making things harder.

A quarter-century of research on poverty and early childbearing has yielded some solid leads on ways to reduce early pregnancy and childbearing. But because the young people involved have multiple problems, the solutions aren't cheap. In order to reduce the number of teenagers who want babies, society would have to be restructured so that poor people in the United States would no longer be the poorest poor people in the developed world. Early childbearing would decrease if poor teenagers had better schools and safer neighborhoods, and if their mothers and fathers had decent jobs so that teens could afford the luxury of being children for a while longer. If in 1994 the United States had finally succeeded in creating a national health care system (becoming the last industrialized country to do so), this change alone would have had a dramatic impact on poor people generally and poor women specifically. Providing wider access to health care, for example, would have eliminated some obstacles to contraception and possibly even to abortion. More fundamentally, it would have meant that young women and men, even if they did have babies and even if they did have them out of wedlock, could have afforded to raise them without going on welfare.

This is no time to be advocating expensive social programs, however. These days, policymakers seem inclined to shred what remains of the safety net, so the best that teenage mothers and potential teenage mothers can hope for is that programs which make life easier will not be totally eliminated in the drive to reduce the federal deficit. If the few employment programs that exist in the United States survive the budget cutting and if they can increase their outreach to young women, greater employment opportunities may reduce pregnancy rates. A 1978 evaluation of the federally funded Job Corps, for example, revealed that young men and women who were enrolled in the program tended to postpone childbearing and had fewer out-of-wedlock babies. And women who found jobs through other federally funded programs seemed to have lower birthrates than women living in similar communities that had no such programs. Some evidence also shows that macroeconomic forces can affect the rates of early childbearing: communities whose job markets are open to young women tend to have fewer teenage mothers.

ADDRESSING THE RANGE OF PROBLEMS

More programs are needed to expand life-planning options, build self-confidence, improve school performance, increase literacy, and strengthen vocational skills. Additional support is necessary for scholarships and bilingual assistance. These initiatives must be coordinated with other opportunities for vocational training, job placement, and higher education, so that participants can see ways to achieve status and self-worth apart from early parenthood. We cannot respond effectively to teenage motherhood without responding also to the broader range of social problems that make motherhood seem to be a teenager's best option. Nor can we address the inadequacy of paternal support without also addressing the inadequacy of employment, education, and drug treatment opportunities.

Deborah L. Rhode, *Political Science Quarterly*, vol. 108, no. 4, 1993–1994.

A widespread misconception is that many poor women live on welfare instead of finding a job. In fact, most women on welfare use their grants to supplement the low wages they earn in the work force and to see them through periods of unemployment or poor health. The kinds of jobs they have usually pay very little and provide no benefits; even if they worked full time and year round, their incomes would still be below the poverty level. Recent expansions in the Earned Income Tax Credit made life a little easier for those at the bottom. Now, the cessation of AFDC [Aid to Families with Dependent Children] as an entitlement program and inevitable cutbacks in the Earned Income Tax Credit will make life on the bottom much harder. Their effects on early childbearing are unknown, but they are unlikely to reduce it. Although it is a cherished belief among conservatives that the level of available welfare affects childbearing among teenagers, and among unmarried teens in particular, if this were true the rate of such childbearing would have declined dramatically over the past twenty years as the real value of welfare plummeted.

Society could also do a number of other things that, although they would not reduce early childbearing, would make the children of teenage parents better off, thereby reducing the ranks of disadvantaged and discouraged people at risk of being the next generation's teenage parents. These measures, too, have come to seem hopelessly utopian in the current political climate. For example, most other industrialized nations provide high-quality, publicly subsidized daycare for poor children; in the best of all possible worlds, the United States would, too. A national childcare and preschool system would ideally be part of the public schools, as is the case in France. Daycare workers would be trained like teachers and paid at similar levels. In this way, children born to young or poor parents would be challenged and educated from their earliest years. As things stand now, most poor mothers rely on a relative to provide daycare for their children. But this family-oriented system might actually motivate teens to have babies at an early age, since a young mother's claim on her female kin—usually her own mother—seems much more reasonable if she is sixteen than if she is twenty-four. If she knows that someone other than her mother will be able to help care for her children, she may wait a few years before having her first baby.

A PUNITIVE AND COERCIVE TREND

The political scientist Hugh Heclo once noted, speaking of antipoverty policies, that what Americans want they can't have, and what they can have they don't want. This dictum seems particularly apt in connection with early pregnancy and childbearing. Americans want teenagers to wait until they are "mature" before they have sex, to wait until they are "ready" before they get pregnant, and to wait until they are married and financially secure before they have children. But there is no consensus on what it means to be "mature," out-of-wedlock births are common throughout the industrialized world, and a great many teenagers will be poor throughout their lives and hence never really "ready" to be parents. Society could conceivably become so punitive and coercive that poor teenagers would be discouraged from ever having babies, but only a few countries such as China have been able to impose this kind of control. It's even

171

doubtful that the draconian welfare-reform policies proposed by the Republicans will make much of a difference. Since teenagers who live in states with generous benefits do not have more out-of-wedlock babies than teens in states with low benefits, and since out-of-wedlock childbearing has been increasing as welfare benefits decline, a radical reduction in welfare benefits for teenagers will probably have a negligible overall effect. Myriad factors affect the way in which young people make decisions about sexual activity, relationships, and childbearing; whether or not they are eligible to receive a welfare check is unlikely to alter their behavior. Most will continue to have babies, hoping that things will somehow work out and that their families will rearrange scarce resources to provide for the newcomers.

BRIGHTER OPPORTUNITIES

The more one knows about early pregnancy and childbearing, the more skeptical one becomes that they correlate with poverty in any simple way. Poverty is not exclusively or even primarily limited to single mothers; most single mothers are not teenagers; many teenage mothers have husbands or partners; and many pregnant teenagers do not become mothers. The rates of pregnancy and childbearing among teenagers are a serious problem. But early childbearing doesn't make young women poor; rather, poverty makes women bear children at an early age. Society should worry not about some epidemic of "teenage pregnancy" but about the hopeless, discouraged, and empty lives that early childbearing denotes. Teenagers and their children desperately need a better future, one with brighter opportunities and greater rewards. Making the United States the kind of country in which—as in most European countries—early childbearing is rare would entail profound changes in public policy and perhaps even in American society as a whole. Such measures would be costly, and some of them would fail.

Any observer of the current scene would have to conclude that these days the chances of implementing costly social programs are extremely small. Americans seem bent on making the lives of teenage parents and their children even harder than they already are. Society has failed teenage parents all along the line—they are people for whom the schools, the health care system, and the labor market have been painful and unrewarding places. Now, it seems, young parents are being assigned responsibility for society's failures. Young parents have never needed help more, yet never have Americans been less willing to help and more willing to blame.

Periodical Bibliography

The following articles have been selected to supplement the diverse views presented in this chapter. Addresses are provided for periodicals not indexed in the *Readers' Guide to Periodical Literature*, the *Alternative Press Index*, the *Social Sciences Index*, or the *Index to Legal Periodicals and Books*.

J. Lawrence Aber,
Jeanne Brooks-Gunn,
and Rebecca A. Maynard
"Effects of Welfare Reform on Teenage Parents and Their Children," *Future of Children*, Summer/Fall 1995. Available from 300 Second St., Suite 102, Los Angeles, CA 94022.

David Broder
"Pregnancy Prevention a Big Step Toward Welfare Reform," *Liberal Opinion Week*, July 4, 1994. Available from 108 E. Fifth St., Vinton, IA 52349.

John Leo
"Learning to Say No," *U.S. News & World Report*, June 20, 1994.

George Marlin
"Adolescent Sexual Behavior and Childbearing," *Women's Health Issues*, Summer 1994. Available from 409 Twelfth St. SW, Washington, DC 20024.

Lynn Martin
"Facing the Realities of Teenage Motherhood," *Responsive Community*, Spring 1994. Available from 2020 Pennsylvania Ave. NW, Suite 282, Washington, DC 20006.

Robert McCarty
"On the Abstinence Front," *Issues and Views*, Summer 1994. Available from PO Box 467, New York, NY 10025.

George Miller
"Should Congress Halt Welfare Benefits for Unwed Teenage Mothers?" *American Legion*, May 1995.

Kristin A. Moore
"Welfare Bill Won't Stop Teenage Pregnancy," *Christian Science Monitor*, December 18, 1995. Available from One Norway St., Boston, MA 02115.

David Nyhan
"The Insidious Enemy No. 1," *Liberal Opinion Week*, July 4, 1994.

Betsy Wacker and
Alan Gambrell
"Welfare Reform and Teen Parents: Are We Missing the Point?" *SIECUS Report*, June/July 1994. Available from 130 W. 42nd St., Suite 2500, New York, NY 10036.

For Further Discussion

CHAPTER 1

1. Charles Murray argues that teenage pregnancy is the source of many of society's most pressing problems. Janine Jackson counters Murray's argument, claiming that it constitutes another case of "blaming poverty on the character faults and bad decisions of the poor themselves." Do you agree with her assessment of Murray's views? What does Jackson blame for high illegitimacy rates? Whose analysis do you find more convincing? Why?

2. Charles Murray reports an illegitimacy rate of 68 percent of all births to black women, but he says that "the black story . . . is old news." Because the illegitimacy rate has reached 22 percent of all births for whites, Murray contends society needs to take immediate action. Why does he believe the dramatic rise in white illegitimacy constitutes grounds for action while the black rate does not? Do you agree with his distinction? Why or why not?

3. Lloyd Eby and Charles A. Donovan examine the definite link between single-parent households and poverty, and they note the health costs, suffering, and deprivation associated with families headed by unwed teenage mothers. In contrast, Mike Males contends that though unwed teenage mothers may not be better off economically, their lives actually may improve physically and emotionally because of their pregnancy. Which argument do you find more persuasive? Explain your answer.

CHAPTER 2

1. Charles Krauthammer and Donald Lambro agree that if society takes the welfare check away from single teenage mothers, "the society built on babies having babies cannot sustain itself," as Krauthammer phrases it. Based on your reading of these viewpoints, do you agree with the argument that teenagers will stop becoming pregnant if there are no more welfare benefits to support them? Why or why not?

2. Both Joe Klein and Linda Villarosa remark on the high percentage of adult men involved in teenage pregnancies and the high percentage of pregnant teens who have been sexually abused by adult males. But these two writers draw vastly different conclusions about this problem. Identify the differing solutions offered by Klein and Villarosa. Which do you find to

be more promising? Why? Can you think of other solutions not mentioned or stressed by these authors? Explain.

3. Kay S. Hymowitz argues that nothing prevents teenage pregnancy nearly as well as the presence of a loving father living at home. What evidence does she provide in support of this view? Do you find her argument reasonable? Why or why not?

CHAPTER 3

1. According to Jane Mauldon and Kristin Luker, sex education helps to keep down the teenage pregnancy rate, though they argue that specific programs need to be modified to emphasize those measures that actually work. What do these authors find to be successful initiatives in sex education? Which approaches should be discarded as ineffective, in their view?

2. Barbara Dafoe Whitehead observes that New Jersey, a state using comprehensive sex education, has the nation's fourth highest rate of births to unwed teenagers. In Whitehead's view, how should sex education programs like New Jersey's be modified? How do her proposals compare with those of Mauldon and Luker?

3. The Alan Guttmacher Institute report contends that contraceptives are largely successful in preventing teenage pregnancy, while Charmaine Crouse Yoest cites research showing that "condoms have a failure rate of 15.7% at preventing pregnancy over the course of a year." Yoest contends that contraceptives provide a false sense of security and that the risks involved in their use are unacceptable. Do you agree more with the Guttmacher Institute report or with Yoest? Why?

CHAPTER 4

1. The welfare reform bill passed by Congress in August 1996 gives states the option of cutting off or reducing benefits to unwed teenage mothers. James M. Talent and Mona Charen contend that states should end these benefits, arguing that the result will be a decline in teenage pregnancy rates. Mike Males insists that the result of cutting welfare will be higher poverty rates, not lower pregnancy rates. Which view do you find more persuasive, and why?

2. George W. Liebmann contends that unwed teenage mothers who need welfare benefits should either marry, place their babies for adoption, or be required to live in a supervised maternity home. Katha Pollitt believes such homes are not necessarily a bad idea, as long as they are available on a voluntary basis. In your view, should such homes be required or op-

tional for pregnant teenagers who wish to keep their babies and receive welfare benefits? Which approach would be more likely to reduce teenage pregnancy? Explain your answers.

3. Both Arnold Beichman and Regina T. Montoya examine the statistics concerning the role played by adult men in the rising incidence of teenage pregnancy, and both consider the implications of enforcing statutory rape laws. What reservations does Montoya have about such enforcement? Based on your reading of these viewpoints, do you think strict enforcement of such laws would be helpful? Would it serve to reduce teenage pregnancy? What problems, if any, do you foresee with enforcing these rape laws?

4. Douglas J. Besharov believes that making welfare difficult for unwed teenage mothers to obtain will serve to reduce pregnancies among this group. He contends that unwed teenage mothers on welfare should be subjected to a mandatory work or work training requirement. Is this a reasonable proposal, in your view? Why or why not?

ORGANIZATIONS TO CONTACT

The editors have compiled the following list of organizations concerned with the issues debated in this book. The descriptions are derived from materials provided by the organizations. All have publications or information available for interested readers. The list was compiled on the date of publication of the present volume; names, addresses, phone and fax numbers, and e-mail and Internet addresses may change. Be aware that many organizations take several weeks or longer to respond to inquiries, so allow as much time as possible.

Advocates for Youth
1025 Vermont Ave. NW, Suite 200, Washington, DC 20005
(202) 347-5700 • fax: (202) 347-2263

Formerly the Center for Population Options, Advocates for Youth is the only national organization focusing solely on pregnancy and HIV prevention among young people. It provides information, education, and advocacy to youth-serving agencies and professionals, policymakers, and the media. Among the organization's numerous publications are the brochures "Advice from Teens on Buying Condoms" and "Spread the Word—Not the Virus" and the pamphlet *How to Prevent Date Rape: Teen Tips*.

The Alan Guttmacher Institute
120 Wall St., New York, NY 10005
(212) 248-1111 • fax: (212) 248-1951
e-mail: info@agi-usa.org

The institute works to protect and expand the reproductive choices of all women and men. It strives to ensure people's access to the information and services they need to exercise their rights and responsibilities concerning sexual activity, reproduction, and family planning. Among the institute's publications are the books *Teenage Pregnancy in Industrialized Countries* and *Today's Adolescents, Tomorrow's Parents: A Portrait of the Americas* and the report "Sex and America's Teenagers."

Child Trends, Inc. (CT)
4301 Connecticut Ave. NW, Suite 100, Washington, DC 20008
(202) 362-5580 • fax: (202) 362-5533
Internet: http://www.childtrends.org

CT works to provide accurate statistical and research information regarding children and their families in the United States and to educate the American public on the ways existing social trends, such as the increasing rate of teenage pregnancy, affect children. In addition to the annual newsletter *Facts at a Glance*, which presents the latest data on teen pregnancy rates for every state, CT also publishes the papers "Next-Steps and Best Bets: Approaches to Preventing Adolescent Childbearing" and "Welfare and Adolescent Sex: The Effects of Family History, Benefit Levels, and Community Context."

Concerned Women for America (CWA)
370 L'Enfant Promenade SW, Suite 800, Washington, DC 20024
(202) 488-7000 • fax: (202) 488-0806

CWA's purpose is to preserve, protect, and promote traditional Judeo-Christian values through education, legislative action, and other activities. It is concerned with creating an environment that is conducive to building strong families and raising healthy children. CWA publishes the monthly *Family Voice*, which periodically addresses issues such as abortion and promoting sexual abstinence in schools.

Family Research Council
801 G St. NW, Washington, DC 20001
(202) 393-2100 • fax: (202) 393-2134
Internet: http://www.frc.org

The council seeks to promote and protect the interests of the traditional family. It focuses on issues such as parental autonomy and responsibility, community support for single parents, and adolescent pregnancy. Among the council's numerous publications are the papers "Revolt of the Virgins," "Abstinence: The New Sexual Revolution," and "Abstinence Programs Show Promise in Reducing Sexual Activity and Pregnancy Among Teens."

Family Resource Coalition (FRC)
200 S. Michigan Ave, 16th Fl., Chicago, IL 60604
(312) 341-0900 • fax: (312) 341-9361

The FRC is a national consulting and advocacy organization that seeks to strengthen and empower families and communities so they can foster the optimal development of children, teenagers, and adult family members. The FRC publishes the bimonthly newsletter *Connection*, the report "Family Involvement in Adolescent Pregnancy and Parenting Programs," and the fact sheet "Family Support Programs and Teen Parents."

Focus on the Family
Colorado Springs, CO 80995
(719) 531-3400 • fax: (719) 548-4525

Focus on the Family is a Christian organization dedicated to preserving and strengthening the traditional family. It believes that the breakdown of the traditional family is in part linked to increases in teen pregnancy, and it conducts research on the ethics of condom use and the effectiveness of safe-sex education programs in schools. The organization publishes the video "Sex, Lies, and the Truth," which discusses the issue of teen sexuality and abstinence, as well as *Brio*, a monthly magazine for teenage girls.

Girls, Inc.
30 E. 33rd St., New York, NY 10016-5394
(212) 689-3700 • fax: (212) 683-1253

Girls, Inc., is an organization for girls aged six to eighteen that works to create an environment in which girls can learn and grow to their full potential. It conducts daily programs in career and life planning, health and sexuality, and leadership and communication. Girls, Inc., publishes the newsletter *Girls Ink* six times a year, which provides information of interest to young girls and women, including information on teen pregnancy.

The Heritage Foundation
214 Massachusetts Ave. NE, Washington, DC 20002
(202) 546-4400 • fax: (202) 546-0904

The Heritage Foundation is a public policy research institute that supports the ideas of limited government and the free-market system. It promotes the view that the welfare system has contributed to the problems of illegitimacy and teenage pregnancy. Among the foundation's numerous publications is its Backgrounder series, which includes "Liberal Welfare Programs: What the Data Show on Programs for Teenage Mothers"; the paper "Rising Illegitimacy: America's Social Catastrophe"; and the bulletin "How Congress Can Protect the Rights of Parents to Raise Their Children."

The Manhattan Institute
52 Vanderbilt Ave., New York, NY 10017
(212) 599-7000 • fax: (212) 599-3494

The institute is a nonpartisan research organization that seeks to educate scholars, government officials, and the public on the economy and how government programs affect it. It publishes the quarterly magazine *City Journal* and the article "The Teen Mommy Track."

National Asian Women's Health Organizations (NAWHO)
250 Montgomery St., Suite 410, San Francisco, CA 94104
(415) 989-9747 • fax: (415) 989-9758

NAWHO is a community-based advocacy organization dedicated to improving the overall health of Asian women and girls. It believes that teenage pregnancy is a pressing problem facing all communities, and it is committed to addressing the issue in a culturally sensitive and appropriate manner. It publishes a quarterly newsletter and the report "Perceptions of Risk: An Assessment of the Factors Influencing Use of Reproductive and Sexual Health Services by Asian American Women."

National Organization of Adolescent Pregnancy, Parenting, and Prevention (NOAPP)
1319 F St. NW, Suite 401, Washington, DC 20004
(202) 783-5770 • fax: (202) 783-5775
e-mail: noappp@aol.com

NOAPP promotes comprehensive and coordinated services designed for the prevention and resolution of problems associated with adolescent pregnancy and parenthood. It supports families in setting standards that encourage the healthy development of children through loving, stable relationships. NOAPP publishes the quarterly *NOAPP Network Newsletter* and various fact sheets on teen pregnancy.

Planned Parenthood® Federation of America (PPFA)
810 Seventh Ave., New York, NY 10019
(212) 541-7800 • fax: (212) 245-1845

PPFA is a national organization that supports people's right to make their own reproductive decisions without governmental interference. In 1989, it developed First Things First, a nationwide adolescent pregnancy prevention program. This program promotes the view that every child has the right to secure an education, attain physical and emotional maturity, and establish life goals before assuming the responsibilities of parenthood. Among PPFA's numerous publications are the booklets *Teen Sex?*, *Facts About Birth Control*, and *How to Talk with Your Teen About the Facts of Life*.

Progressive Policy Institute (PPI)
518 C St. NE, Washington, DC 20002
(202) 547-0001 • fax: (202) 544-5014
Internet: http://www.dlcppi.org

The PPI is a public policy research organization that strives to develop alternatives to the traditional debate between the left and the right. It advocates economic policies designed to stimulate broad upward mobility and social policies designed to liberate the poor from poverty and dependence. The institute publishes *Reducing Teenage Pregnancy: A Handbook for Action* and the reports "Second-Chance Homes: Breaking the Cycle of Teen Pregnancy" and "Preventable Calamity: Rolling Back Teen Pregnancy."

Religious Coalition for Reproductive Choice
1025 Vermont Ave. NW, Suite 1130, Washington, DC 20005
(202) 628-7700 • fax: (202) 628-7716

The coalition works to inform the media and the public that many mainstream religions support reproductive options, including abortion, and oppose antiabortion violence. It works to mobilize pro-choice religious people to counsel families facing unintended pregnancies. The coalition publishes "The Role of Religious Congregations in Fostering Adolescent Sexual Health," "Abortion: Finding Your Own Truth," and "Considering Abortion? Clarify What You Believe."

The Robin Hood Foundation
111 Broadway, 19th Fl., New York, NY 10006
(212) 227-6601 • fax: (212) 227-6698
handnet: hn5773handnet.org

The Robin Hood Foundation funds and provides technical assistance to organizations serving New Yorkers with very low incomes. The foundation makes grants to early childhood, youth, and family-centered programs located in the five boroughs of New York City. It publishes the report "Kids Having Kids: A Robin Hood Foundation Special Report on the Costs of Adolescent Childbearing."

Sexuality Information and Education Council of the U.S. (SIECUS)
130 W. 42nd St., Suite 350, New York, NY 10036-7802
(212) 819-9770 • fax: (212) 819-9776
e-mail: SIECUS@siecus.org

SIECUS develops, collects, and disseminates information on human sexuality. It promotes comprehensive education about sexuality and advocates the right of individuals to make responsible sexual choices. In addition to providing guidelines for sexuality education for kindergarten through twelfth grades, SIECUS publishes the reports "Facing Facts: Sexual Health for America's Adolescents" and "Teens Talk About Sex: Adolescent Sexuality in the 90s" and the fact sheet "Adolescents and Abstinence."

Teen STAR Program
Natural Family Planning Center of Washington, D.C.
8514 Bradmoor Dr., Bethesda, MD 20817-3810
(301) 897-9323 • fax: (301) 897-9323

Teen STAR (Sexuality Teaching in the context of Adult Responsibility) is geared for early, middle, and late adolescence. Classes are designed to foster understanding of the body and its fertility pattern and to explore the emotional, cognitive, social, and spiritual aspects of human sexuality. Teen STAR publishes a bimonthly newsletter and the paper "Sexual Behavior of Youth: How to Influence It."

BIBLIOGRAPHY OF BOOKS

Alan Guttmacher Institute	*Sex and America's Teenagers.* New York: Alan Guttmacher Institute, 1994.
Shirley Arthur	*Surviving Teen Pregnancy: Your Choices, Dreams, and Decisions.* Buena Park, CA: Morning Glory Press, 1991.
Claire D. Brindis et al.	*Adolescent Pregnancy Prevention: A Guidebook for Communities.* Palo Alto, CA: Health Promotion Resource Center, Stanford Center for Research in Disease Prevention in Cooperation with the Henry J. Kaiser Family Foundation, 1991.
Center for Population Options	*Condom Availability in Schools: A Guide for Programs.* Washington, DC: 1993.
Patricia L. East and Marianne E. Felice	*Adolescent Pregnancy and Parenting: Findings from a Racially Diverse Sample.* Mahwah, NJ: Lawrence Erlbaum Associates, 1996.
Linda Gordon	*Pitied but Not Entitled: Single Mothers and the History of Welfare.* New York: Free Press, 1994.
Lingxin Hao	*Kin Support, Welfare, and Out-of-Wedlock Mothers.* New York: Garland Press, 1994.
Irving B. Harris	*Children in Jeopardy: Can We Break the Cycle of Poverty?* New Haven, CT: Yale University Press, 1996.
Debra Hauser	*Teen Pregnancy Prevention and the School-Based and School-Linked Health Center Model.* Denver: Women's Network, 1993.
Frances Hudson and Bernard Ineichen	*Taking It Lying Down: Sexuality and Teenage Motherhood.* New York: Macmillan, 1991.
John Kingdon	*Agendas, Alternatives, and Public Policies.* New York: HarperCollins, 1995.
Annette Lawson and Deborah L. Rhode, eds.	*The Politics of Pregnancy: Adolescent Sexuality and Public Policy.* New Haven, CT: Yale University Press, 1993.
Michael Lind	*Up from Conservatism: Why the Right Is Wrong for America.* New York: Free Press, 1996.
Kristin Luker	*Dubious Conceptions: The Politics of Teenage Pregnancy.* Cambridge, MA: Harvard University Press, 1996.
Mike Males	*The Scapegoat Generation: America's War on Adolescents.* Monroe, ME: Common Courage Press, 1996.
Jane Mauldon and Kristin Luker	*Contraception Among America's Teens: The News Is Better than You Think.* Berkeley: Graduate School of Public Policy, University of California, 1995.

Rebecca A. Maynard, ed. *Kids Having Kids: Economic Costs and Social Consequences of Teen Pregnancy.* Washington, DC: Urban Institute Press, 1996.

Josh McDowell *The Myths of Sex Education: Josh McDowell's Open Letter to His School Board.* San Bernardino, CA: Here's Life Publishers, 1990.

Kristin A. Moore et al. *Adolescent Pregnancy Prevention Programs: Interventions and Evaluations.* Washington, DC: Child Trends, Inc., 1995.

Kristin A. Moore et al. *Adolescent Sex, Contraception, and Childbearing: A Review of Recent Research.* Washington, DC: Child Trends, Inc., 1995.

Judith S. Musick *Young, Poor, and Pregnant: The Psychology of Teenage Motherhood.* New Haven, CT: Yale University Press, 1993.

Constance A. Nathanson *Dangerous Passage: The Social Control of Sexuality in Women's Adolescence.* Philadelphia: Temple University Press, 1991.

Margaret K. Rosenheim and Mark F. Testa, eds. *Early Parenthood and Coming of Age in the 1990s.* New Brunswick, NJ: Rutgers University Press, 1992.

Sarah E. Samuels and Mark D. Smith, eds. *Condoms in the Schools.* Menlo Park, CA: H.J. Kaiser Family Foundation, 1993.

Mercer L. Sullivan *The Male Role in Teenage Pregnancy and Parenting: New Directions for Public Policy.* New York: Vera Institute of Justice, 1990.

Kathleen Sylvester "Preventable Calamity: Rolling Back Teen Pregnancy." Policy Report No. 22. Washington, DC: Progressive Policy Institute, 1994.

Maris A. Vinovskis *An Epidemic of Adolescent Pregnancy?* New York: Oxford University Press, 1988.

Patricia Voydanoff and Brenda W. Donnelly *Adolescent Sexuality and Pregnancy.* Newbury Park, CA: Sage Publications, 1990.

Ruth Ellen Wasem *Adolescent Pregnancy: Programs and Issues.* Washington, DC: Congressional Research Service, Library of Congress, 1992.

Constance Willard Williams *Black Teenage Mothers.* Lexington, MA: Lexington Books, 1991.

Lois Ann Wodarski and John S. Wodarski *Adolescent Sexuality: A Comprehensive Peer/Parent Curriculum.* Springfield, IL: C.C. Thomas, 1995.

Barbara L. Wolfe and Maria Perozek *Health and Medical Care Costs to Society of Teen Pregnancy: Children from Birth to Age 14.* Madison: Institute for Research on Poverty, University of Wisconsin, 1995.

Laurie Schwab Zabin   *Adolescent Sexual Behavior and Childbearing.* Newbury Park, CA: Sage Publications, 1993.

Ann Creighton Zollar   *Adolescent Pregnancy and Parenthood: An Annotated Guide.* New York: Garland Publishing, 1990.

INDEX

HIV, 118-20
housing, subsidized, 31, 37, 143
Howard, Marion, 110
Hymowitz, Kay S., 82

illegitimacy
    and blacks, 28-29, 34, 38, 43, 65,
        86, 142, 162
    and crime, 29, 136
    economic penalties for, 31
    and education, 28-30, 136
    and income, 28-29
    increases in, 141
    is society's worst problem, 22, 27-34
        con, 35-40, 49, 56
    remedies for, 31-34
    statistics on
        adults, 28, 115, 141
        blacks, 28, 38
        education, 28
        income, 29
        national, 28, 44, 60, 62, 136
        teens, 37, 38, 42, 68, 83, 115, 141,
            156
        whites, 28, 29
    stigma of, 31, 32, 37, 70, 138, 143
    and whites, 28-31, 42-43, 162

Jackson, Janine, 21
Job Corps, 170
jobs, low-wage, for women, 23, 61,
    170
Johnson, Lyndon, 64, 65

Kantor, Leslie M., 114, 130
Karwan, Angie, 50
Kaul, Donald, 23
Kaus, Mickey, 61, 62
Kennedy, Ted, 57
Kerrey, Bob, 144
Kirby, Douglas, 100-101, 108-11
Klein, Joe, 24, 73, 151-53
Krauthammer, Charles, 24, 59

Lambro, Donald, 63
Larsen, Leonard, 163
Lewis, Jerry Lee, 19
Liebmann, George W., 145
Lind, Michael, 38, 56
Losing Ground (Murray), 37, 60, 140
Loving and Caring, Inc., 148
Luker, Kristin, 56, 57, 95, 167

Males, Mike, 24, 47, 79, 139
Manpower Demonstration Research
    Corporation (MDRC), 163, 165
marriage
    and adolescents, 37, 88

and blacks, 38, 91
early, 88, 98
and government, 33
as irrelevant, 85
is necessary to society, 30-31
rewards for, 33-34
sex rates outside of, 98
shotgun, 32, 88
will reduce poverty, 136
Martin, Lynn, 147
maternity homes
    as alternative to welfare, 69, 72
    as help for teens, 48, 74, 76
    would deter teen pregnancy, 136,
        145-49
    would punish pregnant teens, 150-53
Mauldon, Jane, 95
Mayden, Bronwyn, 75
media, exaggerates teen pregnancy, 22-
    26
men
    inner-city, sex codes of, 60, 119
    older
        cause teen pregnancy, 18, 24, 50,
            74, 78, 80, 143, 151, 156-57, 159
        as predators, 18, 28, 74-75
        and sexual abuse, 19-20, 24, 74-75,
            78-80, 143, 151, 155-57
Montoya, Regina T., 158
Moore, Kristin, 39, 71
mothers
    single
        divorced, 166
        eliminating government support
            for, 31, 37
        family support for, 31-32, 49
        intergenerational, 44, 83, 85, 136,
            163
        lack control of children, 85
        most not teens, 56, 115, 172
        and poverty, 23, 61
        statistics on, 91
    teenage
        black, 142
        disadvantaged, 114
        economic incentives, 24, 136
        ending welfare will devastate, 139-44
        homes for, 48, 69, 72, 74, 76, 136
            would deter pregnancy, 136,
                145-49
            would punish, 150-53
        number on welfare, 43, 56, 69-70,
            153, 162
        poverty is not caused by, 22-23,
            50-51, 57-58, 169
        remaining with family, 20, 24,
            48-50, 75-76, 78, 137, 152
        as society's scapegoats, 36, 49, 51,

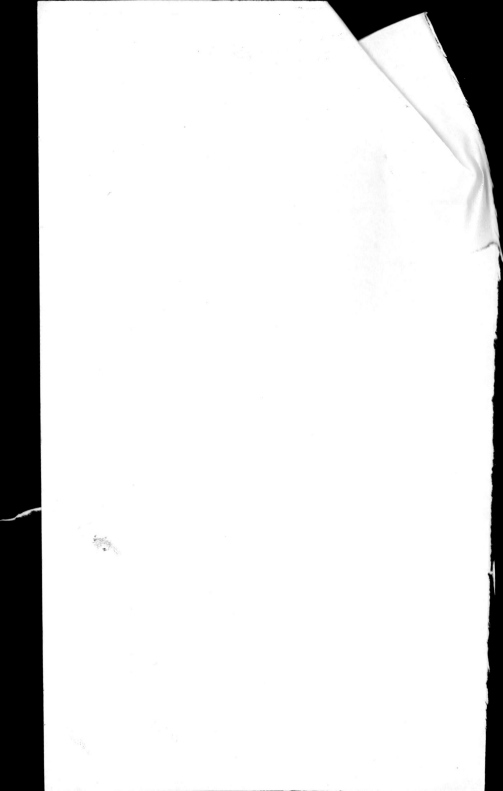

AMERICA'S OLDER POPULATION

AMERICA'S OLDER

POPULATION

Paul E. Zopf, Jr.

Dana Professor of Sociology
Guilford College

Cap and Gown Press, Inc.
Houston

Copyright © 1986 by Cap and Gown Press, Inc.

Cap and Gown Press, Inc.
Box 58825
Houston, Texas 77258 - U.S.A.

Library of Congress Catalog Card Number 84-71505

Library of Congress Cataloging in Publication Data

Zopf, Jr., Paul E.
    America's older population.

    Bibliography
    Includes indexes.
    1. Aged—United States—Social conditions. 2. Aged—
United States—Statistics. I. Title.
HQ1064.U5Z67 1986   305.2'6'0973   84-71505
ISBN 0-88105-055-5
ISBN 0-88105-056-3 (paper)

Printed in the United States of America

Dedicated to

Eric and Mary

CONTENTS

List of Figures

List of Tables

xiii

Preface

America's Older Population examines the characteristics of older people and the ways in which those characteristics are interwoven, using data for 1980 and later years. The book is concerned, too, with the combined effects of fertility, mortality, and migration in aging America's population and shaping its major features. The study is also comparative, contrasting America's elderly population with those in other societies. Within the United States it compares men and women, blacks and whites, Hispanics and non-Hispanics, and rural and urban people. Moreover, the work assesses the social, economic, political, and other results of the process of aging in America's population, basically along two lines: (1) the impact that the elderly and their characteristics have on society, and (2) the consequences that those characteristics have for the elderly themselves.

The book also has a pervasive humanistic component, for it deals with the welfare and rights of older people and their relationships with younger ones. The roles that the elderly have played historically in American society are also accounted for, traced by using the trends to which the older population has been subject.

Overall, the book emphasizes social demography, which brings together the data and methods of the demographer, the analyses of the sociologist, and the insights and concerns of the humanist. Therefore, I hope the work will be useful as a text or collateral reading for teachers who approach the subject from any of those perspectives, and that it will serve as a reference work for other professionals in gerontology.

America's Older Population also examines the stereotypes about elderly people and submits those assumptions to as factual an examination as possible. Thus, the book confronts the belief that most elderly are abandoned by their adult offspring, that large proportions live in nursing homes, that most older persons are poor, senile, and sexless, and other commonly held misconceptions about those aged 65 and older.

Finally, most chapters of the book offer projections, meant to be a contribution to rational social planning for the numbers and proportions of older people who will be part of American society well into the next century, and for the needs they and the working population will have.

Twentieth century trends and their potential changes allow one to infer much that will apply in the twenty-first century, despite the risks inherent in making projections. I hope those conclusions will prove useful and reasonably accurate.

The topics in *America's Older Population* are as follows: (1) number and distribution of older people; (2) age composition; (3) sex composition; (4) marriage and family status; (5) educational status; (6) work characteristics; (7) retirement; (8) income and poverty status; (9) mortality levels, differentials, and trends; (10) internal migration; and (11) some implications of America's aging population.

I am deeply indebted to the many people who have contributed so significantly to knowledge and insight in the fields represented in this work. Their numbers are so large that I can only acknowledge them collectively here, while I cite them individually in my references. Their work has been invaluable, as have the data collected and published by the U.S. Bureau of the Census, the National Center for Health Statistics, the United Nations, and other agencies. Without those very significant materials I could not have prepared a study such as this. I hope those persons and agences will accept my gratitude for their major contributions to demography and gerontology, and that they will forgive any misinterpretations of their work that mine may contain.

My colleagues at Guilford College, as always, deserve special thanks for moral support in my research endeavors, and I am indebted to the college itself for a study leave that provided the time to do this research and for several grants that helped underwrite its costs. In particular, I appreciate the encouragement of Vernie Davis, Cyrus Johnson, William Rogers, Sam Schuman, and other friends at this institution. I am also deeply indebted to my students, who helped me develop and refine many of the ideas that are in this volume.

There is no way I can express my full appreciation to Evelyn Zopf for her patience as I dash off to meet deadlines, come home late because of my research projects, and rely repeatedly on her for help. But she has my heartfelt devotion nonetheless. So does Eric Zopf, whose own career is now unfolding and who is also supportive of my work.

PAUL E. ZOPF, JR.

Chapter 1

Number and Distribution
Of Older People

Introduction

America's older population is larger than at any time in history, and so is its proportional representation in the total population. This is one of the fundamental facts shaping American society and its economic system, tax structure, and human relationships, and it calls for substantial social innovation to accommodate the aging of its population. Moreover, stereotypes and misconceptions abound about the roles that elderly people play in the social drama, the strains they endure, and how they mesh with the rest of us. Most serious is the tendency to lump all elderly together as sick, poor, senile, sexless, and generally unproductive, while we also sometimes venerate their wisdom and experience. Either attitude, however, places the whole group on the fringes of the society and denies the very integration that makes social life useful, for as Simon de Beauvoir argues, "either by their virtue or by their degradation they stand outside humanity."[1]

Perhaps these attitudes are less significant where the proportion of older people in a population is relatively small; certainly they are minimal or absent in traditional societies that integrate the elderly fully into social life. But America's older population is large numerically and proportionately and promises to become more so; we are not a traditional society and we do tend to isolate and stereotype our older people, partly because Americans see death as an enemy to be eluded and don't want the presence of their elderly to remind them of their own mortality. In turn, that mindset helps to create a youth-oriented culture and to convert the elderly into a minority group whose ranks eventually will include all those younger people who manage to avoid dying prematurely. Given present age-specific death rates and life expectancy, about 77 of each 100 babies born today will reach age 65, so the chances are good that any one of us will enter what has become one of America's largest minorities. Therefore, considering the demographic realities and the perceptions about "old age," we need to take both an objective and a compassionate look at the size of the enlarging group of older persons, the reasons for its growth, the composition of that population, its migratory patterns and death rates, the probable size of the elderly group in the next century, and some of the consequences of an aging population. All of this adds up to a demographic profile that includes insights from formal demography, sociology, psychology, economics, health research, and other fields that help enlighten the realities of America's aging population in the 1980s and 1990s.

Master Trends

Demographers are concerned with three related aspects of aging in the United States:

(1) The absolute numbers of older persons in the population, the extent to which those numbers are increasing, and the demographic characteristics of the older group; (2) the proportion of people who are defined as elderly, which reflects the aging of the population; and (3) the longevity of individuals, which shows up as declining death rates and increases in the expectation of life at specific ages. Therefore, while these aspects are closely linked, it is important to remember that the number of older people, the aging of a whole population, and the aging of individuals are not the same thing.[2] Moreover, while the aging of a whole population is largely a socially determined process, the aging of individuals is primarily a physiological one.[3]

Given these strategic variations, the demographic circumstances of America's elderly are being shaped by several major trends that contribute to the continuing growth of this older group, their larger proportional representation in the total population, their greater average life expectancy, and their changing demographic relationships with the rest of the population. In these master trends appear some of the basic processes that produce America's aging and the complex relationships between those processes, along with some of the more significant socioeconomic implications.[4]

1. Continuing a long trend, life expectancy at birth has increased markedly since 1940 — about 9 years for males and 12 years for females. Consequently, male babies born today can expect to live an average of 71 years, female babies approximately 78 years. Everyone does die of something, of course, but the much larger number of people who now live longer gives the country a rapidly growing elderly population, while the average person who reaches 65 has many additional years of life remain-

ing. The man who attains that age can expect an average of 14 additional years, the woman an average of 18 more years.[5]

2. The nation's birth rate, which was high during the baby boom after World War II, began to fall significantly in 1960, and by 1976 it was lower than ever before. Though the rate has climbed a little since then, it is still so low that the infant and child population is a comparatively small share of the total. Consequently, older groups, especially people 65 and over, are becoming a larger percentage of the nation's total. This shows clearly that fluctuations in the birth rate are ordinarily more important than any other factor in determining the percentage of people aged 65 and over, or of those in any other age range.

3. The huge baby boom of 1945-1960 will show up as an unusually large elderly population in the years after 2010, and 40 years later people 65 and over will be about 22 per cent of the entire population, as compared with just over 11 per cent in 1980. By 2050 the nation will have at least 67 million older citizens, or more than two and half times the number living in 1980.[6]

4. The survivors of the great waves of foreign immigration, which reached most of its highest peaks between 1905 and 1914, are a relatively old population, with fully a third of them 65 or more. Only a fraction of their original ranks have been replenished by younger legal immigrants, however, because of restrictive legislation, so the elderly foreign-born group also contributes somewhat to the aging of the population. But given the average age of foreign-born people — now over 52 years compared with 30 years for the total population — that group will become continually smaller, and the major cause of aging will be the balance between birth and death rates. That process is already far along, for the impact of the aging immigrant population was greater two or three decades ago than it is now.

5. Despite greater life expectancy, people tend to retire from their jobs younger than they did earlier, even though the mandatory retirement age was raised in 1978 from 65 to 70. Earlier retirement means additional years of reliance on Social Security and various private pension plans, some of which are already seriously strained by the growing retired population, built-in cost-of-living increases, and inflation rates in the whole economy.

6. As the postwar baby-boom population ages, the proportion of active workers will decrease dramatically while that of older people rises, and the ratio of workers to retirees will decline steadily for some time. Therefore, while 1980 saw about five people aged 20-64 for each person over 65, 2050 will see less than three in the younger age group for each one in the older category. So the cost of retirement, a large share of which is borne by the employed population, will increase and the proportion of people available to carry it will shrink. At the same time, however, the overall support burden will be lightened by a small number of children per

worker, so there will be significant compensations for increases in the elderly support burden, though part of it will continue to shift from private to public funds.

These are some of the basic trends involved in the steady increase in the percentage of people who are aged 65 and older. The trends will promote substantial social change, new stresses for the older and younger populations, and more demands for a decent old age for all citizens, including those who are now young. Moreover, the aging process and the expanding elderly population will have a powerful impact on all sorts of social services, especially medical care, and on America's family systems, concepts of marriage, and ability to care for retired people, particularly the oldest ones.

Factors That Affect the Age Profile

The master trends show that the only thing which can alter a nation's age profile is the balance between rates of fertility, mortality, and migration — the three components of all population change. If birth and death rates remained constant and there were no net gains or losses by migration in particular age groups, a country's age profile eventually would consist of unchanging proportions of children, the elderly, and younger adults.[7] But those three demographic processes rarely stay the same over long periods, and most populations have abnormally large percentages of people in some ages that reflect increases in fertility at one time, relatively small percentages in other ages that mirror low rates of reproduction at other times, and variations from heavy net gains or losses by migration in given years.

Changes in death rates at various times also affect the age profile, but unless they are concentrated heavily among one group, they exert far less impact on the age profile than do fertility rates. Even the general decline in death rates that enlarged the *number* of older people has not raised their *proportion* in the United States recently, because the improvements in mortality have been greater at the lower end of the age scale than at the upper end, and have actually served to increase the percentage of children, not the elderly.[8] That pattern could change, but at present the aging of America's population results primarily from long-term fluctuations in the birth rate and lower proportions of children now than in the past, because that drop makes older people a much larger share.

Given these relationships among the population processes, current growth in the number of America's elderly people reflects high birth rates 65 and more years ago and the decreasing death rates since then, while growth in their proportion reflects both the earlier high birth rates and the lower ones that prevail now.[9] Moreover, the fluctuations in the numbers of older people that will occur until the year 2050 or so can be projected with reasonable accuracy, for they will result largely from past birth rates that obviously cannot change, though the projection rationale does as-sume no drastic increases in the death rate because of epidemics, wars, or other massive causes, nor major decreases because of new life-saving events. The percentages of older people are less easy to project, however, for a new baby-boom could expand the child population and thus decrease the proportional importance of the elderly. In addition, a spectacular decrease in mortality is possible because we will learn to control cancer, heart disease, or other major killers of older people, and it could reduce their death rates markedly and raise both their numbers and proportions.[10] But although such advances could raise life expectancy several years and experiments in cell biology and other areas could even increase the biological limits of the human life span — now estimated at about 100 years by some — they would simply shift the older population upward in the age scale. The death rates of the elderly would still be relatively high as compared with other age groups, and membership in their age category would still be comparatively short, though it might be useful to raise the generally accepted threshold of "old age" from 65 to 75 or even 85 years.

Immigration has its impact, too, though it affects the age profile less now than formerly. When the volume of immigration is heavy and consists mostly of young adults, it contributes to a relatively large number of elderly people about 45 or 50 years later; that fact accounts for a consider-able amount of the growth in America's elderly population until about 1960. But when immigration falls off sharply, as it did in the United States after 1914, though with a few important increases in the early 1920s, its later impact on the aging of the population is far less.

In fact, the relative youthfulness of the present large illegal immigration to the United States, coupled with that of the smaller group of legal entrants, will tend to slow the demographic aging of the whole population, though the actual impact is difficult to measure. But even if we know relatively little about the size and demographic composition of the illegal group, it is clear that most of the new immigrant populations do consist heavily of young adults and children, and they will keep the percentage of older people from increasing even faster than it is already, at least for a time. Considering the patterns of the twentieth century, however, the largest impact of immigration on the aging of the population has probably passed, and future changes in age composition will depend even more heavily on fertility than they have many times in the past.

Organization of the Book

Give these basic conditions, the purpose of this book is to explore the demographic realities of the older population and some of the meanings of those realities for the entire society and for the elderly themselves.

The remainder of this chapter considers the past, present, and projected size and proportion of the aging group and the way in which they are distributed geographically throughout the country. Included are variations by metropolitan and nonmetropolitan residence and some of the redistribution now underway because of variations from place to place in net migration and fertility.

Chapter 2 looks at the age breakdown of the overall elderly group, and at the changing ratio of older people to younger adults and what that means for support burdens. There the study explores the demographic relationships between the declining percentages of children and the increasing proportions of elderly people as components of the total dependency burden that producing adults must carry.

Chapter 3 turns attention to the balance between men and women and what it means for older people who have lost their mates and for their ability to deal with solitude, diminished income, and other unhappy realities that affect many. That chapter also focuses on the male-female differences in death rates and longevity that distort the sex balance and create a superabundance of women in the older ages.

Chapter 4 deals with the marital status and family characteristics of the older population, particularly the effects of widowhood and its aftermath. The loss of a mate is predominantly a problem of women because of sex differences in life expectancy, and calls for a careful look at the impact of widowhood on them.

Chapter 5 assesses the educational standing of older people and the reasons why it averages below that of younger people. Included, too, are the patterns of re-education among some of the many older people who remain viable and optimistic.

Chapter 6 considers the work characteristics of older people, including the extent to which they continue in the labor force, the occupations they hold, the industries that employ them, and their problems with unemployment.

Chapter 7 concerns retirement, including the composition of the retired population, why people retire and how they adjust, and changes in the nature of retirement. The study examines the trend toward early retirement and how inflation, recessions, and high unemployment rates affect that trend.

Chapter 8 is an account of income distribution and poverty status, and deals with the degree of income equitability that exists between elderly people and other groups. Important also are income differences by race and sex, the principal sources of income for the elderly, and the features of the older segment that falls below the official poverty line.

Chapter 9 explores the mortality levels and differentials among older people and the principal causes of death that finally end their lives. That chapter examines life expectancy and mortality differences by race and sex, the long-term reduction in the death rates of older people, and changes in the importance of various causes.

Chapter 10 concerns the relatively small share of America's older people who migrate after they reach age 65, especially those who move from place to place within the United States in search of retirement opportunities. Included are the movements to Florida, Arizona, California, and other Sunbelt states, and the way in which migration selects for certain characteristics. The reasons for elderly migration and its basic trends are also explored.

Chapter 11, which concludes the book, is an account of some social consequences of America's aging population, both for the elderly and the larger society. Some aspects are the role ambiguity, isolation, minority group status, and other problems faced by some elderly, and the adjustment, productivity, and good health enjoyed by many others. Included, too, are the prospects to intervene in the aging process, thereby increasing both life expectancy and life span itself.

Why 65 and Over?

Even though biological aging takes place at very different rates for individuals, this book uses 65 and over as the ages defining the older population. It is an arbitrary choice that should not imply uniformity in people's social and economic performance, for the category does include people well past age 65 who are not old physiologically and others who have just turned age 65 but who are very old biologically. Moreover, 65 marks the popularly accepted threshold of the older ages simply because it was arbitrarily selected as the forced retirement age in Germany's social welfare system that was created in 1889 by Chancellor Otto von Bismarck.[11] Bismarck actually set retirement at 70, but it was dropped to 65 in 1916,[12] partly because the German government assumed few people would live past that age to collect benefits from a program that was created in the first place to offset the appeals of socialism.

The U.S. Census Bureau also defines the elderly as those aged 65 and older and reports its data on that basis, and if those valuable data are to be useful, there is little choice but to accept its classification. In addition, the Social Security Administration uses 65 as the point for beginning to pay full benefits, and many other agencies employ that age in their operations. Therefore, it is simply practical for this study to use 65 as the threshold for becoming "elderly," even though the mandatory retirement age is now 70 and the average retirement age at this writing is actually lower than 65.

The most accurate measure would really be *functional age,* which reflects the person's ability to work, engage in intellectual activity, and be self-maintaining.[13] But there is little agreement on how to assess functional age, and because it varies from person to person the index is difficult to use as a standard or to represent statistically. Furthermore, in large groups of people, such as the nation, "the aging process, functional age, and physiological age follow chronological age closely,"[14] though there are wide individual variations within those large populations. In this search for an ideal index, however, it is most important to avoid any implication that the elderly are all alike and all share poverty or affluence, good health or illness, social disengagement or integration, or any other features that encourage stereotyping and thus obscure the group's great diversity. The older contingent is nearly as heterogeneous as many others in American society, except that all of its members are at least age 65.

The analyses in the following chapters refer mainly to people aged 65-84, because they are the vast majority of the elderly group. In 1980, for example, they made up 91 per cent of the whole category 65 and over, though the proportion 85 and over is increasing rapidly. In addition, there are serious distortions in the data beyond age 84, basically for two reasons: (1) The numbers in some categories beyond that age are so small that a few individuals more or less can change the statistical pattern significantly; and (2) because it is prestigious to be a centenarian and one receives attention as a curiosity if not a respected elder, there are substantial distortions in age-reporting among people approaching the century mark; some are not even sure of their correct age. Therefore, the data for people aged 85 and older need to be used cautiously, though some things about that group can be reported separately, especially the large sex imbalance.

Numbers and Proportions of Elderly People

Numbers

In 1980 there were 25.5 million people aged 65 and older in the United States. They were a larger number than ever before and they are continuing to increase. That group is more than eight time as large as the one in 1900, because birth rates were high when today's elderly generation was born, death rates have fallen off dramatically during their lifetimes, and the survivors of the large immigrant populations of the early twentieth century are now quite old.[15] Thus, the large numbers of older people are the collective result of the aging process among increasing millions of individuals. This is not the same thing, however, as the "aging" of the nation's whole population, which occurs when elderly people grow not just in numbers, but as a percentage of the total.

Proportions

In 1980 the nation's older people were 11.3 per cent of the whole population, which is a higher proportion than ever in the past and which is certain to increase markedly over the next several decades, probably to level out only after the middle of the next century. There will also be a brief leveling and perhaps even a slight proportional decline just after the turn of the century, however, when the small baby crops of the 1930s are elderly.

The major statistical relationships between various age groups appear in the 1980 portion of Figure 1-1, which is an age-sex pyramid that portrays the percentages of males and females by five-year age ranges. In that diagram the present relative abundance of older people is easily apparent, as is the comparative scarcity of children. All of this contrasts sharply with the situation in 1870, when older people were a far smaller share of the total population, young people a much larger part. Moreover, the aging of the whole population, represented by more than a century of dramatic change in the proportions of people at various age levels, has created new implications for the nation's ability to absorb older people into satisfying roles, including occupations, and for family structure, the political process, investment policies, and other basic social matters that tend to differ from one age group to another.[16]

Despite the high percentage of elderly people in America's present population, however, they do not come close to being a world record. In fact, the United States ranks only twentieth in the proportions of those aged 65 and older; the other 19 countries are all European and have had extremely low birth and death rates for a considerable time. (See Table 1-1.) Most are in Western Europe, though several other Eastern European countries would join those already on the list if the partial success of recent pro-natalist policies had not increased their percentages of children and caused their proportions of older people to fall, at least temporarily.[17]

These aging populations in the developed countries contrast sharply with the much younger ones in most developing nations, where relatively high birth rates and declining death rates, especially among infants, elevate the percentages of children and depress those of elderly people. In Mexico, for example, the elderly are less than 3.5 per cent of the population, as they are in Indonesia, Brazil, and most other developing nations with recent population explosions and life expectancies well below those of the industrialized countries. Thus, by world standards the United States has a very high percentage of older people, though a fairly low one by European standards.

Growth Trends in America's Older Population

Even though fluctuations in fertility, mortality, and migration have made the population of the United States younger at certain times and older at others, the long-term trend has been toward a larger number and

10

higher proportion of elderly people. That is true of most industrialized nations, where the percentages of children have fallen and those of elderly inhabitants have risen substantially in recent decades. Furthermore, as America's proportion of children has shrunk, the percentages of people in many of the age groups between 20 and 64 have grown, but not as rapidly as the share of the elderly. As a result of these patterns, the median age in the United States went from less than 17 years in 1820, to 23 years in 1900, to 30 years in 1980. The average age was even a bit higher in 1940 and 1950 than in 1980, for it reflected the very low birth rates of the 1930s and

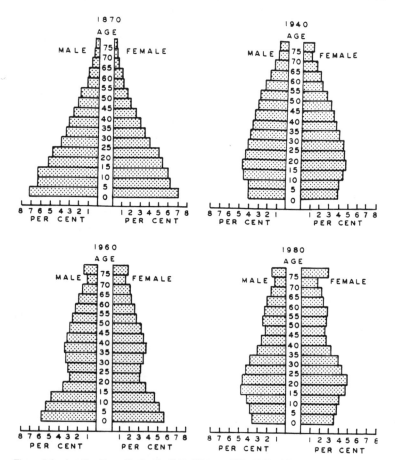

Figure 1-1. Age-Sex Pyramids for the United States: 1870, 1940, 1960, and 1980
Sources: U.S.Census Office, *Ninth Census of the United States, Vital Statistics of the United States* (1872), table 22; U.S.Bureau of the Census, *U.S. Census of Population: 1960, Characteristics of the Population, U.S. Summary* (1964), table 47; *1980 Census of Population, Supplementary Reports,* PC80-S1-1, *Age, Sex, Race, and Spanish Origin of the Population by Regions, Divisions, and States: 1980* (1981), table 1.

early 1940s and the aging immigrant population. Then in 1960 and 1970 the median age was down some because of the high post-World War II fertility levels, though the reductions proved to be temporary. These changes also reflect the rapid growth in the numbers of older people from 1900 to 1952 or so, followed by somewhat slower increases in their ranks. Despite the fluctuations, however, the long-term aging of the population resumed after 1970, and the 11.3 per cent of America's population who were aged 65 and older in 1980 contrasted markedly with the 3 per cent in 1870.

Table 1-1. Elderly Population of Countries Having 1 Million or More Inhabitants and Higher Percentages of Elderly Than the United States

Country	Year	Total Population (000)	Population 65+	
			Number (000)	Per Cent
Sweden	1980	8,310	1,354	16.3
East Germany	1980	16,737	2,661	15.9
Austria	1980	7,505	1,162	15.5
West Germany	1980	61,566	9,550	15.5
England & Wales	1980	49,244	7,424	15.1
Norway	1980	4,086	603	14.8
Denmark	1980	5,123	739	14.4
Belgium	1979	9,855	1,410	14.3
France	1980	53,583	7,535	14.1
Scotland	1980	5,153	724	14.1
Switzerland	1980	6,314	872	13.8
Italy	1980	57,070	7,676	13.5
Hungary	1980	10,711	1,438	13.4
Greece	1979	9,449	1,233	13.0
Czechoslovakia	1978	15,137	1,892	12.5
Finland	1980	4,780	572	12.0
Bulgaria	1980	8,861	1,051	11.9
Netherlands	1980	14,091	1,616	11.5
Northern Ireland	1978	1,539	175	11.4
UNITED STATES	1980	226,505	25,544	11.3

Sources: United Nations, Demographic Yearbook, 1979, table 7; 1980, table 7; 1981, table 7.

The proportion of older people actually grew rather slowly between 1870 and 1930, but then their rate of increase picked up considerably for several reasons. (See Table 1-2.) (1) Many older people were products of a large fertility increase after the Civil War, and by 1935 much of their sizable age cohort had reached age 65. (2) Decreases in the birth rates between 1900 and 1935 made children and young adults proportionately less abundant in the population and elderly people more so. (3) By the last quarter of the twentieth century the millions of immigrants who had arrived early in the 1900s had aged past 65, and because they were not fully replaced by young immigrants, the average age of the foreign-born population was significantly higher than that of the native-born group. (4) The increases in life expectancy that occurred after 1930 allowed more infants to survive and more people of other ages to live longer.

Table 1-2. People 65 and Over in the American Population, 1870-1980

Year	Total Population (000)	Population 65+	
		Number (000)	Per Cent
1870	38,558	1,154	3.0
1880	50,156	1,723	3.4
1890	62,622	2,417	3.9
1900	76,212	3,084	4.0
1910	92,229	3,954	4.3
1920	106,022	4,940	4.7
1930	123,203	6,645	5.4
1940	132,165	9,036	6.8
1950	151,326	12,295	8.1
1960	179,323	16,560	9.2
1970	203,212	20,066	9.9
1980	226,505	25,544	11.3

Sources: U.S. Bureau of the Census, Sixteenth Census of the United States: 1940, Characteristics of the Population, U.S. Summary (1943), table 8; U.S. Census of Population: 1970, General Population Characteristics, U.S. Summary (1972), table 53; 1980 Census of Population, Supplementary Reports, PC80-S1-1, Age, Sex, Race, and Spanish Origin of the Population by Regions, Divisions, and States: 1980 (1981), table 1.

These four conditions that favored aging of the population were augmented by significant fertility reductions after 1960. Therefore, between 1870 and 1980 the number of people 65 and over grew 2,114 per cent, while the total population increased only 487 per cent. The group of children under 15 was 239 per cent larger in 1980 than in 1870, and the group aged 15-64 was 572 per cent greater. All of these changes contributed to the gradual aging of the American population. In fact, just in the twentieth century the elderly population has increased more than three and a half times as fast as the population of all ages. Figure 1-1 shows how this process has appeared on the age-sex pyramid at particular times.

State-to-State Increases

Elderly people are most numerous, of course, in the states with the largest total populations. Therefore, in 1980 California had the largest number, followed in order by New York, Florida, Pennsylvania, Texas, Illinois, and Ohio. In fact, those seven states accounted for 11.6 million elderly people, or 45 per cent of the nation's total.

The number of people aged 65 and older increased in each of the 50 states and the District of Columbia between 1970 and 1980 and, therefore, in each of the regions and divisions, but the rates of increase varied widely, with some far below the national average of 27 per cent, others substantially above. (See Table 1-3 and Figure 1-2.) The proportions grew only slightly in the District of Columbia and modestly in New York, Iowa, Nebraska, South Dakota, and Massachusetts. At the same time, the percentages of elderly people increased tremendously in Nevada, Arizona, Hawaii, and Florida, though the 1980 populations were relatively small in all except Florida, and even modest numerical increases produced high rates of growth in some states. Other states that experienced at least 40 per cent increases in the elderly population are Alaska, New Mexico, South Carolina, North Carolina, Utah, and Georgia. The largest numerical increases occurred in Florida, California, and Texas. California registered a proportional increase of only 34 per cent and Texas one of 38 per cent, however, because their total populations and influxes of younger people are so large that even the addition of huge numbers of older people produces fairly modest proportional increases overall.

In every state except Wyoming, the elderly population grew faster than the total population. In most states of the Northeast and North Central regions, the older group increased several times more rapidly than the total, and it even grew substantially where the total populations declined — Rhode Island and New York. In the Southern and Western States, whose overall growth rates were unusually high, the older population also grew more rapidly than the total, even expanding modestly in the nation's capital despite an overall population decrease of 16 per cent. Rates of increase among older Americans in the states of the South and West were often two or three times higher than the rates for total populations, though Wyoming's elderly increased at only about half the state's overall rate.

Some Projections

The nation's elderly population is certain to become substantially larger than it is now, because the people who will enter this category in the next

Table 1-3. Percentage Change in the Elderly and Total Populations of Each Region and Division, 1970-1980

Region and Division	Population 65+, 1980 (000)	Per Cent Change, 1970-80	
		65+	All Ages
United States	25,544	27.3	11.4
Northeast	6,072	16.8	0.2
New England	1,520	19.7	4.2
Middle Atlantic	4,551	15.8	-1.1
North Central	6,691	16.8	4.0
East North Central	4,492	17.9	3.5
West North Central	2,199	14.8	5.2
South	8,484	40.4	20.0
South Atlantic	4,363	48.6	20.4
East South Central	1,657	30.5	14.5
West South Central	2,463	34.2	22.9
West	4,298	38.8	23.9
Mountain	1,060	52.5	37.1
Pacific	3,237	34.8	19.8

Sources: U.S. Bureau of the Census, U.S. Census of Population: 1970, General Population Characteristics, U.S. Summary (1972), tables 57 and 72; 1980 Census of Population, Supplementary Reports, PC80-S1-1, Age, Sex, Race, and Spanish Origin of the Population by Regions, Divisions, and States: 1980 (1981), table 2; Statistical Abstract of the United States: 1981 (1981), table 9.

15

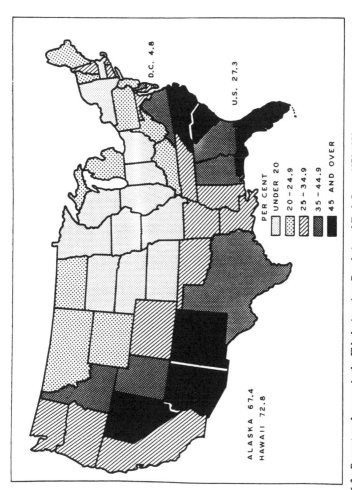

Figure 1-2. Percentage Increase in the Elderly American Population of Each State, 1970-1980

Sources: U.S. Bureau of the Census, *U.S. Census of Population: 1970, General Population Characteristics, U.S. Summary* (1972), table 62; *U.S. Census of Population, Supplementary Reports, PC80-S1-1, Age, Sex, Race, and Spanish Origin of the Population by Regions, Divisions, and States: 1980* (1981), table 2.

16

several decades are already alive and subject to age-specific death rates that have been predictable so far. The rate of growth, however, will vary substantially over time, and the numbers and proportions of elderly people will even fall now and then because of fluctuating birth rates in past years.

Table 1-4 shows the probable patterns, based on Series II projections of the population made by the U.S. Bureau of the Census. It should be made clear, however, that those data depend on several assumptions about rates of fertility, mortality, and net immigration, any of which could be altered by unpredictable events, such as a new baby boom that would increase the infant population significantly, or some major disaster or health improvements that would alter the death rate drastically. In particular, Series II projections assume a level of fertility intermediate between the highest (Series I) and the lowest (Series III) that seem possible in light

Table 1-4. Projected Numbers and Percentages of People 65 and Over, 1980-2050

Year	Total Population (000)	Population 65+	
		Number (000)	Per Cent
1980[a]	226,505	25,544	11.3
1985	238,648	28,673	12.0
1990	249,731	31,799	12.7
1995	259,631	34,006	13.1
2000	267,990	35,036	13.1
2025	301,022	58,636	19.5
2050	308,856	67,060	21.7

Sources: U.S. Bureau of the Census, 1980 Census of Population, Supplementary Reports, PC80-S1-1, Age, Sex, Race, and Spanish Origin of the Population by Regions, Divisions, and States: 1980 (1981), table 1; "Projections of the Population of the United States: 1982 to 2050" (advance report), Current Population Reports, P-25, no. 922 (1982), table 2.

[a]Census data.

Projections based on Series II assumptions.

of the American demographic experience and the social, cultural, and economic factors that influence population processes. Moreover, all of the projections assume that future mortality levels will decline but that the balance between immigration and emigration could add from 250,000 to 750,000 people each year. Series II projections assume annual net immigration of 450,000, although that figure does omit the large undocumented immigration to the United States, much of it from Latin America.[18] In addition, legal immigration is sometimes higher than 450,000 (in 1981 it was 597,000), although between 1970 and 1980 it did average 450,000 annually.

If Series II assumptions do prove reasonably accurate, the combination of fertility, mortality, and migration will raise the nation's elderly population by about 3 million per year until 1995, when that group will represent about 13 per cent of the total population. Then the proportion of older inhabitants will stop growing and their numbers could even drop some, because the low birth rates before World War II will appear around the turn of the century as comparatively stable numbers of people aged 65 and older. But when the products of the postwar baby boom move into the older ages, the numbers and percentages will increase once again. By 2030 the large elderly group, which in its younger years has already caused great expansions in school systems that are now having to reduce operations and which has placed heavy burdens on the job market, will have one last major impact on society as it reaches the ages 65 and beyond.[19] Eventually, if fertility and mortality rates do not change much, the proportions of children, younger adults, and older people will approach a stable equilibrium. Such a population would not have severe indentations or large bulges anywhere in the age profile, and the aging of the population would stop. While all of this is going on, Series II projections imply that the proportion of children under age 15 will drop to 21 per cent of the total population by 2000 and to 17 per cent by 2050.

Projections are risky, however, and there is still the possibility of a significant fertility increase in the 1980s or 1990s that would raise the percentages of children in the nation's population and thereby reduce the share of older people. Some demographers predict just such a baby boom, ironically because of the relatively small cohort who will be in their most fertile years. Richard Easterlin, for instance, suggests that when the small baby crops of the period after 1965 reach their most fertile stage about two and a half decades later, those people will experience fewer economic pressures than some earlier cohorts, because their small numbers will put them in demand in the job market. Their incomes will be relatively high as a result and will allow them to get material things and also raise somewhat larger families than their parents,[20] other influences being equal. If so, the percentage of children will rise and that of the elderly will be lower than expected. In the same vein, Easterlin interprets the low birth rates of the late 1960s and the 1970s as a reaction to the relative deprivation felt by the large age cohort that achieved its peak reproductive potential during that period. They reduced their fertility levels, he argues, because of the employment squeeze, inflation, and other economic constraints generated in part by the relatively large size of their age group. Therefore, as fertility and the proportion of children dropped in response to these conditions, the percentage of older people was able to rise sharply. If any new increase in fertility comes, it will change the age profile by broadening the base of the age-sex pyramid and slowing proportional growth at the apex, at least temporarily. Even if fertility levels were to rise, however, the proportion of older people would still increase between 2010 and 2020, when the huge baby boom of the late 1940s and the 1950s becomes 65 and over. Therefore, while the aging of the population could slow in that decade, the massive new baby boom that would be required to reverse it seems highly unlikely.[21]

We shall have to see what happens, although the constraints imposed on fertility by inflation, unemployment, energy shortages, changes in women's roles and opportunities, and other realities are all variables in the equation, and they will probably cause relatively small cohorts to give birth to other relatively small cohorts in the foreseeable future. If fertility and mortality then come into equilibrium and neither changes appreciably over a long period, the proportions of people in the major age groups will stabilize and the percentage of elderly people will stop growing; the progressive aging of America's population will then be over, at least for a time. It is worth noting also, however, that even at low rates of reproduction, large cohorts produce other large cohorts who will later reach the older years.

Geographic Distribution

The distribution of elderly people in the United States is far from even, with the largest percentages to be found in New England and the Middle Atlantic division, the Great Plains area, and a few sections of the South. The older group is underrepresented in several other parts of the South, various industrialized districts of the North Central region, and almost all of the Mountain and Pacific divisions. The parts of the country with high percentages of elderly often have low birth rates, which help increase the proportional importance of older age groups. Some places, especially in the Sunbelt, have received relatively large migrations of the elderly. Still other "aging" sections are quite rural and have lost large proportions of young adults by net migration, which not only reduces their proportional significance, but also that of the children they bear. Conversely, the places with comparatively few older people either have high birth rates or large migratory influxes of people under age 65, though fertility and migration frequently act in concert.

Patterns by States

As in the case of the regions and divisions, the 50 states vary widely in their proportions of people aged 65 and older, ranging from a 1980 high of 17.3 per cent in Florida to only 2.9 per cent in Alaska. (See Figure 1-3.) As is well known, Florida receives a large retired population by migration, though younger adults are also part of the massive flow and help keep the elderly group from being an even larger percentage than it is. The movement to Alaska, on the other hand, consists chiefly of young adults, often with children, and very few older people are part of that migration. A large share of Alaska's population growth has also been quite recent, so those people have not yet had a chance to become 65. Furthermore, some people in that state's population who do reach the older ages migrate to warmer places, sometimes those from which they came. The other chief cause of Alaska's youthful age profile is its relatively high fertility level, for in 1980 its birth rate was exceeded only by those of Utah and the District of Columbia.

In addition to Florida, the elderly group is 13 per cent or more in Arkansas, Rhode Island, Iowa, South Dakota, and Nebraska, and is between 12 and 13 per cent in Pennsylvania, Kansas, Massachusetts, Maine, Oklahoma, New York, North Dakota, West Virginia, and Wisconsin. Several of these states, such as the ones in the Northeast, have comparatively low birth rates that account for their relatively large shares of elderly people, whereas other states, such as those in the Midwest, have high birth rates but also comparatively large rural populations with fairly sizable numbers of older people. In fact, in 1980 the influences of farm and nonfarm residence at the national level were such that older people made up 12.3 per cent of the farm population but only 10.9 per cent of the nonfarm group.[22] Furthermore, the farm population is the nation's only major residence segment in which the number of elderly men exceeds that of elderly women, though by a far smaller margin than in the past.

The states with unusually low percentages of older people, besides Alaska and Utah, are Hawaii, Wyoming, Nevada, Colorado, and New Mexico, each of which had less than 9 per cent elderly in 1980. All have birth rates above the national average. In addition, such states as Michigan, Maryland, Virginia, South Carolina, Georgia, Louisiana, Texas, and Idaho have between 9 and 10 per cent older people. The last five have birth rates well above the national average, but they and the others also have unusually large groups of working-age people, because they are either highly industrialized or suburbanized and do not draw or retain abnormally large elderly groups.

These cases all underscore the fact that the causes of high or low proportions of older people are extremely complex. If one considers only the migration component, for example, a particular state may have had a

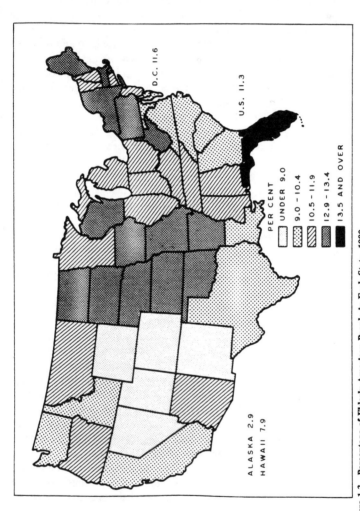

Figure 1-3. Percentage of Elderly American People in Each State, 1980
Source: U.S. Bureau of the Census, *1980 Census of Population, Supplementary Reports*, PC80-S1-1, *Age, Sex, Race, and Spanish Origin of the Population by Regions, Divisions, and States: 1980* (1981), table 2.

great economic boom 40 or 50 years ago that attracted many young adults who have aged but stayed put. Another may have a high proportion of elderly because large numbers of immigrants settled there in the early twentieth century. In some states, such as Alaska, the population migrating in now is quite young and also relatively fertile, and those realities help keep down the percentages of older people. In California, whose total and elderly populations are the nation's largest, the age composition of in-migrants has been so mixed that, while the number of older people increased 34 per cent between 1970 and 1980, their proportion only rose from 9 to 10.2 per cent. These are a few of the ways migration affects the state-to-state differences in the share of older people. The influences of birth and death rates are equally complex and usually even more significant than migration.

Metropolitan-Nonmetropolitan Patterns

In many instances, the degree to which an area is rural or urban shapes the ways that birth, death, and migration affect its age structure. Therefore, we need to consider how the proportions of older people differ between the metropolitan and nonmetropolitan areas of the nation.

Metropolitan elderly. The bulk of the nation's people of all ages, including the elderly, live in metropolitan areas, but older people are still underrepresented there because of their relative scarcity in some of the sections just outside the central cities. On the other hand, older people are fairly heavily represented within those large central cities, especially those with 1 million or more inhabitants. (See Table 1-5.) Middle-aged people are more apt to avoid those places, and in that sense, the elderly are more like young adults, who are disproportionately represented in large urban centers, though usually for different reasons. At the same time, the elderly account for a relatively small share of the people residing outside the central cities of metropolitan counties. Therefore, a comparatively large percentage of the elderly is highly urbanized, living amidst the advantages and disadvantages of the nation's great cities, even though that tendency is not as strong as it was in the past. Some were born in the places where they reside, others are first-generation immigrants, and still others have moved to the cities from other parts of the nation; many of them were part of the huge rural-to-urban migration that shifted more than 55 million people off the farms between 1933 and 1970.[23]

Certain parts of the central cities often contain dense concentrations of the elderly, sometimes because their incomes are too low to allow them to migrate elsewhere, or because they choose to remain in familiar neighborhoods among friends, particularly those of the same ethnic background and age.[24] Many of those elderly are simply left behind as younger family members flee poor educational and occupational opportunities, deterioriating housing, high crime rates, and other conditions that the elderly who remain must endure. The older people then may form "gerontological enclaves,"[25] and because they tend to succumb more readily to the role of "victim" in such places, the loss of younger people also represents a decreasing level of protection for many elderly. As a result of these residential dynamics, the relatively high overall proportions of older people in many large central cities often reflect specific concentrations here and there within those centers, sometimes troubled by problems that intensify as the elderly concentrate more heavily and younger people become even scarcer.[26] These enclaves often degenerate into "gray ghettos" in some sections of nearly all central cities, usually the aging and deteriorating parts of the urban core.[27]

Suburban elderly. The older people who inhabit the suburgs have been a comparatively small group historically, but more elderly now live there than in the central cities. Therefore, suburban groups are aging along with the rest of the population, and the percentages of people 65 and over are growing there just as they are in the cities and the countryside.

Table 1-5. Proportional Representation of Persons in Various Residence Classes, by Selected Age Groups, 1980

Residence Class	Age Group				
	25-34	35-44	45-54	55-64	65+
All Classes	16.4	11.3	10.1	9.6	11.3
Metropolitan	16.9	11.5	10.2	9.5	10.7
In Central Cities	17.3	10.3	9.6	9.6	11.9
Outside Central Cities	16.6	12.3	10.6	9.4	9.9
Nonmetropolitan	14.9	10.7	9.7	9.8	13.0
Farm	10.0	11.8	13.2	13.3	12.3

Sources: U.S. Bureau of the Census, State and Metropolitan Area Data Book, 1982 (1982), p. 357; "Farm Population of the United States: 1980," Current Population Reports, P-27, no. 54 (1981), table 2.

In some cases, gerontological clusters are appearing in the suburbs, too, though some of them are related to the location of nursing homes, retirement condominiums, and other developments that are not really part of "natural" neighborhoods. In other instances, suburban populations are aging because relatively high percentages of younger people are migrating out to opportunities elsewhere, especially in times of high unemployment. The aging process is also hastened by the high cost of homes and mortgage money, which tends to keep many young couples from moving into the types of suburban housing that their parents were once able to afford more easily and where they still live. Moreover, the average age of a suburban population tends to rise as the suburb itself ages, creating substantial proportions of people 65 and over in many older suburban communities.

Small-town and farm elderly. Another large group of elderly people can be found in the more rural nonmetropolitan parts of the nation. They are heavily represented in the counties with no urban places and in all other types of nonmetropolitan territory, including farms. They have a special affinity, however, for the villages and hamlets with 1,000-2,500 inhabitants, and only a slightly lesser attraction to towns and small cities having between 2,500 and 25,000 inhabitants. Some of those small-town people have simply remained in the places they were born, while others have left nearby farms and moved into these centers, perhaps after a farm has been sold or transferred to an adult son or daughter. Still other elderly residents of the towns have migrated longer distances to find better climatic and other conditions, often leaving large cities as they move. Very few of the elderly people in these nonmetropolitan areas are an aging immigrant group, however, for the small towns attracted far less than their fair share of foreign-born people, while the cities drew relatively large proportions.

The nation's most rural elderly people as a group tend to be especially disadvantaged and to have more than their share of poverty, poor health, deteriorated housing, and psychosocial isolation.[28] This is so partly because the rural areas lost services and income during the huge twentieth-century migration to cities, and partly because subsequent increases in rural incomes and services have not kept pace with the significant regrowth that has occurred in nonmetropolitan places since 1970. Therefore, on the average the most isolated rural people of all ages have fewer advantages than other groups, and older people have the least advantages of the rural segment. Consequently, the rural elderly have lower average incomes than their urban counterparts and are more apt to suffer from chronic illnesses and disabilities, partly because poor public transportation in rural areas keeps many from visiting the health-care facilities that do exist.

The rural elderly also have lower average levels of education than the urban and suburban elderly, are more likely to occupy substandard housing, and are less apt to have joined pension funds and other plans that provide retirement income; even Social Security coverage has been poorer historically for rural than for urban workers. However, elderly rural workers who are self-employed, principally in farming and small-town businesses, may have more discretion in choosing when or even whether to retire than do people employed by someone else, though financial realities influence most of those decisions.[29] As expected, these problems all tend to be more serious for elderly women than for elderly men in the rural areas, and those women probably have fewer alternatives available to them than virtually any other segment of the population.[30]

Race and sex patterns. The patterns of rural-urban distribution by race are similar to the ones just described for the total elderly population. That is, both black and white elderly people, along with those of Spanish origin, are heavily represented in large central cities but are relatively scarce in the metropolitan sections just outside those cities. They are especially abundant in the nonmetropolitan counties, particularly the ones with sizable towns and small cities. The only exception is the relative scarcity of elderly Spanish-origin people in nonmetropolitan counties with places of 25,000 or more inhabitants. Furthermore, only in the rural-farm residence category do elderly men outnumber older women regardless of race or ethnic origin. The sex imbalance is greatest in central cities, where there are only 63 men aged 65 and over for each 100 women in those ages. But even in the nonmetropolitan counties collectively, where the sex imbalance is less, there are only 78 men for every 100 women. In the farm population, however, the ratio is still 112.[31]

The geographic patterns emphasize the heterogeneity of the elderly population and show that some residence groups in the United States are aging somewhat faster than others. Nonetheless, the birth rate has fallen so significantly in virtually all parts of the nation, that the aging of the population is one of its universal demographic phenomena. Therefore, while the average age is a bit higher in the central cities and the more rural nonmetropolitan places than in the suburbs and is substantially higher in the farm population than any other aggregate, most of the differences are narrowing. Consequently, the graying of America's population pervades all of the major residence categories.

Redistribution

As a result of the variable growth patterns from one section to another, the nation's major regions and divisions have added older people at very different rates. In turn, those variations are redistributing the older group more evenly throughout most of the nation, though not necessarily by physical movement. Thus, the Northeast, which has long had higher proportions of older people than the national average, has been witnessing below-normal growth in their numbers, which is bringing the share of older people in that region closer to the national figure. The North Central region, which also has had more than its fair share of elderly during most of the present century, now has approximately the national average because of comparatively slow growth between 1970 and 1980. On the other hand, the South and the West, which historically have had less than their shares of older people, are adding them rapidly. The South is now at the national average, while the West is coming closer to it. Many of the individual states in those regions, however, are still far below the national figure, partly because their birth rates are comparatively high, and partly because of influxes of young adults.

While the elderly population is becoming somewhat more evenly distributed among the major regions, it is also concentrating more heavily in a handful of states in the South and West, largely because of net in-migration. At the same time, the states whose populations show exceptionally low rates of growth among the elderly generally have lost many of them by net out-migration. Migration affects redistribution in other ways, too, however, for many states with extremely high percentages of older people are losing young adults by net migration, while those aged 65 and older stay behind and their proportion remains high.[32] This is going on in parts of the Midwestern farm belt, such as Iowa, where the number of elderly is growing rather slowly (11% between 1970 and 1980), while they also remain a comparatively high proportion of the total (13% in 1980) because of the exodus of younger adults, some of them accompanied by children. Much the same is true in Kansas, Nebraska, South Dakota, and other states with percentages of older people well above the national average, but whose numbers of elderly are growing at rates far below the national norm.

Despite their various movements from place to place, older people don't shift around nearly as much as young adults, for while as many as 25 per cent of the people aged 20-24 change residence in a given year, it is rare for more than 6 per cent of the elderly to do so. Moreover, the moves that most older people do make tend to be of relatively short distance, despite the well-known treks to Florida, California, and other Sunbelt areas. And if they are going to move any considerable distance, older people generally do so in their early or mid-60s, often as part of the adjustment that accompanies retirement. Those past age 75, on the other hand, are much less likely to leave their present homes for faraway sections of the nation, though some may move short distances, perhaps to live near their children or to enter retirement or nursing homes. Others, especially recent

26

widows, return to the local area they may have left a few years earlier.

These dynamics raise the proportions of elderly people slowly in some places and rapidly in others, though it is noteworthy that since 1900 the elderly contingent has grown at least twice as fast as the total population in every state, including Alaska and Hawaii. Clearly, it is possible for the proportion of older people to rise significantly in a state even if practically no increase occurs by net migration of the elderly themselves. Therefore, the changes in the states underscore the intricate interplay of fertility, mortality, and migration which affects numbers, proportions, and growth rates of the elderly population, both directly and indirectly, and which redistributes them throughout the nation's population.

Summary

The United States has never had a larger number of people aged 65 and older than it does now, nor has that group ever been a greater percentage of the total population. Furthermore, the average individual can expect to live longer than his/her counterpart in any previous generation. These basic facts have major implications for many aspects of American life and for the elderly themselves as individuals and as a group.

The three population processes — fertility, mortality, and migration — are variously involved in these basic changes. The *absolute number* of older people is large now because of the high fertility rates when they were born, the reductions in the death rate during their lifetimes, and the huge immigrations of the early twentieth century. The relatively high and climbing *percentage* of elderly people, which "ages" the nation's population, is primarily the result of recent low birth rates that decrease the proportions of children and young adults in the population, though the aging of the immigrant population has also played a part in the process. Death rates, however, have been dropping faster for infants and children than for the elderly, so this actually helps depress the percentage of the latter. Finally, the greater longevity of individuals does depend on long-term reductions in the death rates of all age groups and consequent increases in life expectancy.

Both the numbers and proportions of the elderly will continue to grow until well into the next century, because the group from which they will come is already alive and subject to fairly predictable death rates. Then, numbers and percentages will level out or even drop for a time, only to rise again, provided the nation experiences no major wars or epidemics, unexpected life-saving miracles, baby booms, mass immigrations or emigrations, or other events that would drastically alter the statistical relationship between the age categories.

The elderly population is not distributed evenly throughout the nation, despite a trend in that direction, but shows high concentrations in New England and the Middle Atlantic states, the Great Plains, and a few sections of the South, most notably Florida. Older people are somewhat underrepresented in metropolitan areas as a whole, though they are overrepresented in certain parts of central cities and in the towns and on the farms of nonmetropolitan counties. They have increased in the suburbs, and their percentages are rising there. Moreover, the proportion of older people is growing virtually everywhere, and their rate of increase between 1970 and 1980 was greater than that of the total population in 49 of the 50 states; Wyoming was the only exception. These changes suggest the pervasive nature of the aging that now typifies America's population and raise strategic questions about its economic and political implications, the needs for medical and retirement provisions, and the form and dynamics of the nation's future social system.

NOTES

1. Simon de Beauvoir, *The Coming of Age.* New York: Putnam's Sons, 1972, p. 4.

2. For a discussion of these aspects, see Matilda White Riley and Anne Foner, *Aging and Society,* v. 1, *An Inventory of Research Findings.* New York: Russell Sage Foundation, 1968, pp. 15-35.

3. Joseph J. Spengler, *Population and America's Future.* San Francisco: Freeman, 1975, p. 90.

4. Some of the trends are adapted from Joseph A. Califano, Jr., "The Aging of America: Questions for the Four-Generation Society," *Annals of American Academy of Political and Social Science* 438 (1978): 97-98.

5. Data are from the U.S. Bureau of the Census, *Statistical Abstract of the United States: 1982-83.* Washington, DC: U.S. Government Printing Office, 1982, table 107.

6. U.S. Bureau of the Census, "Projections of the Population of the United States: 1982 to 2050," *Current Population Reports,* P-25, no. 922 (1982): 13; *1980 Census of Population, Supplementary Reports,* PC80-S1-1, *Age, Sex, Race, and Spanish Origin of the Population by Regions, Divisions, and States: 1980* (1981), table 1.

7. Charles B. Nam and Susan O. Gustavus, *Population: The Dynamics of Demographic Change.* Boston: Houston Mifflin, 1976, p. 190.

8. Henry S. Shryock and Jacob S. Siegel, *The Methods and Materials of Demography,* v. 1. Washington, DC: U.S. Government Printing Office, 1973, p. 248. Cf. U.S. Bureau of the Census, "Demographic Aspects of Aging and the Older Population in the United States," *Current Population Reports,* P-23, no. 59 (1978), pp. 10-11.

9. U.S. Bureau of the Census, "Demographic Aspects of Aging...," *ibid.,* p. 4.

28

10. See Ansley J. Coale, "The Effects of Changes in Mortality and Fertility on Age Composition," *Milbank Memorial Fund Quarterly,* 34 (1956): 79-114.

11. J. John Palen, *Social Problems.* New York: McGraw-Hill, 1979, p. 388.

12. Harrison Givens, Jr., "An Evaluation of Mandatory Retirement," *Annals, op. cit.,* p. 52.

13. Beth J. Soldo, "America's Elderly in the 1980s," *Population Bulletin,* 35 (1980): 5.

14. U.S. Bureau of the Census, "Demographic Aspects of Aging...," *op. cit.,* p. 1.

15. Riley and Foner, *op. cit.,* p. 16.

16. *Ibid.,* p. 21.

17. For a discussion, see Henry P. David, "Eastern Europe: Pronatalist Policies and Private Behavior," *Population Bulletin,* 36 (1982).

18. For a discussion of the projection method, see U.S. Bureau of the Census, "Projections of the Population...," *op. cit.,* pp. 2-3.

19. Leon F. Bouvier, "America's Baby Boom Generation: The Fateful Bulge," *Population Bulletin* 35 (1980): 30.

20. Richard A. Easterlin, "What Will 1984 Be Like? Socioeconomic Implications of Recent Twists in Age Structure," *Demography* 15 (1978): 397-421. Cf. Ronald D. Lee, "Demographic Forecasting and the Easterlin Hypothesis," *Population and Development Review* 2 (1976): 459-468. See the discussion of Easterlin's work by Glenn Collins, "The Good News About 1984," *Psychology Today* 12 (1979): 34-48.

21. Soldo, *op. cit.,* p. 10.

22. For the data, see U.S. Bureau of the Census, "Farm Population of the United States: 1980," *Current Population Reports,* P-27, no. 54 (1981), table 2.

23. For an account of the rural-to-urban migration, see T. Lynn Smith and Paul E. Zopf, Jr., *Demography: Principles and Methods,* 2nd ed. Port Washington, NY: Alfred, 1976, pp. 498-513.

24. Jacob S. Siegel, "On the Demography of Aging," *Demography* 17 (1980): 353. Cf. Donald O. Cowgill, "Residential Segregation by Age in American Metropolitan Areas," *Journal of Gerontology* 33 (1978): 446-453.

25. Siegel, *op. cit.,* p. 353.

26. On this matter, see Stephen M. Golant, ed., *Location and Environment of the Elderly Population.* New York: Wiley, 1979.

27. Soldo, *op. cit.,* p. 13.

28. National Council on the Aging, "Special Concerns II," *Perspective on Aging,* v. 9 (1980), p. 20.

29. For a study of this matter, see Norah Keating and Judith Marshall, "The Process of Retirement: The Rural Self-Employed," *The Gerontologist* 20 (1980): 437-443.

30. National Council on the Aging, *op. cit.,* p. 24.

31. U.S. Bureau of the Census, "Farm Population of the United States," *op. cit.,* table 2.

32. U.S. Bureau of the Census, "Some Demographic Aspects of Aging in the United States," *Current Population Reports,* P-23, no. 43 (1973): 9.

Chapter 2

Age Composition of the Older Population

America's elderly are far from a homogeneous group, for the aging process is based on such a wide range of environmental causes and individualized physiology and heredity, that persons go through it at very different rates.[1] In addition, at any given moment a person's aging represents a unique accumulation of experiences that also affect his/her remaining life expectancy. Therefore, while 65 is the accepted threshold of the older ages because American society causes several things to happen to most people then, the group that has crossed the threshold is tremendously varied, with quite different individual prospects for good health and additional years of life. Even the elderly themselves often do not fully appreciate the heterogeneity of their own age category. This was reflected in the 1974 survey by the National Council on the Aging which found that most tend to overestimate the seriousness of problems faced by their group and believe their own individual maladies to be more common than they actually are, while the ones with relatively few problems tend to believe they are rather rare exceptions.[2] Therefore, the great majority of elderly "who said they faced very serious problems imputed that same experience to most of the other elderly."[3] The end result is often a misleading assumption of homogeneity within and about the older population concerning not only health and finances but many other aspects as well.

Given these perceptions and the stereotypes widely held by younger people, it is important to emphasize the substantial variations that exist within the group aged 65 and older, and that the problems associated with the aging of a population depend as much on the composition of the elderly group as they do on its size.[4] One reflection of the variability is the way the elderly population is distributed among its several age categories from 65-69 to 85 and older and the features that tend to accompany each of the narrower age groupings. No matter what the patterns or indexes used to explore them, however, the key to a view of the people 65 and over is heterogeneity in terms of employment, income, sexual activity, and other factors, though homogeneity does increase gradually as the elderly age.[5] Moreover, there tends to be considerable continuity among older people in the sense that levels of happiness, activity, life satisfaction, and other features neither improve nor deterioriate dramatically relative to those of other cohort members with whom individuals have reached the older years.[6]

Distribution of Ages

Within the elderly population the great majority are concentrated relatively close to age 65, whereas those aged 85 and older are a small minority, though they are increasing as a proportion. (See Table 2-1.) Thus, the present percentages represent less concentration at the lower end of the 65-and-over scale than in the past. In 1900, for example, 71 per cent of the elderly were between 65 and 74 and only 4 per cent were 85 and older. The recent tendency for people to be more heavily represented in the oldest ages is not yet due primarily to any significant increases in the human life span, which is regarded by some as a biological attribute of the species and only now on the verge of significant extension. Changing age distribution has resulted instead from the larger proportions of people who survive to the older ages of that life span.[7] In addition, the higher percentages of very elderly people who appear at certain times are due to high fertility levels when their cohort was born, as was the case with the group born just after the Civil War. The survivors of that cohort were in their late 70s and 80s in the decade after World War II, when the proportion of people aged 75 and older rose to about a third of the entire elderly group. Finally, the aging of people who immigrated in the early 1900s also contributed to the size of the group 75 and over, for by 1980 an abnormally large share of those foreign-born people still surviving were in the oldest categories, though migration is usually less important than fertility and mortality in shaping a nation's age profile.[8]

Differences by Sex and Race

Females have a greater survival potential than males at all ages, from the newborn to centenarians, for the death rates of females are substantially lower than those of males across the entire age spectrum. Therefore, men in the older ages are more likely than women to cluster near 65, whereas the women are distributed more evenly among the age ranges. In 1980, for instance, only 34 per cent of the nation's older men but 42 per cent of the women were aged 75 and older. (See Table 2-1.)

In general, elderly black people concentrate more heavily in the ages near 65 than do white people, and they are less represented in most of the older years. At fault is the higher death rate that has prevailed among blacks throughout America's history and which is still in evidence, though less dramatically than it was. Nevertheless, if a black person is able to survive the relatively high death rates until age 75 or 80, his/her survival potential actually is somewhat better than that of a white person. Thus, while the death rates of white males are lower than those of black males at all ages until 75, the reverse is true beyond that age. This "crossover"

Table 2-1. Percentages of Older People in Specific Age Groups, by Sex, Race, and Spanish Origin, 1980

Race and Sex	Per Cent				
	65-69	70-74	75-79	80-84	85+
All Races	34.4	26.5	18.9	11.4	8.8
Male	37.9	27.7	17.9	9.9	6.6
Female	32.0	25.9	19.3	12.6	10.2
White	34.0	26.6	18.8	11.7	8.9
Male	37.8	27.7	17.9	10.0	6.7
Female	31.6	25.8	19.4	12.8	10.4
Black	37.2	27.0	18.6	9.6	7.6
Male	39.1	27.7	18.1	8.9	6.3
Female	35.9	26.5	19.0	10.1	8.5
Spanish Origin[a]	37.3	27.3	19.2	9.3	6.9
Male	37.9	27.8	19.3	9.0	6.1
Female	36.7	26.9	19.2	9.7	7.5

Source: U.S. Bureau of the Census, 1980 Census of Population, Supplementary Reports, PC80-S1-1, Age, Sex, Race, and Spanish Origin of the Population by Regions, Divisions, and States: 1980 (1981), table 1.

[a]May be of any race.

also occurs for women, but at a somewhat older age than for men. As a result of the reversal, the white man who reaches age 85 has an average of 5.3 years remaining, the black man an average of 7.8 years; the figures for women are 6.7 years and 9.9 years, respectively.

Despite the crossover effect in the oldest ages, however, the higher birth rates of black people and their higher death rates at most ages cause only 8 per cent of all American blacks to be aged 65 and older, contrasted with about 12 per cent of all whites. Those proportions are shaped, too, by the fact that immigrants are a far smaller share of the black than of the white population, while those black immigrants who do enter the country now tend to be significantly younger on the average than the white immigrants.

When age and sex are accounted for together, white women are far more likely than any other group to show up in the 75-and-over category, whereas black men are the most poorly represented in those ages. But none of the racial discrepancies is as great as in the past, for the death rates of black people have been falling faster than those of whites and the distributions of the races within the older age ranges are slowly growing more alike. At the same time, death rates have fallen faster for women than for men in both racial groups, so the distribution of the sexes throughout the elderly ages is less similar than in the past. Those dynamics all contribute to the substantial majorities of older women, both black and white.

The Role of Mortality

The preceding comments suggest that differential death rates by race and sex powerfully affect how the various age groups appear in the 65-and-over category, though other significant factors are also involved. The influence of mortality can be examined by looking briefly at differences in the proportion of people who survive to particular ages and at the average number of years of life remaining to those who do make it to age 65, 75, and the older years. The appropriate data appear in Table 2-2 on the percentages of survivors and Table 2-3 on life expectancy. Both sets of data use the racial categories "white" and "other races," who have been at least 90 per cent black in all years.

Proportion of survivors. In 1980 about 77 per cent of all races collectively could expect to survive from birth to age 65, compared with only 41 per cent at the turn of the century, when the first national life tables were compiled. This remarkable improvement has been most impressive among women, for about 85 per cent of the whites and 75 per cent of the blacks can now expect to reach age 65. Naturally, beyond that age the comparatively high death rates for all race and sex groups reduce the percentages who reach the older years, but the current figures all represent substantial improvements over 1900-1902, especially for black women, who fared much worse relative to white women than they do now.

The situation has been and still is less favorable for men, and the rate of improvement in their survival potential has been slower than that among women. Thus, in 1980 about 72 per cent of the white men and only 58 per cent of the blacks could plan to see age 65. Moreover, just 17 per cent of the white men and 14 per cent of the blacks could anticipate reaching age 85 — proportions which are less than half those for women in each race. In 1900-1902, however, the sexes were more nearly alike in their probability to attain the older ages, while the races were less alike than they are now. This change shows that the nation's older population is becoming increasingly female in the sense that a growing share of the whole group aged 65 and older consists of women. At the turn of the century they made up 50

Table 2-2. Percentages of Persons Surviving to Specified Ages, by Race and Sex, 1901 and 1980

Race and Sex	Per Cent Surviving to					
	Age 65		Age 75		Age 85	
	1901[a]	1980	1901[a]	1980	1901[a]	1980
White						
Male	39.2	72.3	21.4	47.5	5.2	18.3
Female	43.8	84.7	25.4	68.5	7.1	38.4
Other Races						
Male	19.0	58.0	8.9	35.5	2.0	13.9
Female	22.0	75.0	11.1	55.7	3.6	29.6

Sources: National Center for Health Statistics, Vital Statistics of the United States: 1978, vol. 2, sec. 5, Life Tables (1980), table 5-4; "Advance Report of Final Mortality Statistics, 1980," Monthly Vital Statistics Report, vol. 32, no. 4 (1983), table 2.

[a]Average of data for 1900-1902 in the death-registration states.

per cent of the total, while in 1980 they were 60 per cent. Particularly striking is the fact that improvements in life expectancy for black men lag far behind those for black women. On the other hand, the proportions of black and white men who survive to age 65 are now more nearly alike than they were in 1900-1902, as are those of black and white women. So while the races have converged in this respect, the sexes have diverged.

Table 2-3. Average Number of Years of Life Remaining at Specified Ages, by Race and Sex, 1901 and 1980

Race and Sex	Remaining Life Expectancy at					
	Age 65		Age 75		Age 85	
	1901[a]	1980	1901[a]	1980	1901[a]	1980
White						
Male	11.5	14.2	6.8	8.8	3.8	5.0
Female	12.2	18.5	7.3	11.5	4.1	6.3
Other Races						
Male	10.4	13.5	6.6	8.9	4.0	5.3
Female	11.4	17.3	7.9	11.4	5.1	7.0

Sources: National Center for Health Statistics, Vital Statistics of the United States: 1978, vol. 2, sec. 5, Life Tables (1980), table 5-4; "Advance Report of Final Mortality Statistics, 1980," Monthly Vital Statistics Report, vol. 32, no. 4 (1983), table 2.

Remaining life expectancy. Americans aged 65 and older can expect an average of 16.4 additional years of life, though individuals range widely around that norm. This compares with an average of 11.9 years in 1900-1902. But while the changes during the century did add about 4.5 years of life expectancy for the elderly, it is a fairly small increase, given the huge improvements in health and nutrition that have lowered general death rates and infant mortality levels so drastically. Therefore, the relatively small magnitude of the change suggests that reductions in the death rates of older age groups have not been as great as those of younger ages.[9] In turn, it shows that the death rates of older people continue to be high relative to those of other age groups and that their time in the 65-and-over category is really quite brief, though more people do survive over a longer portion of the age span than ever before.[*10*] Once again, females have a marked advantage over males, for the average life expectancy of elderly women in both major races has improved considerably more than that of elderly men.

Some Trends and Projections

Age composition within the elderly group keeps changing because of variations in fertility, mortality, and net migration, but a few long-term trends have remained relatively constant. In particular, the whole group has grown less concentrated near 65 and an increasing share is in the oldest ages. (See Figure 2-1.) But the major increases in the proportion 75 and over came after 1940, for in each decade prior to that year only about 29 or 30 per cent fell into that age group. Conversely, seven-tenths or so of all elderly appeared in the ages under 75. The familiar factors involved in

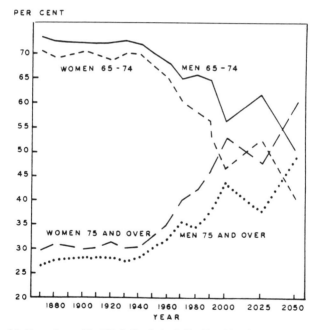

Figure 2-1. Percentages of the Elderly Population in Two Broad Age Groups, by Sex, 1870-2050
Sources: U.S.Bureau of the Census, *Sixteenth Census of the United States: 1940, Characteristics of the Population, U.S. Summary* (1943), table 8; *U.S. Census of Population: 1970, General Population Characteristics, U.S. Summary* (1972), table 53; *1980 Census of Population, Supplementary Reports*, PC80-S1-1, *Age, Sex, Race, and Spanish Origin of the Population by Regions, Divisions, and States: 1980* (1981), table 1; "Projections of the Population of the United States: 1982 to 2050" (advance report), *Current Population Reports*, P-25, no. 922 (1982), table 2.

preserving the lopsided distribution were relatively high rates of death that allowed comparatively few people to reach the oldest ages, high birth rates that enlarged the lower end of various cohorts 65 years later, and an immigrant population that was still relatively youthful early in the century.

By 1950, however, the proportion 65-74 had begun to decline significantly and those 75 and older had started to rise, thereby accelerating a trend which had slow beginnings much earlier and which seems likely to persist into the twenty-first century. In fact, given the age groups of people already alive and their probable death rates, it is likely that by 2050 people 75 and over will be considerably more than half the entire elderly population. This represents a remarkable change since 1940, when people in the 65-74 age bracket outnumbered those 75 and over by more than two to one, and is still another reflection of the aging of America's population.

The group aged 85 and older has grown especially rapidly while the elderly population as a whole has been increasing in numbers and proportions. Between 1950 and 1980, for example, people aged 85 and older increased from about 600,000 to 2.2 million, or 288 per cent. At the same time, the number aged 65-74 increased 85 per cent and those aged 75-84 expanded 136 per cent. As a consequence, people aged 85 and older went from 4.7 per cent of the total elderly population in 1950 to 8.8 per cent in 1980. Given these rates, they promise to number at least 16 million by 2050, or more than seven times the figure in 1980, and to be about 24 per cent of all elderly.

Figure 2-1 also indicates that women have long been more heavily represented than men in the oldest age group and that they will continue to be so; even in 1870 about 30 per cent of the elderly women but only 27 per cent of the men were 75 and over. Moreover, given the differential death rates by sex, the gap will widen, and by 2050 it is likely that 60 per cent of America's elderly women but only 49 per cent of the men will be aged 75 and older.

We can expect some temporary reversals in the overall trends, however, which correspond to earlier variations in fertility. For example, in 2000 the percentages of both sexes aged 74-75 will drop significantly, for that comparatively small group will consist of the survivors of the small baby crops born in the 1920s and 1930s. The decline will enhance the statistical importance of people 75 and over and their percentages will grow. By 2025, though, the large baby boom of 1945-1960 will have reached the elderly ages and the percentage of people 65-74 will rise dramatically as that of older ones falls. In the two decades to follow the trends will again reverse, as the much lower birth rates after 1960 show up in the form of smaller percentages of people aged 65-74 and consequent increases of those 75 and over.

These dynamics all have significant implications for the kinds of facilities American society must provide in the next half century or so. We will need to focus rather heavily on medical care, nursing homes, and other services for extremely old people and on their social and emotional needs. On the whole, that group begins to develop quite a different health profile than people who have just become 65, because many of the older ones suffer the ravages of illness and disability that most of the younger ones can still avoid for a decade or so. Therefore, it is not enough to plan for an expanding group 65 and over, which is certainly on its way. The nation has to account for the proportions who will be over 75 and 85 and for the things that happen to those older people. For example, while 41 per cent of the women aged 65-74 are already widowed, 69 per cent of those 75 and over have lost their mates, and the proportion reflects a great

Table 2-4. Percentages of the Elderly Population in Two Broad Age Groups, by Race and Sex, Selected Years

Age and Year	All Races		White		Other Races	
	Male	Female	Male	Female	Male	Female
65-74						
1910	71.8	69.7	71.9	70.0	71.2	65.9
1940	71.9	69.6	71.5	69.3	76.2	72.7
1980	65.6	57.9	65.4	57.4	66.7	62.4
2000[a]	56.5	46.6	56.2	45.8	59.5	52.7
75+						
1910	28.2	30.3	28.1	30.0	28.8	34.1
1940	28.1	30.4	28.5	30.7	23.8	27.3
1980	34.4	42.1	34.6	42.6	33.3	37.6
2000[a]	43.5	53.4	43.8	54.2	40.5	47.3

Sources: U.S. Bureau of the Census, U.S. Census of Population: 1970, General Population Characteristics, U.S. Summary (1972), table 53; 1980 Census of Population, Supplementary Reports, PC80-S1-1, Age, Sex, Race, and Spanish Origin of the Population by Regions, Divisions, and States: 1980 (1981), table 1; "Projections of the Population of the United States: 1982 to 2050" (advance report), Current Population Reports, P-25, no. 922 (1982), table 2.

[a]Projections based on Series II assumptions.

number of personal tragedies in the oldest years.

Also, the death rates for males and females aged 75-84 are more than double those for people aged 65-74, and while the higher levels do result in part from many sudden, relatively painless deaths, they also reflect a large number of people who suffer prolonged illnesses marked by physical and emotional pain and deterioration. Therefore, the growing abundance of people in the oldest ages calls for a heavy focus on hospice facilities, home care for invalids, and warmth and understanding for those whose lives are ebbing slowly and who are easy to pity, resent, or neglect. These and other realities suggest the great differences a society confronts when it has either an abundance of older people near age 65 or a heavy concentration in the upper 70s and beyond.[11]

The proportion of people in the 75-and-over group is increasing among both blacks and whites. (See Table 2-4.) Early in the twentieth century the percentages aged 75 and older in both races tended to be only half or less those of people aged 65-74 — a situation that persisted until 1940. That was the census year when the large number of people born just after the Civil War were aged 65-74, and while both races tended to concentrate in that category, it was more true of blacks than whites. Since 1940, however, the proportions of elderly people who are 75 and older have been increasing in both racial groups, while the percentages of those 65-74 have been dropping. Moreover, the extremely old, especially women, will continue to become a larger share of both racial groups and will stand in marked contrast with the proportions in 1910, when both blacks and whites clustered close to 65 and very old people of either race were quite scarce.

If Series II projections prove accurate, the changes will probably leave the nation with at least 17 million people aged 75 and older in 2000 and 37 million by 2050. Moreover, nearly two-thirds of the latter group will consist of women, most of them widows. In the ages 85 and older, increases will be especially rapid and the number of women in those ages will be nearly the same as that in the group aged 75-84. The oldest women will outnumber men by about 2.5 to one. But the very existence of these large groups of the old-old reflects improvements in health and longevity and a prolonged ability to be useful in American society. At the same time, however, increasing percentages of the elderly have been leaving responsible roles in jobs and the economy in general, whether voluntarily or involuntarily, and many more are apt to be perceived as the wards of a welfare state that expects its oldest citizens to withdraw from full productivity. Therefore, while the older population has higher levels of education and better average health than ever before, the society makes it more difficult for them to perform constructively, while it also grows more resentful about the cost of their support. Aggravated by the pressures of high unemployment rates among the baby-boom generation now become adult, the failure to make fully productive use of the elderly is a problem for the nation and for many elderly themselves, especially those 65-74.[12] It is this combination of circumstances that deprives some older Americans of purpose and meaning, and the one that stems not from changes in fertility, mortality, and migration, but from restrictive social attitudes. We have added several years to the lives of many more Americans but tend to make those years less useful; in the process we have converted numerous contributing people into dependents. Therefore, the analysis now turns to some aspects of that dependency.

Dependency Ratios

An evaluation of the average burden of support for elderly people, carried essentially by younger adults, logically accompanies the assessment of age distributions and their underlying population processes. In a broader sense, demographers are also concerned with the child-support burden, for many questions about population pressures involve the proportions of people available to look after those whose age and its social correlates keep them from caring fully for themselves and who make up the dependent population. The latter group consists of people aged 0-19 and those 65 and older,[13] and while this study focuses on the elderly, it must also account for the youth support burden as part of the total responsibility that falls on people aged 20-64. In that connection, it is important to emphasize that in all industrialized countries the child support burden has dropped very significantly as that for the elderly has risen, thus producing a net decrease in the total dependency burden.

One principal index of support burdens is the *dependency ratio*, calculated as follows:

$$\text{Dependency ratio} = \frac{\text{Population aged 0-19 and 65 and over}}{\text{Population aged 20-64}} \times 100$$

It is expressed as the number of dependents for each 100 producers. People aged 15-19 could also be considered part of the producing population, especially in any study of the developing countries where many enter the labor force at those younger ages, but in the United States so many people aged 15-19 are still in school that the majority are not self-supporting. In addition, some people under 65 are not producers and many older ones are; indeed, one of the judgments in this book is that more older people should be allowed to produce more fully if they wish and are able. Whether or not a particular person is really dependent is affected by health, financial standing, occupational involvement, the cultural definitions that surround age, and other factors.[14] But a demographic study can only deal with categories of people, not individuals, and the decision was made earlier to use 65 as the threshold of the older ages. In fact, occupational involvement does drop substantially by that age and drastically afterwards. In 1980, for example, about 91 per cent of the men aged 45-54, 72 per cent of those aged 55-64, and only 19 per cent of the ones 65 and older were in the labor force; for women the decline was from 60 per cent, to 41 per cent, to 8 per cent.[15] Nor is official inclusion in the labor force the only way for older people to be productive. Nonetheless, while there is much variation in what dependency means socially and individually, the Census Bureau reports the majority of its age data for five-year ranges, and it seems most useful to classify Americans aged 0-19 and 65 and over as dependents and those aged 20-64 as producers.

Use of the dependency ratio could also imply that the support burden is distributed evenly among people aged 20-64, which is not so in any society. Nor does the index allow for the levels of living at which the support burden is carried in various populations.[16] Thus, while the dependency ratio does describe the statistical relationship between the older population and younger adults over time and in different places, its variations should not be taken to reflect differences in levels of living. Moreover, when the ratio can be refined to relate the elderly who actually do not work to the group aged 20-64 who do, it is more accurate than when it is based only on age categories,[17] though the data rarely permit such refinements by sex, race, and other characteristics.[18]

Some International Comparisons

In 1980 there were about 76 Americans aged 0-19 and 65 and over for each 100 aged 20-64, which is a relatively low figure compared with many earlier periods and with the bulk of the world's countries now. (See Table 2-5.) The dependency ratio for the elderly (20) accounted for a quarter of the overall support burden, the youth ratio (56) for the other three-quarters, and while the former is continuing to grow and the latter to shrink, the two together do not represent a particularly heavy burden of support. In fact, relatively few of the world's countries have smaller youth dependency ratios, though not many have larger elderly ratios either.

The youth dependency ratios are low and the elderly ones high in the urban-industrial countries, because fertility and mortality rates have been quite low for some time and the populations in those places are aging ones in the sense that people 65 and over range between 11 and 16 per cent of the total in most cases. About 20 countries have higher elderly dependency ratios than the United States, and all are European. As shown by the 10 representative ones in Table 2-5, almost all are highly industrialized, though other factors are also at work in such nations as Bulgaria and Hungary, where the percentages of workers engaged in agriculture are still relatively high, while elderly dependency ratios are also about 20. In fact, the aging of those populations demonstrates that effective fertility control can exist where levels of industrial development are substantially below those in the more urbanized nations. Despite the large elderly populations and comparatively small youthful segments in the representa-

Table 2-5.   Selected Countries With Low and High
             Dependency Ratios, 1980

Country	Dependency Ratio			Number 20-64 for each One 65+
	Elderly	Youth	Total	
Sweden	28.5	46.2	74.7	3.5
East Germany	28.4	50.4	78.8	3.5
Austria	28.0	52.6	80.6	3.6
England & Wales	27.0	52.0	79.0	3.7
West Germany	26.8	46.1	72.9	3.7
Norway	26.6	53.9	80.5	3.8
Scotland	25.4	55.3	80.7	3.9
Denmark	25.3	50.1	75.4	4.0
France	25.3	54.7	80.0	4.0
UNITED STATES	19.9	56.4	76.3	5.0
Nicaragua	8.0	154.3	162.3	12.6
Ecuador	7.9	138.7	146.6	12.6
Bolivia	7.6	123.1	130.7	13.2
Thailand	7.5	118.0	125.5	13.3
Brazil	7.4	113.3	120.7	13.5
India	7.4	109.3	116.7	13.5
Guatemala	6.8	130.2	137.0	14.7
Zaire	6.1	138.7	144.8	16.3
Sudan	5.9	111.3	117.2	16.9
Gambia	4.7	113.0	117.7	21.2

Sources: United Nations, Demographic Yearbook, 1980, table 7; 1981, table 7;   U.S. Bureau of the Census, 1980 Census of Population, Supplementary Reports, PC80-S1-1, Age, Sex, Race, and Spanish Origin of the Population by Regions, Divisions, and States: 1980 (1981), table 1.

tive developed countries, however, people under age 20 still outnumber those aged 65 and older in every case, though the two groups are much nearer the same size than they are in all of the developing nations with recent or present high birth rates. Paradoxically, therefore, the industrialized countries best able to support large numbers of children have the smallest proportions of them, whereas the heaviest youth support burdens occur in the developing countries least equipped to carry them. At the same time, while the developed countries have the largest percentages of older people, most also use mechanisms that either force or encourage the elderly to be less than fully productive or even fully integrated into their societies.[19]

Though the least developed nations have the lowest elderly dependency ratios, those for youth are so high that the two combine to produce high overall support burdens.[20] Those societies are concentrated largely in Africa, parts of Asia, and all but the temperate sections of Latin America. In fact, the 10 representative countries with extremely high rates shown in Table 2-5 have such youthful age profiles that the elderly group is only 4 per cent or less of the total population in each case. In some of them the birth rate has dropped in very recent years; in others it has risen a bit; and in the rest it has remained fairly static at a high level. But in all of the countries the basic cause of the huge child burdens and the small elderly ones is the high level of fertility coupled with recent precipitous declines in mortality, especially among infants. The populations in those places have become more youthful in the past few decades as they incurred their population explosions, and child care is a tremendously larger concern than is support for the small percentage of elderly, many of whom must keep working and fill economically useful roles anyway. In the future, however, the number of elderly people is likely to increase faster than that of children in most parts of the world, so the elderly segment will gradually become a larger part of the dependent population, children a somewhat smaller part.[21] Nevertheless, the latter will still account for the great bulk of the world's dependency situation, particularly in the developing countries.[22]

Some other countries not listed in Table 2-5 have moderate overall support burdens, but the relative importance of young and elderly people varies widely among them. One group consists of developing countries with relatively high youth ratios but low ones for the elderly; most have experienced drastic reductions in mortality and about half also have declining birth rates. These changes in the vital processes are comparatively new, however, and the percentages of children are still fairly high, those of older people relatively low. The countries in another group with moderate burdens have fairly low youth ratios but rather high elderly indexes; they include Canada, Australia, New Zealand, some temperate parts of South America, and a few European nations. There the birth and death rates have been low enough long enough for the elderly to become increasingly large parts of the total populations, though they are still below the proportions in the United States and most of Europe. Those countries are unlikely to experience reductions in infant and youth mortality comparable to earlier decreases, and if fertility rates hold at a relatively low level, the proportions of producers and older people will rise and the elderly support burdens will grow.[23]

Ratio of workers to older people. Given the dependency ratios for the elderly in the United States, there are now about five people aged 20-64 for each person aged 65 and older. That figure closely resembles those in the other urban-industrial nations, whereas the developing countries have relatively large numbers of workers for each older person. (See Table 2-5.) But when the ratio of workers to each child is added, the great strains in the developing countries become obvious. For example, while there are 13 producers for each 10 dependents in the United States, there are only 6 in Nicaragua. Thus, the vast child population, not the growing elderly group, imposes the large majority of the support burden in most countries, as it did earlier in the United States. The present huge group of children in the developing nations also imperils levels of living and the world ecosystem far more than do dependent elderly people, for today's child population will draw from the earth's resources for many decades, and even at relatively low birth rates they will still produce huge numbers of children of their own. Eventually, the large child populations will also become large elderly populations and will still impose heavy support burdens on the producing population and strains on the ecosystem. Thus, past high birth rates make their effects felt for the better part of a century, even if a society has managed to achieve low ones recently.

Racial and Ethnic Differences in the United States

The total dependency ratio in the white population is low compared with that among blacks and is much below those of other races and Spanish-origin people. (See Table 2-6.) The components of those various ratios also differ widely, because whites have a comparatively light support burden for youth and a relatively heavy one for the elderly, while blacks bear a heavier burden for children and a lighter one for the elderly. As birth and death rates become more alike for the two races, however, the component ratios also grow more similar. The group of "other races" and the people of Spanish origin have especially high youth dependency ratios and low ones for the elderly. As a result of these variations, the number of workers for each elderly person is lowest among whites and rises successively for blacks, Spanish-origin people, and other races. But the population of white children is now so small relative to the group of producing adults, that even when those aged 0-19 are compared with the group of white elderly, there are more workers for each dependent person among whites than among blacks, other races, and the Spanish-origin population.

The youth dependency ratio would be even higher for Spanish-origin people and their elderly dependency figure would be lower if it were not for the Cuban contingent, because their proportion of children is far smaller than those of people with Mexican, Puerto Rican, or Central and South American backgrounds. Thus, while the Spanish-origin group as a whole has a relatively high support burden for youth and a comparatively low one for the elderly, the reverse is true for Cubans, many of whom came to the United States in 1960 or so and who are now an aging population.[24]

Even though these patterns underscore the greater weight of child care and the lesser burden of older people that tend to be borne by blacks and Spanish-origin people, the statistical situation should not imply that the actual support burdens of blacks are all carried exclusively by blacks, any more than those of whites are carried entirely by their race. American society is far more complex than that, with many mechanisms that both disperse and concentrate income irrespective of average dependency ratios by race.

Nonetheless, the statistical differences do have fundamental implications for social and economic conditions, particularly when they are coupled with the fact that median per capita family income is still significantly higher for whites than for blacks and Spanish-origin people. That is particularly true among elderly people, which means the average older black or Spanish-background person has a greater financial struggle to be self-supporting than does the older white, though family ties and other sources of assistance do alter the situation in many individual cases. But on balance and because of the combination of age patterns and income-distribution mechanisms, the average black wage earner carries a much heavier total support burden than does his/her white counterpart, and still does so at a substantially lower level of income. The fact that elderly dependency ratios are lower for blacks than for whites doesn't change that basic condition, because the relative scarcity of older blacks is more than offset by the numbers of children. Therefore, the data on dependency ratios also underscore the differences in fertility and mortality that still persist between racial and ethnic groups, even though the rates have become more alike for blacks and whites.

Some Changes and Projections

The various changes in age composition in the United States, produced

Table 2-6. Dependency Ratios in the United States, by Race and Spanish Origin, 1980

Race	Dependency Ratio			Number 20-64 for each One 65+	Number 20-64 for each Dependent[a]
	Elderly	Youth	Total		
All races	19.9	56.4	76.3	5.0	1.31
White	21.2	52.7	73.9	4.7	1.35
Black	15.1	76.6	91.7	6.6	1.09
Other Races	8.1	82.5	90.6	12.4	1.20
Spanish Origin[b]	9.3	82.5	91.8	10.8	1.09

Source: U.S. Bureau of the Census, 1980 Census of Population, Supplementary Reports, PC80-S1-1, Age, Sex, Race, and Spanish Origin of the Population by Regions, Divisions, and States: 1980 (1981), table 1.

[a]Dependents are those aged 0-19 and 65+.

[b]May be of any race.

by fluctuations in the three population processes, have decreased the overall dependency ratio very significantly, though not without some temporary increases reflected in the censuses of 1950, 1960, and 1970. (See Table 2-7.) Moreover, the youth ratio has fallen continually, except for those three times, while the elderly ratio has risen in each succeeding decade. In fact, the youth burden has been cut nearly in half since 1870, while the elderly support burden has more than tripled, though the net result in 1980 was a total dependency ratio little more than two-thirds that in 1870. This has happened because fertility declined in the long run and reduced the proportional significance of the child population, mortality decreased significantly and raised life expectancy for all age groups, and immigration introduced progressively fewer young adults. These factors changed the age profile so much that the upward surge in the birth rate after World War II was neither great enough nor sustained enough to offset fully the far longer period when both vital rates fell rapidly and immigration dropped off drastically. Consequently, there have been only a few temporary reversals in the trend toward a higher median age and a lower overall support burden, and no halt at all in the movement toward a higher elderly dependency ratio.

It seems likely that the elderly dependency ratio will continue to increase gradually until 2000 or so, when the relatively small birth cohorts of the Depression will be in the older years. At the same time, barring any new baby boom the youth dependency ratio should continue to fall steadily, until it is only half that in 1880. Therefore, the overall dependency ratio will also fall between now and 2000. By 2025, however, the elderly dependency ratio will leap upward as the postwar baby boom inhabits the older ages, the youth ratio will continue to fall gradually, but the total ratio will rise because of the large group aged 65 and older. Those trends will continue until at least 2050, when the youth and elderly dependency ratios won't be far apart. But the total ratio will still be lower than the one in 1970, even though the relative importance of its components will have changed dramatically.

Table 2-7 also shows the steady decline in the ratio of workers to elderly people and indicates that the figure in 1980 was less than a third that in 1870. But the great decline in the proportion of children actually increased the ratio of workers to all dependents. As Americans enter the twenty-first century, the number of workers for each older person will continue to decline, which will certainly increase the average cost per worker for Social Security taxes, Medicare and other health payments for older people, and similar services. But the reductions in child-care responsibilities will compensate partly for increases in those for the elderly, so we can expect more of a realignment in expenditures than vast increases for both dependent parts of the population combined. In addition, there is more opportunity for the elderly than for young children to be self-supporting,

Table 2-7. Dependency Ratios in the United States,
1870-2050

Year	Dependency Ratio			Number 20-24 for each One 65+	Number 20-64 for each One 0-19 and 65+
	Elderly	Youth	Total		
1870	6.3	105.0	111.3	15.8	0.90
1880	7.1	99.2	106.3	14.1	0.94
1890	7.7	92.2	99.9	12.9	1.00
1900	7.9	86.3	94.2	12.7	1.06
1910	8.0	78.2	86.2	12.5	1.16
1920	8.6	74.7	83.3	11.7	1.20
1930	9.7	69.6	79.3	10.3	1.26
1940	11.7	58.6	70.3	8.6	1.42
1950	14.0	58.7	72.7	7.1	1.38
1960	17.7	73.6	91.3	5.7	1.10
1970	18.9	72.5	91.4	5.3	1.09
1980	19.9	56.4	76.3	5.0	1.31
1990	21.7	48.9	70.6	4.6	1.42
2000	22.2	47.3	69.5	4.5	1.44
2025	34.8	43.7	78.5	2.9	1.28
2050	39.5	42.5	82.0	2.5	1.22

Sources: U.S. Bureau of the Census, Sixteenth
Census of the United States: 1940, Characteristics
of the Population, U.S. Summary (1943), table 8;
U.S. Census of Population: 1970, General Population
Characteristics, U.S. Summary (1972), table 53; 1980
Census of Population, Supplementary Reports, PC80-S1-1,
Age, Sex, Race, and Spanish Origin of the Population
by Regions, Divisions and States: 1980 (1981),
table 1; "Projections of the Population of the United
States: 1982 to 2050" (advance report), Current
Population Reports, P-25, no. 922 (1982), table 2.

Projections based on Series II assumptions.

and while all infants do have to rely on someone else for survival, many elderly do not. The group of self-sufficient older people certainly can be enlarged by more imaginative social and economic arrangements that provide better access to jobs and other opportunities, especially as the small birth cohorts of the 1970s and subsequent years finally shrink the proportion of younger workers and put skilled older ones in greater demand. If the cost of living can be kept reasonable, the tradeoff of a heavier elderly support burden for a much lighter youth burden should be manageable for the working population, though not without problems and even potential intergenerational conflict.

Naturally, the numbers and proportions of people aged 20-64 also affect the size of the dependency ratio, for they are the base group to which the two dependent ones are related statistically. Therefore, changes in that category are just as strategic as fluctuations among younger and older people. The absolute numbers of people in the group 20-64 have grown sevenfold since 1870 and the group increased from 47 per cent of the total population in that year to 57 per cent in 1980. The increases that took place at more specific times during that period generally represent the movement of progressively larger birth cohorts into the 20-64 category, while periodic decreases, especially in 1960 and 1970, reflect new growth spurts in the child population. The numbers aged 20-64 promise to continue increasing until about 2020, to decline temporarily, and then to increase slowly once again. By 2050 those people will number about 170 million and will be about 56 per cent of the total population.

The total dependency ratio has fallen at various times in the past because a given child population was proportionately smaller than several which preceded it, and because those earlier large cohorts entered the group of producers. Therefore, if the birth rate remains reasonably stable at a low level, the large cohorts that eventually will age into the 65-and-over category will raise the elderly dependency ratio for a time and then will die. If fertility and mortality both remain comparatively stable, the three large age groups will come into equilibrium with each other, the dependency ratio will neither rise nor fall markedly, and the nation will be able to count on fairly stable support burdens, at least demographically. That outcome is not guaranteed, of course, given the historical capriciousness of the birth rate and potential increases in the average life span; nor does it imply anything about the financial ability of people to carry even a demographically stable support burden. But the size and age composition of future populations may be more predictable than many in the past, which should make certain social and economic planning easier. It will still be a long time, however, before families and the society can expect the elderly support burden to stop fluctuating, and during most of the next half century it will still grow substantially and the locus of financing will shift more from private to public funds.[25]

Aged-Child Ratios

One infrequently used but sensitive index of aging in a population is the *aged-child ratio,* which accounts simultaneously for the numbers of people and changes at both ends of the age scale.[26] In using this index and to be sure it refers to children, the data are based on the numbers of those aged 0-14 rather than 0-19, and on those aged 65 and older. The index is computed as follows:

$$\text{Aged-child ratio} = \frac{\text{Number of persons 65 and over}}{\text{Number of persons 0-14}} \times 100$$

In societies with large proportions of children, such as India, Thailand, and other so-called developing countries, the aged-child ratios are commonly under 10 older people for each 100 children, whereas in the developed nations with relatively large shares of older people, the index is often 50 or higher. (See Table 2-8, which uses the same countries as Table 2-5.) Indeed, increases in the aged-child ratio are actually an index of aging in a population.[27] For example, India, with a total population nearly three times that of the United States, has more than five times as many children but 3 million fewer elderly. As a result, the aged-child ratio in India is less than 9, while that in the United States is 50. Nonetheless, even though the American child population is much smaller relative to that of older people than it was in the past, the United States still has far from the world's highest aged-child index, for it is surpassed by nine countries listed in Table 2-8 and several others. They are all European, but include some in both the East and the West.

The aged-child ratios in most of the developing countries, on the other hand, are close to the one in the United States in 1870, when the index was only 8 and children were 39 per cent of the total population, elderly people a mere 3 per cent. Thus, the developing countries in Table 2-8, as well as many others not listed, have such huge proportions of children and so few elderly people that their aged-child ratios are commonly only a small fraction of those in the industrialized nations. In India, for example, about 41 per cent of the population consists of children, whereas the elderly are only 3 per cent. In contrast, children are 18 per cent of West Germany's population, older people 16 per cent. The two countries have aged-child indexes of 9 and 85, respectively.

Within the United States the aged-child ratio is highest for the white population, less than half as great for blacks, and even lower for the Spanish-origin contingent. (See Table 2-9.) These data reflect the signifi-

Table 2-8.   Selected Countries With Low and High
              Aged-Child Ratios, 1980

Country	Number 0-14 (000)	Number 65+ (000)	Aged-Child Ratio[a]
West Germany	11,187	9,550	85.4
Sweden	1,628	1,354	83.2
East Germany	3,290	2,661	80.8
Austria	1,540	1,162	75.5
England & Wales	10,289	7,424	72.2
Denmark	1,068	739	69.2
Norway	908	603	66.4
Scotland	1,125	724	64.4
France	11,997	7,535	62.8
UNITED STATES	51,282	25,544	49.8
India	262,656	22,762	8.7
Brazil	49,973	4,140	8.3
Thailand	19,378	1,575	8.1
Bolivia	2,412	184	7.6
Ecuador	3,810	269	7.1
Guatemala	3,201	208	6.5
Nicaragua	1,310	83	6.3
Sudan	8,383	510	6.1
Zaire	12,189	661	5.4
Gambia	252	13	5.2

Sources: United Nations, Demographic Yearbook,
1980, table 7;   1981, table 7;   U.S. Bureau of the
Census, 1980 Census of Population, Supplementary
Reports, PC80-S1-1, Age, Sex, Race, and Spanish
Origin of the Population by Regions, Divisions,
and States: 1980 (1981), table 1.

[a]Number aged 65+ per 100 aged 0-14.

cantly lower proportions of children and higher percentages of elderly people in the white group than in the other two. Moreover, the aged-child ratios in all groups increased very substantially during the twentieth century, and they will probably leap forward in the next century as the population ages rapidly. In fact, by 2025 there will probably be more elderly people than children in the white population, though the numbers in the two age groups will also become more nearly alike among blacks. If Series II projections made by the Census Bureau hold up, in 2050 children should be about 17 per cent of the total population, elderly people around 22 per cent. But the two groups together will be only a little less than they were in 1870 (42%), when children outnumbered elderly people 13 to one.

Table 2-9. Changes in Aged-Child Ratios in the
United States, by Race, 1900-2050

Year	Number Aged 65+ per 100 Aged 0-14		
	All Races	White	Other Races
1900	11.8	12.5	7.6
1910	13.4	14.1	8.2
1920	14.6	15.4	9.2
1930	18.4	19.5	9.6
1940	27.3	29.0	15.6
1950	30.2	32.0	17.7
1960	29.7	31.9	16.3
1970	34.7	37.4	19.5
1980	49.8	57.2	23.3
1990	58.2	65.2	29.4
2000	62.7	70.4	32.9
2025	106.2	118.7	65.5
2050	124.5	134.6	94.3

Sources: U.S. Bureau of the Census, U.S. Census of
Population: 1970, General Population Characteristics, U.S. Summary (1972), table 53; 1980 Census
of Population, Supplementary Reports, PC80-S1-1,
Age, Sex, Race, and Spanish Origin of the Population
by Regions, Divisions, and States: 1980 (1981),
table 1; "Projections of the Population of the
United States: 1982 to 2050" (advance report),
Current Population Reports, P-25, no. 922, table 2.

Projections based on Series II assumptions.

In fact, in 2050 the proportion of the two groups together will be virtually identical to the one in 1900, though the relative shares of children and the elderly will have changed radically.

The aged-child ratios have also changed greatly for whites and blacks in the twentieth century, more than quadrupling between 1900 and 1980 among whites and more than tripling among blacks. But the figure for blacks remained consistently behind that for whites and increased more slowly, basically because of the higher birth rates and larger proportions of children in the black population, along with the higher death rates of black people at most ages and the lower percentage of survivors to age 65. As a result, the black aged-child ratio was 61 per cent of the white ratio in 1900, but only 41 per cent in 1980. But given the rapid rate at which black fertility is now falling and its tendency to approach that of whites even more closely, the black ratio will probably rise considerably faster than the white figure, especially after 2000. To the extent the index represents growing similarity between the races in fertility rates and proportions of elderly people, it also reflects improvements in the socioeconomic conditions that earlier kept the black child population relatively large, the black elderly one comparatively small. In turn, the racial convergence in at least some of these conditions mirrors the impressive growth of the black middle class and its norms, despite the persistence of serious problems for those black people who live in poverty and the ghettos.

Summary

The nation's elderly population contains very different percentages of people in the several age ranges which make up the 65-and-older group, because of variable levels of health and other factors that raise the death rate as people age increasingly beyond 65, and because of the past fluctuations in fertility. Even now most elderly are concentrated fairly close to age 65, though the proportion of those 75 and older is expanding the most rapidly. Consequently, the elderly population is dispersed somewhat more evenly throughout all of the ages, and the young-old are becoming a smaller share of the 65-and-over age group, the old-old a greater share. That is so because larger proportions of people now have more years of life expectancy remaining than did their parents, and because the survivors of large birth cohorts and the last remnants of large immigrations have moved into the oldest ages. Women are more heavily represented than men in those ages and whites are proportionately more abundant than blacks, though with notable exceptions in a few of the oldest years, essentially because of previous fertility patterns and differential death rates by race and sex. These differences among various groups can be measured by the percentages in a birth cohort who survive to the various older years and by the average life expectancy that remains to people who have already reached particular ages.

The dependency ratio also enables a look at how the numbers of elderly people and children relate to the numbers of those aged 20-64 available to support the two dependent groups, though categorical designations of "dependent" and "producer" do ignore many individual variations. In the United States the ratio of children to producers has fallen markedly as the birth rate has dropped, and it will amount certainly continue to decline well into the twenty-first century. At the same time, the elderly support burden has risen significantly and will continue on that course. These changes together, however, have produced an overall dependency ratio which has dropped a great deal since 1870, which will fall even more until about 2010, and which will then rise a bit above the 1980 level. Therefore, while the proportional burden of support for children will shrink and that for the elderly will grow for several decades, the total responsiblity that falls on productive adults won't be much heavier than it is now and will be far less weighty than it was a century ago. Nonetheless, inflation and other problems could turn the relatively stable statistical support burden into one that grows much heavier financially.

The number of elderly people for each 100 children aged 0-14 has increased astonishingly in the twentieth century and promises to rise even more in the twenty-first. Eventually, if birth and death rates stabilize and do not rise or fall significantly over long periods, the aged-child ratio and other indexes of the statistical relationships among various age groups also will not change. But because a given fertility situation continues to have a significant demographic impact for eight decades or more, such stability and the stationary population it would reflect may never occur. If it does, the proportions of children, workers, and elderly people will also approach a stable balance.

NOTES

1. Matilda White Riley, "Introduction: Life-Course Perspectives," in Matilda White Riley, ed., *Aging from Birth to Death.* Boulder, CO: Westview Press, 1979, p. 6.

2. Hubert O'Gorman, "False Consciousness of Kind," *Research on Aging* 1 (1980): 105.

3. *Ibid.,* p. 107.

4. Beth J. Soldo, "America's Elderly in the 1980s," *Population Bulletin* 35 (1980): 11.

5. Erdman Palmore, *Social Patterns in Normal Aging: Findings from the Duke Longitudinal Study.* Durham, NC: Duke University Press, 1981, p. 113.

6. *Ibid.,* pp. 4 and 109.

54

7. Matilda White Riley and Anne Foner, *Aging and Society,* v. 1, *An Inventory of Research Findings.* New York: Russell Sage Foundation, 1968, p. 25. Cf. Philip M. Hauser, "Aging and World-Wide Population Change," in Robert H. Binstock and Ethel Shanas, eds., *Handbook of Aging and the Social Sciences.* New York: Van Nostrand, 1976, p. 65.

8. Hauser, *ibid.,* pp. 64-65.

9. Riley and Foner, *op. cit.,* p. 27.

10. Hauser, *op. cit.,* p. 65.

11. For an account of some of these implications, see *ibid.,* pp. 81-83.

12. Peter Uhlenberg, "Demographic Change and Problems of the Aged, " in Riley, *Aging from Birth to Death, op. cit.,* pp. 157-158.

13. For a discussion of support burdens as a way to evaluate overpopulation, see David R. Kamerschen, "On an Operational Index of 'Overpopulation'," *Economic Development and Cultural Change,* 13 (1965): 169-187.

14. William Petersen, *Population.* 3rd ed. New York: Macmillan, 1975, p. 354.

15. U.S. Bureau of the Census, *Statistical Abstract of the United States: 1982-83.* Washington, DC: U.S. Government Printing Office, 1982, table 626.

16. For a discussion of how consumption norms and labor force participation bear on dependency ratios, see Ephraim Kleiman, "A Standardized Dependency Ratio," *Demography* 4 (1967): 876-893.

17. Jacob S. Siegel, "On the Demography of Aging," *Demography* 17 (1980): 357.

18. Discussions of the dependency ratio as an analytical device appear in Petersen, *op. cit.,* pp. 72-75; and John R. Weeks, *Population: An Introduction to Concepts and Issues,* 2nd ed. Belmont, CA: Wadsworth, 1981, pp. 188-189. See its use in Paul E. Zopf, Jr., "Variations in Support Burdens as Measured by the Dependency Ratio," *Greek Review of Social Research,* no. 19-20 (1974): 29-43.

19. Ansley J. Coale, "How a Population Ages or Grows Younger," in Ronald Freedman, ed., *Population: The Vital Revolution.* Garden City, NY: Doubleday, 1964, p. 54.

20. For a study of this matter in Indonesia, see Nathan Keyfitz, "Age Distribution as a Challenge to Development," *American Journal of Sociology* 70 (1965): 659-668.

21. Council on Environmental Quality and U.S. Department of State, *The Global 2000 Report to the President,* v. 2, *The Technical Report.* Washington, DC: U.S. Government Printing Office, 1980, pp. 16 and 18.

22. Hauser, *op. cit.,* p. 84. See also pp. 83-85 on the social and demographic impact of increases in the numbers of older people in the developing countries.

23. See Kingsley Davis, "Population and Welfare in Industrialized Societies," *Population Review,* 6 (1962): 27.

24. For data on this matter, see U.S. Bureau of the Census, "Persons of Spanish Origin in the United States: March 1980," (advance report), *Current Population Reports,* P-20, no. 361 (1981), table 3.

25. Siegel, *op. cit.,* pp. 356, 357.

26. Henry S. Shryock and Jacob S. Siegel, *The Methods and Materials of Demography.* v. 1. Washington, DC: U.S. Government Printing Office, 1973, p. 234.

27. *Ibid.*

Chapter 3

Sex Composition of the Older Population

One of the most fundamental features of America's elderly population is its large majority of women, because the proportion of males typically declines through the age span, from a small excess of young boys to the massive deficit of men in the oldest ages.[1] In turn, these elements of the sex balance shape other social conditions at various stages in the age scale, for whether a person is male or female helps determine his/her attitudes, activities, and social and economic roles, though these things also are subject to change.

Moreover, the proportions of men and women in the older population affect the tempo of life in that group, particularly as they influence marital status and increase the difficulty older women have in finding male companionship. This reality is underscored by the large statistical surplus of elderly women who are single, divorced, and widowed. In 1980, for example, there were 8.4 million of them, compared with only 2.2 million men who were not married, which left a large surplus of 6.2 million women for whom marriage within their age group was statistically impossible. Translated into innumerable personal adjustments, chances for loneliness, and even individual tragedies, those data reflect one of the sensitive human dimensions of a severe sex imbalance in the older years.[2] The imbalance is especially acute among widows, for while there are less than twice as many single and divorced elderly women as elderly men in those categories, there are five times as many widows as widowers. At the same time, however, the worst problems of old age — poverty and poor health — have improved measurably,[3] so while the pains of widowhood and the problems of altered identity and loneliness do

confront part of our growing population of older women, some other difficulties have improved, especially among well-educated women. Moreover, there is a mounting body of evidence showing that large numbers
of elderly women not only retain but improve their ability to cope effectively with life, while dependence and passivity often decline as various
kinds of creative aggressiveness and adaptive capabilities grow.[4]

Measuring the Sex Balance

The index widely used to measure the sex composition of a population is
the *sex ratio*, which we will use in this chapter and which is computed as
follows:

$$\text{Sex ratio} = \frac{\text{Number of males}}{\text{Number of females}} \times 100$$

A figure over 100, which is rare among older groups, indicates more males
than females; a ratio below 100 reflects the reverse situation — more
females than males — which has become increasingly typical of the
elderly population during the twentieth century.

Factors Affecting the Sex Ratio

Mortality Differentials

The typical pattern of sex ratios in the United States is a general
decrease from birth through extreme old age as males become a progressively smaller share of each succeeding age group, females a larger
proportion. This pattern reflects the relatively high sex ratios at birth,
when there are about 105 male infants delivered for each 100 females,[5]
though even that figure is below the one at conception. But the sex ratio
begins its decline immediately, for even miscarriages take a higher toll of
male than female embryos and fetuses, resulting in the 105 sex ratio at
birth, at least in the nation's white population.[6] (See Figure 3-1.)

The reason for the continued reduction of the sex ratio with age is that
the death rates of males are substantially higher than those of females at
every level from infancy through the oldest years. Moreover, while death
rates have fallen dramatically in the United States over the last several
decades, females have benefited more than males, for their mortality
levels have dropped far faster than those of males. For example, in 1900

57

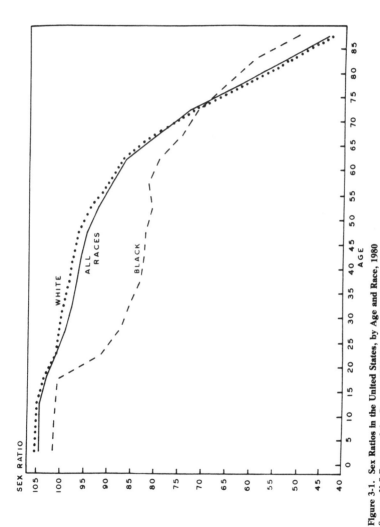

Figure 3-1. Sex Ratios in the United States, by Age and Race, 1980
Source: U.S.Bureau of the Census, *1980 Census of Population, Supplementary Reports*, PC80-S1-1, *Age, Sex, Race, and Spanish Origin of the Population by Regions, Divisions, and States: 1980* (1981), table 1.

58

the age-adjusted death rate of males was 9 per cent higher than that of females, but by 1980 the difference was 80 per cent. Consequently, while life expectancy at birth has increased substantially for both sexes, that for females has climbed far more rapidly, increasing the gap from only 2.9 years at the turn of the century to 7.5 years in 1980. Furthermore, the male-female ratio of age-adjusted rates rose from 1.1 in 1900 to 1.8 in 1980, though the figure did not increase between 1974 and 1980. (See Figure 3-2.) Thus, the growing mortality differential between the sexes, accelerated by reductions in the death rates due to childbirth and other causes that once claimed high proportions of women at younger ages, is the chief reason for the great sex imbalance among the elderly.[7]

The reasons for the lower death rates among women seem largely biological, though social causes, such as higher rates of smoking and greater involvement in dangerous occupations among men, also play a part. But even when we eliminate the deaths from accidents, violence, and other "external" causes that take an especially heavy toll of males, the survival advantage of females remains substantial in all except those few societies where childbirth continues to be particularly dangerous and the low status of women causes an inordinate neglect of females, especially infants. In an effort to uncover the causes of the differential, Madigan

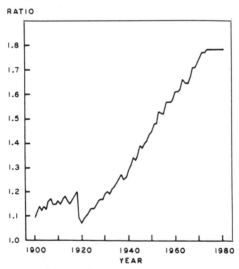

Figure 3-2. Ratio of the Male to the Female Age-Adjusted Death Rate in the United States, 1900-1980

Sources: National Center for Health Statistics, *Vital Statistics of the United States, 1977*, v. 2, *Mortality*, part A (1981), Table 1-2; "Final Mortality Statistics, 1978," *Monthly Vital Statistics Report*, v. 29, no. 6 (1980), table 2; "Advance Report of Final Mortality Statistics, 1979," *Monthly Vital Statistics Report*, v. 31, no. 6 (1982), table 2; "Advance Report of Final Mortality Statistics, 1980," *Monthly Vital Statistics Report*, v. 32, no. 4 (1983), table 9.

learned that when the mortality rates of men teachers in Roman Catholic monasteries were compared with those of women teachers in Catholic convents — both controlled and relatively similar sociocultural environments — the men still had significantly higher death rates at all ages than the women. As a result, he concluded that biological factors have more influence than the exigencies of social life in producing the mortality differential by sex, whereas the social factors that do operate are comparatively minor contributors.[8] Therefore, while we don't know all aspects of the biological advantages that allow far more women than men to reach the older ages, it does seem clear that those factors are chiefly responsible for the great sex imbalance among people aged 65 and older.

One of the major reasons for the lower death rates of women is probably the fact that their extra X chromosome provides more resistance to certain illnesses. Moreover, women are biologically protected during their reproductive span, and because better nutrition and hygiene have lengthened that span, they are protected longer.[9] These factors and some not yet fully understood help produce the divergence in the death rates of the sexes, even while their life styles grow more similar and environmental factors converge to the point where they account for less of the differential. That is particularly apparent in the growing similarity of smoking behavior, for earlier in the century about two-thirds of the death rate differential was due to the fact that many men but few women smoked. The differential has also grown as deaths from infectious and parasitic diseases and childbearing have declined markedly and fatalities from heart disease, cancer, and other "degenerative" illnesses have increased. In the first group of causes the death rates of the sexes are not far apart, so decreases in those causes allow men no great advantage over women. In the group of degenerative causes, however, male death rates are far above those of females, so major increases in the relative importance of those causes strongly disfavor men and favor women. As a result, changes in the importance of certain causes of death have helped produce the large majority of women in the category 65 and over.[10]

In the future, the male-female mortality differential may decrease, for projections to 2050 suggest that the sex ratio of the elderly will stop falling and may even rise a little at times during the period. Some of that leveling will reflect events already past, but it may be that women who get caught up in the "work-or-perish" ethic that drives many men will incur some increases in mortality, or at least will not experience larger reductions than men.[11] Even so, the effect of the biological factors will probably remain largely as it is, and unless we reverse the present immigration pattern and receive large numbers of males, America's older population is unlikely to return to the earlier majority of men.

The steady decline in the sex ratio from birth to the oldest ages is typical of all developed countries, which have comparatively low birth and death rates and mortality differentials that strongly favor the survival of women, though there are some departures from the pattern in the developing nations. Thus, table 3-1 indicates that during early childhood the sex ratios are nearly identical among the representative developed countries and that by age 65 the indexes have fallen well below 80, though the range is far wider then than in the first five years of life. The index for East Germany is particularly low because of the heavy losses of men during World War II. That situation is unusual, however, for even when war kills many men the losses have to be tremendous in youth in order to reduce the sex ratio very much in the older ages. Therefore, the sex differential in the "natural" causes of death is what gives women such a large numerical advantage over men; it is far more strategic than wars in reducing the sex ratio among elderly people in most countries at most times.[12]

Table 3-1. Sex Ratios at Several Ages, Selected Countries, 1980

Country	All Ages	0-4	40-44	65+
East Germany	88.3	105.5	99.7	53.6
West Germany	91.5	105.1	106.1	56.2
Finland	93.6	105.1	102.1	56.4
Austria	89.8	105.2	100.9	56.9
Scotland	92.8	105.8	96.4	60.8
France	96.1	104.8	104.3	64.2
England & Wales	95.0	105.6	102.9	64.5
Switzerland	94.8	104.6	101.1	66.9
UNITED STATES	94.5	104.7	95.8	67.6
Hungary	93.9	105.9	92.9	67.8
Netherlands	98.5	105.1	105.9	70.4
Italy	95.4	105.6	97.5	70.9
Denmark	97.5	105.2	102.0	73.2
Norway	98.3	105.5	102.5	73.8
Sweden	98.2	105.0	104.2	77.0

Sources: United Nations, Demographic Yearbook, 1980, table 7; 1981, table 7; U.S. Bureau of the Census, 1980 Census of Population, Supplementary Reports, PC80-S1-1, Age, Sex, Race, and Spanish Origin of the Population by Regions, Divisions, and States: 1980 (1981), table 1.

Effects of Migration

Immigration, which so greatly swelled the young-adult male population of the United States early in the twentieth century, now plays a less significant part statistically in the balance between older men and women; the role that the aging immigrant group does play affects the segment 75 and over more heavily than it does the one aged 65-74. Moreover, given the heavier representation of women in many recent immigrant groups, the sex ratio of the entire older foreign-born population is moving toward that of the elderly native-born group. A significant difference still remains, but it is diminishing as aged immigrants die and the younger ones with a more nearly even sex balance move into the older ages. In short, despite the impact of early twentieth-century immigration, the balance of males and females in the elderly segment is influenced most strongly by the sex differential in the death rate.[13] In the United States this factor has changed the balance markedly, from a slight surplus of elderly men in 1900 to the large surplus of elderly women at present.[14] This highly significant change and its social implications are yet another consequence of aging in America's population.

Variations in Sex Composition

The sex composition of the older population varies considerably among its component racial and ethnic groups, from state to state, and between rural and urban areas, and there are many significant departures from the average sex ratio. Despite their differences, however, the various groups are all alike in that the populations of women aged 65 and older have been growing much faster than those of men. As a result, between 1970 and 1980 the number of elderly women of all races and ethnic origins grew 31 per cent, while that of men increased only 22 per cent, thereby causing the sex ratio to fall from 72 to 68. This situation, which is most pronounced among whites, puts elderly men in great demand, alters the sex balance in some Sunbelt areas that attract significant groups of elderly migrants, and may even affect investment policy, political processes, and other social structures and dynamics.[15]

Differences by Race and Ethnicity

The proportions of men and women vary between the two major racial groups that make up the nation's elderly population. (See Figure 3-1.) For the most part, these differences result from significantly lower sex ratios at birth among blacks than among whites and from racial variations in mortality by sex.

The number of newborn male infants is closer to the number of females in the black than in the white population, and in 1980 the sex ratios at birth were 102.9 and 105.8, respectively. The black sex ratio at birth has risen faster in recent years, however, and so has that in early childhood, especially as infant mortality rates have fallen, but those ratios are still sufficiently lower than the ones for whites to help reduce the index for blacks at each age up to 70.

The sex ratio at birth isn't the only factor that contributes to the racial difference in the balance of males and females, however, for the death rates of black males and females are also more nearly alike at many ages than are those in the white population. For example, in 1980 the mortality differential between black men and women in all of the ages above 50 was less than in the white group. In addition, there are some distortions in the data, because black males get better coverage than females and the sex ratios recorded in the census reports are a bit higher than the actual ones, though the discrepancy is not great.

These factors interact to produce a sex balance among elderly black people that is more nearly even than the one among elderly whites. Thus, for the group 75 and over in 1980, the sex ratio was 60 for blacks but only 54 for whites. There is still a comparatively large number of widowed black women, however, for the proportion of those who remarry is considerably lower than in the white population; the percentage of black elderly divorced women who do not remarry is also larger than in the white group. Therefore, even though the sex ratio statistically favors remarriage for older black women more than it does for elderly whites, other factors stand in the way. As a result, in 1980 only 14 per cent of the black women 75 and over were classified as married with a husband present, compared with 23 per cent of the whites.

Elderly black women, especially those without mates, make up a "triple minority" insofar as disadvantages are concerned. They experience the social realities of being black, which tends to push their incomes and other indicators of material well-being below those of the white population; they are women, whose various level-of-living indexes compare poorly with those of men; and they are elderly, which intensifies their disadvantages over those suffered by younger people. Furthermore, elderly black women who have lost their mates or who never married tend to be even more seriously deprived than the ones with husbands, though higher percentages do live with other relatives than is true of whites. Older black women are also increasing faster in number than are their white counterparts, so their race will face particularly urgent future needs.

Even though the sex ratios of elderly blacks have been higher than those of whites for many decades, both indexes have also been on their way down for a long time. But the decline with age is less steep and less regular for blacks than it is for whites, producing the higher sex ratios among the black elderly. Even so, elderly people still make up a significantly smaller proportion of the black population than of the white, largely because the birth rates of black people are higher,[16] but also because black mortality historically has reduced the percentages who survive to 65 below those of whites who make it to that age.

The Spanish-origin population has a comparatively small share of elderly people and a relatively high birth rate, and the sex ratio for all ages collectively is fairly high. In 1980 that for elderly Hispanics was 76, contrasted with 67 in the population not of Spanish origin. Death rates and past birth rates play a part in this situation, but the selectivity of migration is a more significant component than in the American population as a whole. That is, men were heavily represented in the immigration from Latin America that brought many of today's elderly Spanish-origin people as young adults, especially from Mexico, Puerto Rico, and certain parts of Central and South America and the Caribbean. The Cuban-origin population, however, which is an aging one, has an unusually large deficiency of elderly men, partly because the post-revolutionary migration from Cuba consisted heavily of families whose elderly women have now outlived their men.

Women also tend to predominate in the recent immigrant population of all national origins collectively, and have done so for several decades. For example, the sex ratio of immigrants of all ages admitted in 1951-1960 was 85; in 1961-1970 it was 81, and in 1971-1979 it stood at 88. Men are still the majority in a few groups of immigrants, such as the refugees from Southeast Asia in the 1970s, but the large preponderance of young men among the earlier arrivals is generally not repeated among the new immigrant populations.[17] As those people age, therefore, the sex ratio of the elderly will fall well below the figure for native-born people and earlier immigrant groups, though presumably their descendants will produce a sex ratio at birth that approximates the national average, and the balance of older men and women in second and later generations will be like that in the total elderly population. In the meantime, however, the sex composition of recent immigrations will help intensify the great surplus of women that already exists among America's elderly, unless some new surge of male immigrants occurs.[18]

State-to-State Variations

All of America's elderly experienced particular historical events that gave them a base of common experiences and produced individual reactions that show up as collective behavior. Those formative events include childhood or young adulthood during World War I, the ravaging influenza epidemic of 1917-1918, the Great Depression, World War II, and the wars and political and economic crises since 1945. Moreover, large proportions of today's elderly have had small-town and farm experience, for in the few decades after 1900 about half the population was still classified as rural. Therefore, the experiences of the nation's elderly, like those of any age cohort, shaped their attitudes and skills, molded their economic pursuits, influenced the size of the families they produced and reared, and affected other patterns of behavior.[19]

The nature of these experiences, however, has varied widely from place to place throughout the nation, especially during the early decades of the century, when urbanization, the automobile, the mass media, and other forces had not yet diminished local and regional differences. The remnants of those differences show up in several forms, one of which is state-to-state variations in the balance of elderly men and women. Most significant is the fact that women substantially outnumber men in every state except Hawaii, where the sex ratio is 102, though Alaska's figure still stands near 100. Everywhere else the indexes range from a high of 85 in Nevada to a low of 58 in the District of Columbia, though it is significant that the elderly in about half the states have sex ratios in the narrow range from 65 to 70. (See Figure 3-3.)

The states that have lower sex ratios than the national average of 68 for all elderly people include several that are highly urbanized and industrialized along lines that attracted women workers who stayed put after retirement. Chief among those places are Washington, D.C., and the states of the Northeast. Many of the Southern states also have less than their fair shares of elderly men, partly because their older small towns and their newer urban centers have drawn elderly women, especially widows, or because those women didn't move when their husbands died. That is not true of Florida, however, partly because the elderly migration to that state consists so heavily of married couples. In addition, when husbands die in Florida, many widows move back to the places from which they came, often to be near adult offspring, though enough remain in Florida to help keep the sex ratio below 100.

Aging men are most heavily concentrated in the states that were still part of the old frontier early in the century, or whose largely "masculine" occupations attracted greater numbers of young men during those decades. Alaska — the last frontier — also has a relative abundance of elderly men, whose concentrations are also well above the national average in most of the Mountain and Pacific states, the Dakotas, and a few states in the South Central division. The last include Michigan and Wisconsin, where the work forces in automobile manufacturing, steel fabrication, dairying, and some other industries consist largely of men. Therefore, because the large majority of elderly people do not migrate after retirement, the present state-to-state variations in the sex balance of older citizens have been influenced by the particular functions that prompted

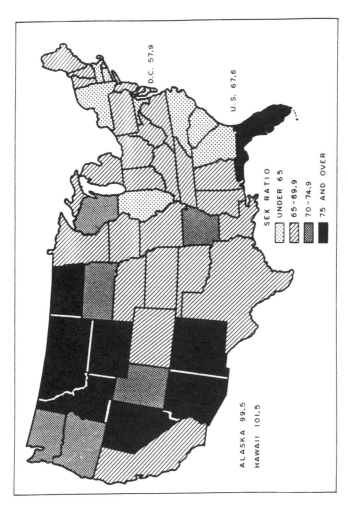

SEX RATIO

UNDER 65
65 - 69.9
70 - 74.9
75 AND OVER

D.C. 57.9

U.S. 67.6

ALASKA 99.5
HAWAII 101.5

Figure 3-3. Sex Ratio of American People Aged 65 and Older In Each State, 1980
Source: U.S. Bureau of the Census, *1980 Census of Population, General Population Characteristics*, reports for states (1981), table 19.

earlier sex-selective migrations.

Certain sections of the country also have variable mortality differentials between males and females, and part of the variation in sex balance in some places is due to those differences in rates of survivorship. Overall, however, this factor is not very strategic, because in the 26 states collectively that have below-average sex ratios, life expectancy for women exceeds that for men to about the same degree as it does in the remaining states with above-average ratios. This similarity reflects the fact that the male-female discrepancy in mortality and life expectancy is almost always greater than are the variations within either sex from state to state or region to region. It is this nationwide differential between men and women that has shifted the sex balance of elderly people to a large predominance of women in every state except Alaska and Hawaii; even there the sex ratios have declined sharply in the twentieth century, just as they have in every other state.

Black-white differences in the states. In most states the sex balance is more nearly even for blacks than for whites, largely because the male-female mortality differential is greater for whites virtually everywhere in the country. Thus, in 1980 black people numbered at least 25,000 in the District of Columbia and 38 states, and 34 of them had significantly higher sex ratios among elderly blacks than elderly whites. For example, the sex ratio among older blacks in Washington, D.C., in 1980 was 63, whereas that for whites was only 51. The social and economic factors shaping the sex balance ordinarily work about the same for both racial groups, though, and those states that have relatively low or high sex ratios in one race usually show the same pattern in the other.

Given these similarities in most parts of the nation, the deficiencies of black and white elderly men are greatest in most of the Northeast and large parts of the South, including the District of Columbia. On the other hand, the smallest deficiencies of men among the elderly of both races are found in the Mountain and Pacific states, some of the industrialized sections of the North Central region, and a few of the Southern states. Older black men are particularly abundant in the places that attracted so many in the heavy migration from the South after 1910, and once drawn by the jobs in industry during both world wars, large numbers of older black men now remain in Ohio, Indiana, Michigan, Wisconsin, Washington, Oregon, and other places that witnessed significant influxes earlier in the century. They are also relatively abundant in Arkansas, Louisiana, and Mississippi, though earlier heavy migratory losses of women help explain those relatively high sex ratios. Furthermore, a sizable share of the small black farm population still lives in those states and elderly men are relatively abundant in that group, though the nation's black farm group has shrunk even more rapidly than the white segment during the last several decades. In fact, while 3 per cent of the nation's white people still lived on farms in 1980, that was true of less than 1 per cent of its blacks,[20] and the average age of the blacks was about four years higher than that of whites.

Rural-Urban Differences in Sex Composition

Elderly women outnumber older men most heavily in the urban parts of the country, especially the central cities, whereas men are relatively abundant in the rural portions, particularly on the farms. Moreover, the comparative abundance of women diminishes and that of men rises from the central cities of metropolitan areas to their suburbs, to small cities outside metropolitan areas, to villages and hamlets, and finally into the open countryside. In part, the sex ratios in the areas outside central cities have fallen because of the aging of the suburban populations that began to move from large cities to outlying districts several decades ago. But even on farms the relative abundance of men has dropped sharply, for the sex ratio of the elderly fell from 134 in 1940 to 112 in 1980. The figure would be considerably lower if many older women did not leave after the death of a spouse, for in the farm population as everywhere else in the nation, death rates are significantly higher for men than for women.[21] But those widows who do stay in farming communities still have a far better chance for remarriage than do their urban sisters.

The two major races differ markedly in the way elderly men and women are distributed among the rural and urban categories. Because they are the large majority, whites follow the national pattern closely and their sex ratios are the lowest in central cities and then rise progressively in the suburbs, the small cities, the towns and villages, and the farming areas. For elderly blacks, however, the situation is almost completely reversed. That is, the highest sex ratios appear in the suburban portions of metropolitan areas, followed closely by the central cities, especially the ones with more than 1 million people. Those were the destinations of many black migrants earlier in the century, and that group contained huge numbers of men fleeing the South in search of better jobs, less punitive race relations, and opportunities of other kinds. Most who have now reached 65 stay put, for while a substantial number of blacks are moving back to the urban South, few of them are elderly men. On the other hand, the sex ratios of elderly blacks are well below the national average for their race in all of the nonmetropolitan sections except the farms, where elderly men still slightly outnumber the women.

The overall sex ratio among older Spanish-origin people is comparatively high in several residential categories. In fact, elderly men make up

68

large majorities in central cities with fewer than 1 million people, nonmetropolitan counties with a city of 25,000 or more, those with no places of 2,500, and on farms. Those patterns are affected by the size of the population clusters than happen to exist in the sections where Hispanic people have settled most heavily, especially the Southwest, but they do represent a different sex balance by residence than is to be found in various other groups. The lowest sex ratios among Hispanics appear in the nation's largest central cities and its suburbs, where elderly women outnumber the men most heavily.

No matter what their race or ethnic background, elderly women living in rural areas often have more socioeconomic disadvantages than the ones in cities and suburbs, though there are many problems in those places, too. The rural women tend to have lower incomes, less education, fewer years of paid work to generate pensions, less access to services and facilities, and more chronic health problems than do the urban women.[22] In the case of whites, the higher rural sex ratio does improve the chance for remarriage and that may solve some of the problems for some women. Among blacks, however, the sex balance lowers the chance of remarriage, and the elderly black woman probably experiences more disadvantages and fewer life alternatives than any other group in American society. That is especially true of the ones living in tiny villages and hamlets and on farms, though the small-town population does not fare much better. Thus, elderly rural women, particularly blacks, often need better services, higher incomes, stronger social ties, and improved health facilities.[23] At present, they are one of the nation's "invisible" groups who share poorly in its affluence.

Trends in Sex Composition

The most striking long-term trend in the balance of older women and men is the extent to which it has tipped strongly toward an abundance of the former. Thus, in 1870, when the census data for people 65 and over were first reported separately by sex, there was a slight overabundance of elderly men and the sex ratio stood near 101. (See Figure 3-4.) It was a little higher in 1880, but lower in both years than it would have been if the Civil War had not taken such a high toll of men of all ages. Then, as the relatively large immigrant groups of the late 1840s and 1850s began to reach age 65, the sex ratio rose to its highest point in 1890 and then began the downward trend still underway, propelled by the growing mortality differential between males and females.

Therefore, the balance between the sexes was again about even in 1930 and dropped off by 1940. (See also Table 3-2.) In the following decades the decline accelerated, especially between 1960 and 1970, partly because so many in the huge immigrant populations admitted before World War II had already died. That group originally contained so many men that in 1910, for example, the sex ratio of the foreign-born population of all ages was a very high 131. By 1940, however, the index for that group had fallen to 112, and by 1960 so many foreign-born people had died that the survivors didn't have much effect on the overall sex ratio of elderly people. The vast majority of the present elderly population is native born and their low sex ratio now reflects earlier fertility patterns and the mortality differential by sex, rather than important results of the sex selectivity in earlier immigrations. Moreover, because recent immigrations from most places contain more women than men, those groups will depress the elderly sex ratio even more when they reach age 65.

Trends by Race

White and black elderly populations have followed roughly similar patterns in that women have increased from slightly less than half of the older group to a large majority. (See Table 3-2.) Thus, women became a majority of the older white population just after 1930 and of the black group shortly after 1940. In later decades that numerical predominance increased rapidly in both races, and while the sex ratios of blacks re-

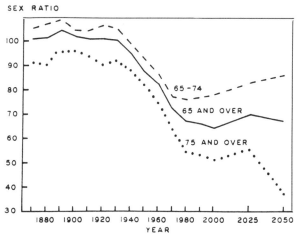

Figure 3-4. Changes in the Sex Ratio of Elderly Americans, by Age Groups, 1870-2050
Sources: U.S.Bureau of the Census, *Sixteenth Census of the United States: 1940, Characteristics of the Population, U.S. Summary* (1943), table 8; U.S. Census of Population: 1970, General Population Characteristics, U.S. Summary (1972), table 53; *1980 Census of Population, Supplementary Reports*, PC80-S1-1, *Age, Sex, Race, and Spanish Origin of the Population by Regions, Divisions, and States: 1980* (1981), table 1; "Projections of the Population of the United States: 1982 to 2050" (advance report), *Current Population Reports*, P-25, no. 922 (1982), table 2.

70

mained above those of whites, the amount of the difference declined. That suggests some convergence between the races in socioeconomic patterns, for when the factors that have historically separated them diminish and disappear, so do most of the major demographic differences.[24]

The sex balance of elderly people in the "other races" category, unlike the situations of blacks and whites, reflected a superabundance of men long before 1910, and until 1950 they became a larger majority with each

Table 3-2. Changes in the Sex Ratio of People 65 and Over, by Race, 1910-2050

Year	All Races	White	Black	Other Races
1910	101.1	100.6	107.7	118.3
1920	101.3	100.6	109.5	155.1
1930	100.5	100.2	103.4	155.4
1940	95.5	95.0	100.6	168.9
1950	87.9	89.2	90.7	191.4
1960	82.8	82.3	86.1	159.0
1970	72.2	71.6	76.5	123.8
1980	67.6	67.2	68.2	84.8
1990	66.1	66.4	61.7	72.9
2000	64.5	65.3	56.1	64.0
2025	70.3	71.8	60.8	65.3
2050	67.6	68.5	64.3	61.8

Sources: U.S. Bureau of the Census, Negroes in the United States, 1920-32 (1935), p. 90; Sixteenth Census of the United States: 1940, Characteristics of the Population, U.S. Summary (1943), table 7; U.S. Census of Population: 1950, Detailed Characteristics, U.S. Summary (1953), table 97; U.S. Census of Population: 1960, Characteristics of the Population, U.S. Summary (1964), table 158; U.S. Census of Population: 1970, General Population Characteristics, U.S. Summary (1972), table 52; 1980 Census of Population, Supplementary Reports, PC80-S1-1, Age, Sex, Race, and Spanish Origin of the Population by Regions, Divisions, and States: 1980 (1981), table 1; "Projections of the Population of the United States: 1982 to 2050" (advance report), Current Population Reports, P-25, no. 922 (1982), table 2.

decade. This reflected patterns of selectivity of immigration in the late nineteenth century, for many of the nonwhite and nonblack racial groups that entered the country consisted mostly of males. Men were an especially large part of the Japanese and Filipino groups and the Chinese contingent that came in the late 1800s to work as various kinds of laborers. Thus, in 1900 approximately 90 per cent of the nation's entire Chinese population of all ages was foreign born, and the sex ratio of that group was a lopsided 189. By 1950 they had grown old, but the sex ratio of Chinese people 65 and over still stood at 191 because of the initial predominance of men among the immigrants. Thirty years later, however, the large majority had died and the sex ratio among elderly Chinese had fallen to 103. Moreover, because most present Americans of Chinese ancestry were born in this country and because women outnumber men among the Chinese who still enter from abroad, the sex ratio of older people in that racial group will soon resemble that of the nation's total elderly population. Much the same is true of Japanese, Koreans, and other groups designated by the U.S. Census Bureau as races, though their initial immigrations also contained large majorities of men.

American Indians, who are also in the "other races" census category, include virtually no immigrants, so their sex ratio has been shaped by fertility and mortality, which have produced a more even balance of elderly Indian men and women than appears in the non-Indian population. Part of that balance results from the poverty in which so many native Americans have lived for so long, because childbirth and various causes of death that are well controlled in other groups have taken an unusually high toll of women. As a result, smaller proportions of Indian women reach old age than is true of blacks and whites. In 1980, for example, less than 6 per cent of all Indian women were 65 and over, compared with 9 per cent of the blacks and 14 per cent of the whites.

Trends by Regions, Divisions, and States

Since the turn of the century, the sex ratios among elderly people have fallen dramatically and the sex balance has become far more similar throughout the nation. (See Table 3-3.) But in 1900, when the sex ratio was 102 for all of the country's elderly people, the District of Columbia and 31 of the present 50 states ranked above that average. Elderly men made up the largest majority in Nevada, where there were 246 of them for each 100 elderly women, but the imbalances were also substantial in all but one of the other Western states, where most sex ratios were 130 or more. The only exception was Utah (sex ratio 98) because the sex balance of older people was still affected by the earlier plural marriage of Mormons — a practice which kept Utah from achieving statehood until 1896.

The majorities of elderly men were also substantial in the Great Plains states, for they, along with most of the West, still embodied many basic elements of the frontier, including an abundance of men. Males were also part of timbering in the Northwest, ranching in the grasslands, "sod busting" in the corn and wheat belts, and fighting in the tragic Indian wars in various parts of the West. Therefore, as the original settlers and adventurers aged, most of the elderly stayed in place and the original majorities of young men became majorities of elderly men.

In 1900 the lowest sex ratios appeared in the Northeast, because so many women had been drawn to the cities from more rural sections. The women, reflecting the historic preponderance of their sex in rural-to-urban migration, remained largely in place after they reached age 65 and caused elderly men to be a proportionately smaller part of the elderly population. In the South — at least the portions most destructively affected by the Civil War — the sex ratios were also relatively low, though they were higher in the border states and those closest to the old Western frontier. In a few cases, such as West Virginia, Mississippi, and Tennessee, elderly men made up slight majorities in 1900, partly because the lives of women had been so precarious that their death rates remained relatively high throughout the 1800s. That was especially true of black women. In addition, Florida had a significant majority of men (sex ratio 110), because it, too, had been a frontier area that attracted many more men than women, not merely in the 1800s but into the early twentieth century as well. The lowest sex ratio of all (84) was in the nation's capital, where governmental functions and related activities have long attracted disproportionately large numbers of young women who tend to remain in and around the city after they reach age 65. New England, however, was the division with the largest majority of elderly women.

By 1980 these early patterns had changed dramatically. The lingering effects of the frontier had virtually disappeared everywhere except Alaska, and the sex balance of the nation's elderly population was subject to certain homogenizing influences that caused the large proportions of women in one state to resemble those in most others. Those forces include a tendency for age-specific death rates to be roughly similar from state to state, the predisposition of most elderly people to stay put rather than to migrate, and the powerful standardizing influences that urbanization, the mass media, and other forces exert over behavior in any urban-industrial society, including much of its rural territory. As a result, the range of sex ratios from region to region and state to state was much narrower in 1980 than it had been in 1900, and the substantial predominance of women was a fact of life in the elderly population almost everywhere.

Some Projections

After 1970 the rate of decline in the proportion of elderly men diminished somewhat and seems likely to slow even more, though additional small reductions are probable until 2000, followed by a series of slight increases and decreases. (See Figure 3-4 and Table 3-2.) Those changes mean that the rapid "feminization" of the nation's elderly population will stop by 2000, though at a level that will make women close to 60 per cent of the older group for at least the half century to follow. This is still a very substantial imbalance, and while it may not intensify much from now on, it will continue to have a profound social effect on the older population, especially the women themselves.

Table 3-3. Sex Ratios in the Elderly Population, by Regions and Divisions, 1900 and 1980

Region and Division	1900	1980
Northeast	88.5	64.0
New England	85.4	62.2
Middle Atlantic	89.9	64.7
North Central	109.9	67.1
East North Central	105.5	66.7
West North Central	118.6	67.8
South	101.1	68.4
South Atlantic	96.4	68.4
East South Central	102.2	67.7
West South Central	110.7	69.0
West	157.5	71.9
Mountain	141.1	76.4
Pacific[a]	164.9	70.4

Sources: U.S. Bureau of the Census, U.S. Census of Population: 1970, General Population Characteristics, reports for states (1971), table 21; 1980 Census of Population, General Population Characteristics, reports for states (1981), table 19.

[a]Includes Alaska and Hawaii.

These patterns will vary some for blacks and whites as their elderly populations are shaped by earlier levels of fertility and mortality. (See Table 3-2.) But by the middle of the next century, the differences in the sex balances of whites, blacks, and other races should be relatively minor, particularly if those groups grow more alike according to various socio-economic criteria and their death rates continue to converge.

It also seems certain that the homogenizing trend of the last 70 or 80 years will continue into the next century, and that the balance of older men and women won't vary much from state to state, given a few exceptions. Most of the states with relatively high sex ratios in 1980 will witness some continuing reductions, whereas those with low indexes in 1980 either will change little or their sex ratios will rise slightly. Consequently, in 2000 most states will have somewhere between 60 and 70 elderly men for each 100 women, though a few states, such as Alaska, Hawaii, and Nevada, may have more. The patterns will also reflect a stabilizing tendency, for the majority of elderly women — already a large majority in nearly every state — won't increase markedly in most of them between now and the end of the century. This projected similarity among the states contrasts sharply with the situation in 1900, when sex ratios covered a range of 167 points. It means that certain demographic conditions that once distinguished one part of the country from another have diminished significantly, though the continuing imbalance of older men and women will produce or intensify certain problems.

Some Consequences of Sex Imbalance

The proportional abundance of women in the elderly population, owing to their greater average life expectancy, is a mixed blessing and even a crisis for many individuals. In particular, when women's greater longevity combines with their tendency to marry men a few years older, it means that large proportions have to expect a prolonged period of widowhood.[25] For that reason, only about a third of the older women are still living with their spouses, compared with about three-quarters of the men. Moreover, when the sex imbalance stabilizes there will be two elderly women for each elderly man, and some living arrangements will reflect that huge imbalance.

Living Alone

Even though most elderly people have adult children, relatively few live under the same roof with them. That fact, coupled with the high incidence of widowhood, means that a large share of America's elderly women live alone.[26] In fact, the likelihood of an elderly woman living by herself is now more than twice what it was in 1950, partly because improved finances make that arrangement possible for a larger percentage,[27] and partly because residence norms have changed in the direction of solitary living for more older people.[28] At present, about two of every three elderly women without a spouse live by themselves,[29] though largely by preference, for most older people choose to maintain residential independence at the same time they try to keep reasonably close social ties with their children and grandchildren. In addition, while the elderly population living in institutions of various sorts has been growing rapidly, that group is still a tiny percentage of all elderly.[30] All of this means that a disproportionately large share of the nation's older population consists of women living by themselves.

It is true that each succeeding generation of widows is somewhat less deprived economically on the average than the preceding one and that their levels of education and marketable skills also tend to be higher. Both improvements contribute to greater self-sufficiency for many older women attempting to acquire life's physical necessities. But those improvements may still leave a residue of stress and loneliness that come from being part of an increasingly large widowed majority, while the share of older men available for companionship and remarriage shrinks. For some older women accustomed to being homemakers and wives and whose fulfillment has been tied up with those activities, the prospect of a long widowhood with no one to care for helps convert the later years into a lonely wait for death. Even that may be made trivial by well-meaning others who attempt to contrive leisure activities and other types of behavior that simply intensify meaninglessness. Therefore, while the much greater life expectancy for women than for men does reflect the former's durability, it has a tragic side, too. Nonetheless, ample numbers of women do have the skills to deal with the death of a spouse, to adapt, and to endure, and most do cope adequately with the realities of widowhood. Whether or not specific ones can do so depends on a range of factors having to do with health, background experiences, emotional support in various social systems, finances, and the ability to find renewed meaning in other social niches. The task of the larger society is to find ways to encourage, sustain, and utilize those women who are unable to transform the tragic aspect of differential longevity into a final span of meaningful life.

Finances

The after-tax income per household member tends to rise gradually with the age of the householder until about age 60. Then it declines slightly for the group 60-64 and falls another 15 per cent or so for those 65 and over.[31] Therefore, while elderly women living alone do fare worse financially than elderly men, it is too easy to stereotype the older woman as poor and lonely and to ignore the sizable numbers who are reasonably well off or even wealthy because of benefits received from their own years of work or inheritances from their husbands. Moreover, that group will grow proportionately, for more women now entering the elderly category are well educated and have held rewarding positions outside the home, though still at wages that average considerably below those of men. These women will probably grow as a force among corporate stockholders and will have a significant impact on investment decisions and other aspects of economic, social, and political life.

But many elderly people living alone still face poverty. In 1980, for example, 24 per cent of the men 65 and over who lived alone fell below the poverty line, as did 32 per cent of the women. Thus, even though the proportion in poverty declined steadily until about 1978, it has risen somewhat since then and still represents almost 2 million elderly women and 354,000 elderly men. Nor do those figures include the elderly who live with other relatives but who are still poor, though their incidence of poverty is below that of solitary individuals. Thus, in 1980 about 11 per cent of all elderly men and 19 per cent of all elderly women, irrespective of living arrangements, ranked below the official poverty line.[32] So even though these proportions are far below those just a few years earlier, the relative economic disadvantage of elderly women still stands out clearly. As expected, black women are at a particular disadvantage.

Part of the problem stems from discrimination against older women in the Social Security system, which, at this writing, still tends to reflect the old assumptions "that women marry once and do not work outside the home."[33] Therefore, a woman who divorces in less than 10 years after marriage cannot claim either a wife's or a widow's benefit, while a married woman who works must settle either for her own retirement benefits or half of her husband's. Ordinarily, the latter is greater because women's working years are generally fewer and their earnings are less, so most women get nothing for their own investment in Social Security.

Competent Older Women

We cannot leave our consideration of elderly women without some attention to the majority whose lives remain viable and who do manage to survive or even thrive financially and emotionally, even though aging is generally perceived more negatively among women than it is among men.[34] That perception, shared by many members of both sexes, tends to obscure the fact that women often enter the older years with skills that enable them to make better adjustments than men to changes wrought by the aging process, including its problems.[35] Indeed, many older women become not passive and dependent but more self-assured, while their husbands tend toward greater dependency, particularly after they retire and when they begin to experience serious health problems. Given the differential death rates by sex, the older woman is far more likely to have the care of an incapacitated mate, and that calls for strength and even aggressiveness that belie the common stereotypes about the older woman. In addition, women generally assume a large part or even all of the effort to survive on a reduced budget, and that, too, calls for inventiveness and competence. Therefore, increasing numbers of studies portray women in the older ages as confident, versatile, and in reasonable control of themselves and the destinies of their relationships.[36] After all, a lifetime of experiences is in place, which, along with the unique demands of the older years, often enhances a woman's ability to deal with life, including solitude. In addition, most older women still do not experience abrupt retirement from a salaried job, and the kinds of things they have been doing with competence tend to carry over without interruption to the later years. The housewife reaching age 65, for example, is apt to incur little of the trauma that may afflict the husband who was a full-time worker one day and a pensioner the next. That continuity of responsibility and role performance also tends to enhance the woman's competence, though the pattern could change as more women retire from salaried jobs in the future.[37]

Summary

Women make up the majority of the elderly population, basically because their death rates are so much lower than those of men, though in the past the large male majorities in immigrant populations offset much of the mortality differential, which was also smaller than it is now. In turn, the significant sex imbalance influences other conditions, including the roles of men and women, the options available to people who have lost their mates, and the kinds of coping mechanisms that widowed people — chiefly women — use to avoid passivity and dependence. In the future, the causal mortality differential, which seems more biological than environmental, will probably not change much and the sex ratio of older people is not likely to drop in the way it did after 1900. Nevertheless, it is unlikely to rise much either, which means that the great superabundance of women will be a permanent feature of America's elderly population.

Within the total elderly population the sex ratios are generally higher for blacks than for whites, though in a few states that isn't true. Moreover, the sex balance is more nearly even among Spanish-origin people than among blacks and whites, partly because men have been the majority in many recent immigrant populations from Spanish America.

The sex ratios of elderly people have become remarkably similar in most of the states, for the frontier conditions and other realities that attracted large majorities of men earlier in the twentieth century have disappeared almost everywhere except Alaska and Hawaii; they are declining there, too. In fact, the only group with more elderly men than women is the one living on farms, whereas the cities, the suburbs, and even the small towns have sizable majorities of women.

The long-term trends reflect a progressive decrease in the sex ratios of the elderly, but the projections suggest a leveling tendency that will leave about 65 or 70 men for each 100 women during the next half century or so. This points to prolonged widowhood for large numbers of women, and that experience, in turn, evokes coping mechanisms to deal with financial matters, solitude, and declining health. Most elderly women do rise to the challenge, however, and counter the stereotype of dependence and passivity, even becoming aggressive and more self-assured as they deal with aging, widowhood, adult children, and other aspects of later life in American society.

NOTES

1. U.S. Bureau of the Census, "Demographic Aspects of Aging and the Older Population in the United States," *Current Population Reports,* P-23, no. 59 (1978): 12.

2. For the data, see U.S. Bureau of the Census, "Marital Status and Living Arrangements: March 1980," *Current Population Reports,* P-20, no. 365 (1981), table 1.

3. Peter Uhlenberg, "Demographic Change and Problems of the Aged," in Matilda White Riley, ed., *Aging from Birth to Death.* Boulder, CO: Westview Press, 1979, p. 164.

4. Carol Boellhoff Giesen and Nancy Datan, "The Competent Older Woman," in Nancy Datan and Nancy Lohman, eds., *Transitions of Aging.* New York: Academic Press, 1980, pp. 59-60.

5. National Center for Health Statistics, "Advance Report of Final Natality Statistics, 1980," *Monthly Vital Statistics Report* 31 (1982), table 7. See the analysis of causes by Gerald E. Markle, "Sex Ratios at Birth: Values, Variance, and Some Determinants," *Demography* 11 (1974): 131-134.

6. I.M. Lerner, *Heredity, Evolution and Society.* San Francisco: Freeman, 1968, p. 120.

7. For an analysis of the differential, see Nathan Keyfitz and Antonio Golini, "Mortality Comparisons: The Male-Female Ratio," *Genus* 31 (1975): 1-33.

8. Francis C. Madigan, "Are Sex Mortality Differentials Biologically Caused?" *Milbank Memorial Fund Quarterly* 35 (1957): 202-223.

9. Jacob S. Siegel, "Prospective Trends in the Size and Structure of the Elderly Population, Impact of Mortality Trends, and Some Implications," in U.S. Bureau of the Census, *Current Population Reports,* P-23, no. 78 (1979): 11.

10. Parts of this analysis are adapted from *ibid.,* pp. 11-13.

11. Jacob S. Siegel, "On the Demography of Aging," *Demography* 17 (1980): 350.

12. For some other international examples, see Organisation for Economic Co-operation and Development, *Socio-economic Policies for the Elderly.* Paris: OECD, 1979, pp. 11-12.

13. Joseph A. Norland, "Measuring Change in Sex Composition," *Demography* 12 (1975): 84.

14. Henry D. Sheldon, *The Older Population of the United States.* New York: Wiley, 1958, p. 14.

15. J. John Palen, *Social Problems.* New York: McGraw-Hill, 1979, pp. 393-394.

16. U.S. Bureau of the Census, "Some Demographic Aspects of Aging in the United States," *Current Population Reports,* P-23, no. 43 (1973): 8-9.

17. The data are from U.S. Bureau of the Census, *Statistical Abstract of the United States: 1982-83.* Washington, DC: U.S. Government Printing Office, 1982, tables 132 and 134.

18. Sheldon, *op. cit.,* p. 14.

19. For this theme, see Beth J. Soldo, "America's Elderly in the 1980s," *Population Bulletin,* 35 (1980): 6.

20. U.S. Bureau of the Census, "Farm Population of the United States: 1980," *Current Population Reports,* P-27, no. 54 (1980), table B.

21. *Ibid.,* p. 2.

22. National Council on the Aging, *Perspective on Aging* 9 (1980): 24.

23. *Ibid.*

24. Paul E. Zopf, Jr., *Sociocultural Systems.* Washington, DC: University Press of Ameria, 1980, p. 423.

25. Uhlenberg, *op. cit.,* p. 161.

26. Siegel, "On the Demography of Aging," *op. cit.,* p. 355. Cf. Sheldon, *op. cit.,* pp. 101-102.

27. Robert T. Michael, Victor R. Fuchs and Sharon R. Scott, "Changes in the Propensity to Live Alone: 1950-1976," *Demography* 17 (1980): 39.

28. Frances E. Kobrin, "The Fall in Household Size and the Rise of the Primary Individual in the United States," *Demography* 13 (1976): 136.

29. Michael, Fuchs and Scott, *op. cit.,* p. 49.

30. Siegel, *op. cit.,* pp. 355-356.

31. For the data, see U.S. Bureau of the Census, "Estimating After-Tax Money Income Distribution Using Data from the March Current Population Survey," *Current Population Reports,* P-23, No. 126 (1983), table 1.

32. See U.S. Bureau of the Census, "Characteristics of the Population Below the Poverty Level: 1980," *Current Population Reports*, P-60, no. 133 (1982), table 15.

33. Soldo, *op. cit.*, p. 39.

34. Giesan and Datan, *op. cit.*, p. 57.

35. *Ibid.*, p. 58.

36. *Ibid.*, pp. 59-60.

37. *Ibid.*, p. 60.

Chapter 4

Marriage and Family Status
Of the Elderly

The personal situation of most older people, like that of most other adults, is strongly influenced by marital status, just as the nature of the whole elderly population is affected by the proportions who are single, married, widowed, and divorced. Beyond the demographic considerations, the marital situation of the elderly has important social ties with family processes, structures, and functions, and especially the roles that people perform. Moreover, the nature and composition of families has much to do with how well the needs of older people are met and with whether they reside in a family setting with a spouse, adult children, or other relatives; outside the family context in an institution or alone; or in some type of quasi-family.

Given these variations, we need to analyze the marital status of America's elderly population in a broad social and demographic context, for the family still has great importance in the lives of older people, including most of those who live alone. Moreover, the marital status and living arrangements of elderly men differ greatly from those of elderly women,[1] basically because of the huge statistical surplus of the latter and the unavoidable solitude of many. In turn, that is a consequence of the differential death rates by sex and the stronger tendency for widowers to remarry, often not just from among the pool of elderly widows, but from the group of younger unmarried women.[2] Therefore, we have to account for the variable marital patterns of the sexes and the consequences that follow. First, however, we need to consider how marital status varies from adolescence to extreme old age.

Age and Marital Status

Any person's marital situation depends so heavily on age, that the proportions of single, married, widowed, and divorced people in a total population are greatly affected by its age profile. Thus, Figure 4-1, which is for the male and female populations aged 14 and over, shows the abrupt decrease in the percentages of single people in young adulthood and the accompanying rise in the proportions married, followed by increases in widowhood with advancing age, especially among women. These general patterns reflect those of most industrialized societies and lead to several conclusions as a context in which to examine the marital characteristics of the elderly.

Married People

By age 15 a few people begin to marry, and from then on the percentage single falls dramatically and that of married people leaps upward, because the average age at first marriage is still in the early 20s. Women, following the tradition that helps prolong widowhood, continue to marry somewhat older men and the marriage curve for women rises sooner, though the time lag is only a couple of years. (See Table 4-1.) The difference has

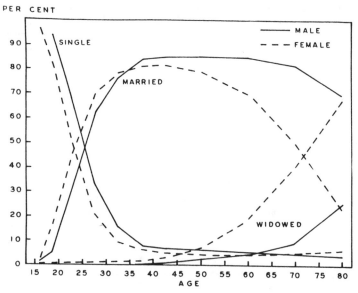

Figure 4-1. The Relationship of Age to Marital Status in the United States, by Sex, 1980
Source: U.S. Bureau of the Census, "Marital Status and Living Arrangements: March 1980," *Current Population Reports,* P-20, no. 365 (1981), table 1.

83

actually diminished by almost two years since 1900, but the reduction has been accompanied by the wide divergence in the death rates of males and females, so the average woman who does marry a man a few years older simply adds to the time she can expect to live as a widow.

As the marriage curve rises with age, eventually it reaches a peak in middle age. Thus, the maximum proportion of women classified as married comes in the ages 35-39, when widowhood begins to increase substantially; the highest percentage of men who are married comes in the ages 45-49. After these peaks have been reached, the percentage married begins to fall off fairly rapidly for women and more slowly for men, and by the time women reach the ages 75 and over, only 23 per cent are still married, compared with 69 per cent of the men.

Widowed People

The proportion of those whose spouses have died are very low in adolescence and young adulthood, but even then more women than men lose their mates to accidents, violence, and other causes. The rate of widowhood among women climbs very significantly after age 45, when the number of widows exceeds that of single women, while a similar situation for men doesn't appear until age 65. Despite these losses for both sexes,

Table 4-1. Median Age at First Marriage, 1890-1980

Year	Male	Female	Difference, in Years
1890	26.1	22.0	4.1
1900	25.9	21.9	4.0
1910	25.1	21.6	3.5
1920	24.6	21.2	3.4
1930	24.3	21.3	3.0
1940	24.3	21.5	2.8
1950	22.8	20.3	2.5
1960	22.8	20.3	2.5
1970	23.2	20.8	2.4
1980	24.6	22.1	2.5

Source: U.S. Bureau of the Census, "Marital Status and Living Arrangements: March 1980," Current Population Reports, P-20, no. 365 (1981), table A.

however, fertility and mortality have changed in such a way that the average young couple who marry today and produce children can expect to live together 14 years longer than their parents could after the last child has left home, barring divorce or separation.[3] Those 14 years represent about a third of the 44 years that people with continuous first marriages can now expect to spend together.[4] Therefore, as tragic as widowhood may be for individuals, its present patterns do represent substantial improvements in longevity and they allow a couple to spend many older years together free of child care. At the same time, there is the huge imbalance between widowed older men and women. For example, among widowed people 65 and over, there are only 19 men per 100 women, and for those in the combined category of single, widowed, and divorced, the figure is just 26. Moreover, the average age of widowers is about three years above that of widows, so most elderly widows who do remarry can expect to become widows again.

Divorced People

Patterns of divorce also vary by age, basically in two ways. First, divorce is most likely to occur for those who marry in their teens, for whom the risk is well over twice as great as it is for those who marry in their 20s. Second, the proportion of people who have divorced and not remarried rises with age until the 30-39 range and then tapers off gradually. This suggests that people aged 30-39 became a pivotal group as divorce patterns changed, for their elders are products of times and circumstances in which divorce was less acceptable and less common, whereas their juniors experience higher divorce rates but are also more apt to remarry. Thus, the pivotal age group experienced a rapid increase in divorce rates when their marriages were new, but as those people grow older they are less and less likely to remarry, especially as the falling sex ratio works increasingly to the disadvantage of women. Therefore, the older women are when they divorce or become widowed or the longer they remain single, the less likely they are ever to marry.

Basic Marital Differences by Sex

A little over half the nation's total elderly people still have a spouse with whom they live and another 2 per cent have a living mate from whom they are separated. Since more women than men survive to the older ages, however, gender has an important bearing on the marital and family status of the elderly.[5] Therefore, we need to consider the circumstances of the sexes separately and account for their relative proportions in each of the marital categories.

Three-quarters of all elderly men are married and living with their spouses, but that is true for little more than a third of the older women, mostly because of widowhood, though somewhat larger shares of women than men are also classified as single. More than half the women are widows, whereas only 14 per cent of the men are widowers. Moreover, these sex differences intensify upward in the age scale, until well over two-thirds of the women aged 75 and older must contend with the realities of being left alone because of a husband's death, having very limited prospects to develop another relationship that will lead to remarriage. Even in those ages, however, more than two-thirds of the men are still married. (See Table 4-2.)

The United States is not alone in these patterns of marital status by age and sex, for the world's elderly populations all share the same general imbalance, though with some variations from country to country. That is, at age 65 and older the large majority of men are still married, usually amounting to three-quarters or more of the total and scarcely ever dropping below two-thirds, while the proportion of widowers is rarely above 25 per cent. Among women the relationship is reversed, for the percentage still married at age 65 and older is always a minority, usually around a third or less of the total, while widows are at least half the total in nearly all countries and over two-thirds in some. Therefore, no matter what the levels of development and despite the somewhat higher percentages of widows in most of the developing countries than in most of the ones already "developed," the large surplus of elderly unmarried women appears nearly everywhere, though the proportional significance of that surplus does vary.

Though the factor chiefly responsible for this pattern is the differential mortality by sex, marriage and remarriage rates also play a part. In turn, they vary according to a society's prevailing religious and cultural norms. But the tendency for women to outlive men is so pervasive that among the 150 or so countries for which the United Nations reported the expectation of life at birth in the late 1970s, there were only six — Bangladesh, Bhutan, India, Nepal, Pakistan, and Sabah in Malaysia — in which male infants could expect longer life than female infants. The greater longevity of women even holds in places where life expectancy at birth is still less than 50 years and women experience unusually high death rates in childbirth. And the phenomenon extends to the few places where the newborn have an average life expectancy of 40 years or less, such as Ethiopia and Yemen. Not one of the reporting countries has greater life expectancy at age 65 for men than for women. Therefore, they all have much higher percentages of widows than widowers in the older ages and far lower proportions of married women than married men, including the few countries where male life expectancy at birth still exceeds that of females.[6]

The patterns of divorce in the United States, unlike those of widowhood, are about the same for both sexes in the older years. People who have divorced and not remarried are found more commonly among the 65-74 age group than in the older ages, but that marital status is significantly less in evidence among all elderly people than it is among the other ages between 25 and 64.

The changes with age in the proportions of men and women who are single, married, widowed, and divorced are also related to the living arrangements of the elderly, for the death of a spouse not only leaves the mate living alone in most cases, but provokes the question of what to do

Table 4-2.   Percentages of Older People in the Marital Status Categories, by Age and Race, 1980

Race and Marital Status	65-74		75+	
	Male	Female	Male	Female
All races	100.0	100.0	100.0	100.0
Single	5.4	5.6	4.4	6.4
Married[a]	79.4	48.1	67.7	22.1
Spouse Absent	2.2	2.0	1.7	1.2
Widowed	8.5	40.3	24.0	68.0
Divorced	4.4	4.0	2.2	2.3
White	100.0	100.0	100.0	100.0
Single	5.3	5.8	4.3	6.5
Married[a]	81.1	49.5	69.2	22.6
Spouse Absent	1.5	1.6	1.1	0.9
Widowed	7.9	39.2	23.5	67.7
Divorced	4.3	3.9	1.9	2.2
Black	100.0	100.0	100.0	100.0
Single	6.1	4.2	5.3	5.1
Married[a]	64.2	35.1	53.1	13.8
Spouse Absent	9.2	5.7	5.8	4.9
Widowed	14.9	49.9	30.4	71.9
Divorced	5.5	5.2	5.4	4.3

Source: U.S. Bureau of the Census, "Marital Status and Living Arrangements: March 1980," Current Population Reports, P-20, no. 365 (1981), table 1.

[a]Spouse present.

after one's marriage has disintegrated. In fact, "the trend in the percentage married as age increases is perhaps the best single index of the cycle of family formation and dissolution."[7] Coming as it does several years after the average couple's last child has left home, the sad occasion of widowhood causes the survivor, usually the wife, to decide in most cases to remain in the home, ordinarily alone, because the vast majority of elderly people do not reside with their children, other relatives, or in institutions. In fact, the last decade or so has seen a decrease in the percentage of elderly people who live in families and an increase in the proportion who maintain their own households, though sometimes with nonrelatives who may help constitute a quasi-family.[8] Therefore, the concept of the three-generation family living under one roof is more fiction than reality, though the family form that does prevail is a logical result of the American tendency to separate the nuclear unit from the larger extended family, at least residentially. Thus, in 1980 about 15 per cent of all American men aged 65 and older and 42 per cent of the women were living by themselves or with nonrelatives, and were designated as "nonfamily householders" (formerly "primary individuals") by the U.S. Bureau of the Census. The percentages are especially high in the groups above age 74. Furthermore, 95 per cent of all nonfamily householders occupied their own house or apartment alone, which points to the nation's substantial share of widows and widowers and its smaller single and divorced elderly populations that carry on their lives in relative solitude.

Variations by Race and Nativity

Race and ethnicity often have strong associations with differences in marital status and familial patterns, largely because of the socioeconomic variations attached to race and nativitiy, particularly when today's elderly people were young and their marital patterns were evolving under the onus of racism and segregation.[9] Therefore, black and white older people differ substantially in the percentages who are single, married, widowed, and divorced, and also in their living arrangements, though none of the variations is as great as in the past.

In general, elderly black men are less likely to be married than are white men but are more apt to be single, widowed, or divorced. (See Table 4-2.) At the same time, however, black men are more likely to be separated from their wives while still legally married to them. Most of the same relationships by race obtain for women, in that smaller percentages of black than white women are married, while higher percentages of blacks are widowed, divorced, or separated. The proportion single is below that among white women, however, and not only are the marriages of blacks dissolved more frequently, but their rates of remarriage are lower than those of whites. As a result, while 61 per cent of the white women aged

65 and older are not living with a spouse for one reason or another, that is true of 72 per cent of the black women. As expected, these conditions intensify with age.

The marital status of elderly Spanish-origin people varies some from those of blacks and whites. Men 65 and over are more likely than black and white men to be single or divorced, while they are intermediate between the two races in the proportions married or separated. Hispanic men are as likely as white elderly men to be widowers, but the proportions in both groups are much smaller than they are in the black segment. Spanish-origin women are intermediate between black and white women in the proportions single, married, or separated, but rank highest in the shares who are widowed or divorced. There are some differences in these patterns, however, between the two age groups that comprise the category 65 and over. There are also several variations among the nationality groups that constitute the Spanish-origin population. Thus, the proportions of single men and women are comparatively low in the Cuban population, relatively high among people with Puerto Rican backgrounds, and a bit above average in the Mexican group. The proportions of married men and women are relatively high in the Cuban group and low among Puerto Ricans, while Cuban and Puerto Rican women are especially likely to be widowed, finding themselves unable to remarry in an unusually large share of cases.

In addition to the rise in the proportion of widowed people in all elderly racial and ethnic categories, the percentages who are divorced or separated are growing in all of the groups, rapidly in some. Therefore, increasing proportions of older people will face living alone or with others who are not spouses or children, for the percentages who live in familes are declining, especially among women. Other things contribute to this tendency as well, such as improved pensions that facilitate independence, various public assistance programs, housing that tends to segregate the elderly from other age groups, and the wish of most adult children to live near but not with their aging parents.[10]

Both blacks and whites contribute to the tendency for elderly people to live alone, for the older members of each race seem to prefer independent arrangements as long as they are physically and economically able. In fact, some people in all racial groups pursue this independence because they cannot always rely on the extended family even when it appears strong, despite the myths about unwavering concern for the elderly in certain ethnic groups, especially the Japanese and Chinese.[11] Moreover, even when financial and other material assistance is available from families, it does not guarantee companionship and emotional support for the elderly, and each race and ethnic group has its minority of elderly parents whose children help provide the former but little or none of the latter, though it is easy to overestimate this problem. In some cases, the children's obligation to supply material assistance may even produce resentments that diminish the more affective types of support, especially as more people come to believe that high Social Security taxes give government the responsiblity for the elderly.

Farm-Nonfarm Variations

In general, city populations contain unusually large percentages of single women, widows and widowers, and divorced men and women, while farm areas have significantly more than their fair share of married people and single men, but relatively low proportions in the other marital categories. Among the elderly population living on farms, these patterns are strongly influenced by the surplus of men. Their group also contains a larger proportion of bachelors than appears in the nonfarm population, for even young men have a poorer statistical chance to marry than do those in cities, because rural-urban migration has taken away large numbers of young women. As these single men age, their statistical marriage prospects do improve somewhat, because the sex ratio declines, though at age 65 and older it is back to 112 in the farm population as compared with one of 68 in the older nonfarm group.

The proportions of widowed people are much lower on farms than they are in the nonfarm group. That isn't because of any mortality advantage in farm populations or because the death rates of men are any closer to those of women than they are in cities. Instead, the woman who becomes a widow in the farm population stands a far better chance of remarriage than her urban sister, owing to the supply of elderly men without wives, though the advantage diminishes fairly rapidly after age 65. In addition, rural norms tend to favor remarriage more strongly than is true in the cities as a whole, and various economic necessities, including the operation of a farm, often pressure a widow toward remarriage. Some of those factors also account for the low proportion of elderly farm people classified as divorced, though the initial divorce rate is also much lower than it is for urbanites.

Sex Ratios and Remarriage Prospects

Just what statistical chances do the elderly have for the remarriage mentioned in the preceding section? How many would actually remarry if the demographic situation allowed it? In order to address the first question we need to consider the categories of men and women who are single, widowed, and divorced, and who are statistical prospects for marriage. The index that allows such an analysis is the familiar sex ratio, which varies significantly by race, residence, and age in the 65-and-over group. The great bulk of this eligible group consists of widowed people, who are 61 per cent of the men who could marry and 85 per cent of the eligible women. Table 4-3 provides the basic data.

The fundamental fact affecting the prospects for marriage and remarriage of elderly people is the great sex imbalance, for as we saw in Chapter 3, in 1980 there was a surplus of 6.2 million women who could not find mates in their age bracket. Moreover, the imbalance intensifies with age. It is also more severe among whites than blacks, for while elderly unmarried white women outnumber men by four to one, black women predominate by just three to one, though the discrepancy is even less in the Spanish-origin population. Partly as a consequence of the sex imbalance among elderly unmarried people, about 18 of each 1,000 men actually do remarry, compared with only two of the women,[12] though unwillingness to establish a new marriage is also a factor for a large number of people. Therefore, the attitudes and the nine-to-one difference in the remarriage rate make remarriage among the nation's elderly people relatively rare.[13] Widowed people make up the majority of those who do remarry, but only because they are such a large share of the unmarried group. Divorced people actually have higher remarriage rates than widows and widowers at all ages including 65 and over. If one is going to remarry at all, it generally happens fairly soon after the first marriage ends, for the status of widowed or divorced person soon becomes part of one's way of life and is not easily relinquished in many cases.

Table 4-3. Sex Ratios of Elderly People Classified as Single, Widowed, and Divorced, by Race and Spanish Origin, 1980

Race and Ethnicity	65+	65-74	75+
All Races	26.1	28.2	23.8
White	25.2	27.3	23.1
Black	33.3	34.8	31.2
Spanish Origin[a]	42.1	43.2	40.3

Source: U.S. Bureau of the Census, "Marital Status and Living Arrangements: March 1980," Current Population Reports, P-20, no. 365 (1981), table 1.

[a]May be of any race.

Because their experiences bear little resemblance to those of divorced people, widows and widowers tend to marry each other, though they have to choose within a fairly narrow age range due to the rigid norms that still keep women from marrying much younger men. Those constraints further limit a widow's choices and discourage many women from marrying no matter what the statistical situation. Many don't want to repeat previous problems, care for another invalid husband, or suffer bereavement once again. Others cherish their independence and guard their finances against loss. Still others are concerned about the impact of remarriage on their children, who may be opposed for various reasons. Some believe the original marriage was so good and the first husband so saintly that neither could possibly be duplicated.[14] Furthermore, the older a woman is when she becomes a widow, the less her chances of remarriage, because the demographic and social factors both conspire against that possibility. Conversely, younger women are the best candidates to remarry, especially if they have worked for wages, are adept at making significant personal adjustments, and had deeply satisfying emotional relationships with their first husbands.[15] Many of these factors help reduce the numbers of elderly people who would remarry even if the sex ratio were closer to 100, so the 6.2 million "surplus" women do not constitute an eager throng who would all choose new husbands if only there were enough to go around.

Remarriage, even when it occurs, also presents certain problems, partly because American culture still includes remnants of the myth that there is only one love for each person, and thereby creates certain conflicts and hazards for the new marriage. In turn, a widowed person who idealizes the first spouse may cause the new mate to feel he/she is second choice, while friends, relatives, and in-laws from the first marriage may make the new relationship difficult to manage.[16] Nonetheless, most widowed people who do marry seem to succeed, partly because the marriage represents an escape from loneliness and other problems and thereby encourages people to adjust to a new mate who may be less than ideal.[17]

The Experience of Widowhood

Inasmuch as the vast majority of elderly people without mates are widows who don't remarry, we can consider some of the aspects of widowhood, though widowers deserve attention as well.

Widowhood is fundamentally different from other ways of ending a marriage, for it is involuntary, it provides the survivor with recognizable status, and it evokes sympathy from friends and relatives, at least for a time. Nor is widowhood perceived as failure in the same sense as divorce, though the widowed person may become a pariah with whom others feel

92

uneasy for different reasons. Despite the more positive attitude toward
widowed people, loneliness is still often a major problem, especially
among women, for they are even less likely now than in the past to move
in with adult children.[18] Therefore, the widow faces a social world
oriented to couples and from which she is suddenly excluded, and her
status is further complicated by the fact she is elderly in a society that
prizes youth; many of the oldest ones also have health and financial
problems. These conditions diminish the chances that a widow can find a
mate in the small pool of widowers, and they contribute to the problems
that can accompany solitude.

Widows and widowers differ in certain respects that make some adjustments more difficult for one group than for the other, though they also
have many problems in common. Some elderly women find marriage the
primary source of status, and the end of a marriage leaves a major gap in a
woman's life. This is not to say, of course, that men are necessarily less
dependent on their marriages, particularly those men who are retired and
lack the occupational status to which they had been accustomed. Moreover, most men and women have other relationships and interests in their
lives, and while the death of a spouse may alter some of them, it rarely
destroys or even changes all of them. Despite these protections, however,
there is a strong tendency for widowed people to feel shunned by friends
and relatives who follow the American tendency to deny death and who
may even assess a kind of blame for it. Therefore, the surviving spouse —
man or woman — generally endures "the pain over being deserted, of
losing a love object, and at least a significant other, of grief and loneliness,"[19] and must often struggle with these things in the absence of
continuing support from friends and relatives. The problems are intensified because the nuclear family is the functioning domestic unit in the
United States, while the potentially supportive network of the extended
family is at least partly fragmented by residence arrangements that discourage the three- or four-generation household. Thus, widowed people of
both sexes have in common the death crisis itself, the loss of someone to
share household responsibilities and emotional ties, and the role-disor-
ganization that may follow.

Widows and widowers can also experience financial problems as the
result of the death, though on the average the women are less well off than
the men, and they may either have to seek public assistance or help from
children or see their levels of living decline. But even that fact fails to
account for the economic loss sustained by a widower when his wife dies,
whether or not she earned wages. Furthermore, widowers seem to suffer
more severe problems of adjustment than widows and are more likely to
be in poor health. Many widowers also appear to have poorer adaptive
skills and find it more difficult to adjust to solitude and to the status of
single in a world of couples. In any case, they suffer from higher rates of

mental illness and suicide than do widows,[20] though their situations are also affected by class standing, level of education, and other factors. In short, even though some problems affect individual widows or widowers differently, the death of a spouse provokes many more common difficulties and adjustments. Therefore, many of the socioeconomic differences between elderly widows and widowers pale beside the fact that the former outnumber the latter by more than five to one.

The living arrangements of widowed people tend to reinforce the problems that some of them face, especially loneliness and the lack of material support. Thus, in 1980 over 64 per cent of the elderly widowers and 67 per cent of the widows were classified as nonfamily householders living alone. Most of the remainder were living in families headed by relatives, principally adult children; but even many of those elderly are there because of financial constraints and would actually prefer to reside independently. The elderly widowed people most likely to live alone are white, especially women, while less than half of the blacks reside by themselves, more often finding homes with relatives or friends. The percentage of widowed people living alone declines somewhat with age, because the oldest people are more likely to be incapacitated and in need of constant companionship, but in their case, too, solitude is more common among whites than blacks.

Living alone has increased markedly in the past several decades, partly because of changes in family relationships. In numerous earlier cases, especially in farming areas, parents accepted a newly married couple into an established household. The aging woman gradually turned its management over to the younger one but continued to reside in the home. Now an elderly widow who wishes to live with adult children must break up her original home and move in with a daughter or daughter-in-law. Because neither she nor the younger woman may really want that relationship, the elderly widow is more apt to remain in and control her own home, even though it may mean solitude. That solitude, however, tends to produce a lower level of life satisfaction for both rural and urban widows than does living with adult children,[21] though it is often modified by continuing contacts with the children.

Families of the Elderly

The older man or woman usually has numerous family roles as spouse, parent, grandparent, relative of other kinds, and more frequently than in the past, even child of a very old parent.[22] These roles cluster into a complex but changing set of relationships that affect the composition of the elderly person's family.[23] Moreover, while the older man or woman finally must adapt to the death of a spouse, for most people aged 65 and older the demanding adjustments to a new marriage, the acquisition of small children, and even the departure of the last child are far in the past. In place of those adjustments are such things as the husband's and perhaps the wife's retirement from a salaried job, reduced income, the appearance of grandchildren, eventual bereavement, and adjustment to the prospect of one's own death. The social network necessary for dealing with these changes is curtailed by the propensity of most older people to live alone or only with their spouses, while a small and declining minority live with their children. Nonetheless, many elderly people do come to depend emotionally, financially, and in other ways on the offspring who once depended on them, and a comparatively large majority do live *near* at least one of their children and visit often. Assistance during illness or incapacity is an especially significant factor in these relationships. In fact, one of the most persistent fictions about the elderly in contemporary American society is that they are largely abandoned by their adult children. That myth has evolved largely from the fact that the vast majority of elderly people do not reside with their children and are assumed, therefore, to be ignored or neglected. The abandonment myth is further sustained by the many elderly who do not receive the attention they would like, by the mistaken notion that the nuclear family is emotionally isolated from the larger kin network, by other beliefs about intergenerational relationships,[24] and by the role that government at many levels has assumed in meeting certain needs of the elderly. In fact, however, significant and productive ties still exist between most elderly people and their families, even though they don't all live under one roof.[25] The more common tendency is for the elderly and their offspring to work out mutually productive and fulfilling contacts that reflect the *modified extended family,* which holds together and provides in certain ways for its members, even though they may be geographically separated. It is a unit typical of urban-industrial societies whose members change residence frequently.[26] Moreover, the modified extended family reflects the persistence of parent-child relationships throughout life, partly because people share certain values and a sense of duty and obligation toward each other.

Family Functions

Aging does alter the nature of the older person's family and the contributions he/she makes to it. But the durability of family relations in some form is largely due to the functions that the family performs for older people and the contributions they make to it.

The elderly may help socialize children and thereby teach them certain elements of the society and create some dimensions of personality and the self-concept, though present-day older people are less likely to serve as authority figures than as benign baby-sitters. Moreover, since the family helps blend one generation into the next, elderly people give children apprenticeship with the oldest group, though that function is compromised when young offspring regard their parents as the older generation and their grandparents as ancient curiosities with little to offer.

The family remains a source of emotional security for many older people, largely because those relationships provide some caring and uncritical acceptance which, in turn, helps people deal with isolation, tension, and stress, and which constitutes the principal protective function of contemporary families that no longer have to overcome natural dangers. But the family also generates conflict and the opportunity for conflict management. The ability to control conflict and to interact productively with elderly members may be a skill that carries over into other relationships. Those functions may be limited, however, by the fact that more than two generations rarely live together, because the geographic separation of the elderly from young family members, even if only by a block or two, keeps many contacts between youth and the elderly artificial and weakly integrative. Nevertheless, the type of interaction in today's modified extended family is better than none at all in helping to moderate the prevailing stereotypes about older people. Even when conflict does occur, it may have a less devastating effect on the elderly than simply being ignored.

Finally, the family provides some links with other social institutions the older person can use, and it provides patterns and mechanisms for property inheritance when the older person dies. For many elderly, the family is an economic support unit and a convenient final step in the economic distribution system of the larger society. As such, it provides a context in which some elderly still operate as producers and all function as consumers of goods and services. Its form and level of income even help determine the nature and amount of those goods and services, especially the ones supplied by government.

These and other fundamental functions suggest that the family, flaws and all, still does strategic things for most of the elderly and that they contribute to the institution, though not always in the same ways or as well as before. Therefore, while changes in family relationships may make it seem that older people are largely isolated from kin contacts, a functional analysis actually indicates that families play vital roles for most elderly.[27]

Composition of Elderly Households and Families

The large majority of elderly men are householders (formerly called heads of households), and each unit usually consists of the man and his wife without children. (See Table 4-4.) Thus, in 1980 three-quarters of the men aged 65 and older headed families that included at least one other person, though the proportion dropped off progressively in the years past 65. The rest either lived alone or in domestic units headed by someone else. Most of the last group were living with middle-aged children and their offspring, though only a small fraction of elderly men actually take up residence with children.

About half the women 65 and over also are householders, but mainly because they are living alone, not because they are heads of families containing at least two people. In turn, that high proportion reflects the large percentages of women who are only reported in the census data as householders after their husbands have died. In 1980 about two-fifths of the elderly women were solitary householders, and the proportion increases with age. At the same time, almost half were living in a family setting with at least one relative, usually an elderly husband or adult offspring. The latter arrangement tends to be created, however, only when the elderly person is incapacitated or too old to manage independently, and then the usual host is a middle-aged daughter or daughter-in-law who carries the principal responsibility for the aged person's care. It is far more common for the elderly person to live near that relative and to receive attention and emotional support while maintaining a separate household, generally by preference, though adult children may also hesitate to take an elderly person into the home and thereby sacrifice potential employment and income, social activities, and privacy.[28] The least likely arrangement of all is for the elderly person to live with nonrelatives.

Blacks and whites differ some in the family settings of older people, though the general patterns are the same. Thus, black men are less likely than white men to be householders and are more likely to live alone or with adult children. Black men are also more apt to be living with friends or other nonrelatives, though the incidence is not great for either race. Black women are more likely than white women to be householders but less likely to be living alone or in families they do not head.

Thus, the living arrangements of the nation's elderly are quite varied — probably more so than in any other age group. Nonetheless, the large majority of elderly men and about half the women can still be found in family groups of one kind or another.[29] No matter what the living arrangements, however, it is clear that Americans don't generally abandon their older people, but instead provide emotional support routinely and money and other help when it is needed. Indeed, about 80 per cent of the home care required by elderly people is given by family members and much of the remainder is supplied by friends. Ignored though these contributions may be, they greatly exceed the assistance provided by public funds and personnel. Moreover, the support role of middle-aged offspring will become increasingly important as the proportion of very old people grows, and it will not be unusual for women who are elderly themselves to be looking after an extremely aged parent. Even now about a fourth of the people who have reached age 60 still have one surviving parent,[30] and given the patterns of mortality and the content of social roles, that situation produces a substantial number of elderly women looking after even older women, usually both of them widows. That type of care will probably grow more difficult, however, because an increasing

Table 4-4. Percentages of People 65 and Over With Various Living Arrangements, by Race and Sex, 1980

Living Arrangement	Male	Female
All Races	100.0	100.0
Householder	90.4	52.3
Family Householder	75.0	10.5
Living Alone	14.6	40.8
Living with Nonrelatives	0.8	1.0
Not Householder	9.6	47.7
Living in Families	8.0	46.6
Not in Families	1.6	1.1
White	100.0	100.0
Householder	91.4	51.8
Family Householder	76.5	9.3
Living Alone	14.2	41.6
Living with Nonrelatives	0.7	0.9
Not Householder	8.6	48.2
Living in Families	7.3	47.1
Not in Families	1.3	1.1
Black	100.0	100.0
Householder	83.4	60.0
Family Householder	61.9	22.6
Living Alone	19.5	35.3
Living with Nonrelatives	2.0	2.1
Not Householder	16.6	40.0
Living in Families	13.1	38.4
Not in Families	3.5	1.6

Source: U.S. Bureau of the Census, "Marital Status and Living Arrangements: March 1980," Current Population Reports, P-20, no. 365 (1981), table 6.

share of the women who look after an aged parent are also in the labor force and are responsible for more than one time-consuming commitment. Furthermore, when the baby-boom cohort is quite elderly, the number of adult offspring to look after them will be relatively small, and the problems of dependency will intensify. Therefore, the realities call for more imaginative governmental participation in meeting the needs of the very old, including more workable Medicare provisions, though the major responsibility seems likely to remain with family members.

These dependency patterns ought not to obscure the fact that husbands and wives have longer lives together than ever before and that dependency comes at a later age than in the past. For more than a century the rate at which marriages are dissolved by death has been declining, and despite the large mortality differential between the sexes, much higher percentages of people live longer as couples and delay entry into widowhood.[31] Therefore, the intact family is subject to aging in the same sense that the nation's whole population is aging, and in a growing percentage of American kin relationships adult children have joined their surviving parents in the 65-and-over group.[32]

Sexual Relations

The sexual interests and behavior of the elderly have been studied since the first Kinsey reports,[33] but many of the studies had various methodological problems that tended to obscure the actual sexual behavior of the elderly. The investigations often relied on voluntary reporting and were scarcely representative of the older population. Until the Duke Longitudinal Study, none of the research on sexuality followed the same subjects over time; most of the studies did not control for marital status and, therefore, for the availability of a partner with whom to have sex.[34] For these reasons and because stereotypes die hard, many Americans still assume that older people lack sexual interest or are vulgar, ridiculous, or even dangerous if they retain it. We often perceive sexuality to be an attribute of the young, to diminish sharply in middle age, and to have virtually disappeared when one reaches age 65 or 70. The biases in advertising and the mass media have much to do with that perception, but it is also perpetuated by adult children who can scarcely visualize their parents in a sexual relationship, let alone one parent in a lover relationship with a new mate or a date. Consequently, the myths that surround sexuality among the elderly help to aggravate the lack of intimacy that already troubles many, and some elderly are denied not only sexual relationships, but other expressions of intimacy as well.[35]

The facts about elderly sexuality indicate that many enjoy marital sex well into old age, even the more advanced years, and that good sex in the younger years can become good sex in the later ones. Deteriorating health certainly inhibits the sexuality of some older people, but even in many of those cases medical corrections are possible. Moreover, sexual fulfillment is more constrained by the loss of one's partner and by social pressures and psychological barriers than it is by physical infirmities. It is especially handicapped by the widespread failure to recognize "that sexuality and sexual expression are integral to the integrity of the personality from infancy through old age."[36] In addition, the sexual capability of elderly men seems to wane more than that of elderly women, but partly because of boredom and the fear of failure and not just from physical decline. Moreover, the men seem to regard sexual performance as a basic factor in their well-being, while the women consider it less central to self-confidence and tend to separate it from other aspects of the self.[37] These attitudes do generate considerable anxiety among elderly men about their sexuality, whereas elderly women are more likely to deny and suppress theirs. Both orientations are also strongly influenced by the social expectations and taboos that were attached to sex when today's elderly were young. As a result of these and other factors, many older people do have less interest in intercourse and get less satisfaction from it than when they were younger, and many simply lack the opportunity; thus far, few seem inclined to seek reconditioning to improve sexuality.[38]

Though it is easy to carry these generalizations too far and to ignore the individuals and couples who remain sexually interested and active well beyond age 65, the Duke studies do show that sexual interest, activity, and enjoyment tend to decrease gradually with advancing age, even among people who are still married. The studies also show, however, that about half the men are still sexually active through their mid-70s, half the women are active through their mid-60s, and the bulk of married couples are certainly not asexual, even until their 80s in many cases. For some older people, sexual activity even increases temporarily after age 65, though with advancing age sexual behavior becomes less variable and more homogeneous in the older population, and its frequency declines. Furthermore, among older people who have the opportunity to be sexually active, the level of health has much to do with actual performance. So does socioeconomic status, because those who rank higher on the social class scale tend to be more sexually active than those who place lower,[39] generally because of the better health, greater longevity, and other advantages that accompany higher social status.

Nonfamily Institutionalization

Despite the common notion that throngs of elderly Americans reside in nursing homes and similar nonfamily settings, less than 6 per cent of all people aged 65 and older actually live in institutions. Moreover, certain age groups are disproportionately represented and most are there because they have no spouse, children, siblings, or other intimates who could help look after their daily needs in the community.[40] Thus, the Census Bureau's 1976 study of the nation's institutional population showed that there were about 1 million elderly people in long-term care institutions, well over nine-tenths of them in nursing homes of various sorts. The remainder — less than 40,000 — were in facilities for the physically or psychiatrically impaired or the mentally handicapped, and in other settings besides nursing homes.[41] By 1980 the number in nursing homes had risen to about 1.4 million.[42] Some 60 per cent of the institutionalized elderly reside in private establishments run for profit, another 30 per cent are in private nonprofit places, and the remaining 10 per cent live in publicly supported institutions, most operated by state and local governments.

Characteristics of the Institutionalized Elderly

The people in nursing homes and other institutions are not a cross-section of the total population aged 65 and older, but a group with special characteristics that led to their institutionalization initially. The very old are heavily represented among this group. In 1976 about 62 per cent were at least 80 years of age, whereas people in those advanced years represented only 20 per cent of the total elderly population. Moreover, women make up more than two-thirds of the elderly institutional population. The group also has a very high rate of physical or mental disability that requires constant attention to meet even basic needs and perform routine tasks on a daily basis; perhaps as many as half the residents of nursing homes suffer from mental impairments of various kinds, many of them potentially correctable.[43] That argues for more research on such problems as Alzheimer's Disease in order to return many older people to the community and reduce the cost of their care and the severity of their problems.

The elderly institutional population is also characterized by a substantial scarcity of family members or others to look after them in the community, which means that those living in institutions are quite likely to be unmarried. In fact, about 64 per cent of the institutionalized elderly are widowed, 15 per cent are single, and 5 per cent are divorced or separated, whereas only 15 per cent are married. Furthermore, at least half have no adult children who could help them, and that group accounts for a large share of the older people who admit themselves to institutions. This suggests that the other half do have children who could be of assistance, but in most cases the offspring have already provided help to the older parent and have chosen the nursing home as a last resort, often when care at home has become impossible.

Some older people in institutions could reside with children if the latter wanted them, but they represent a small minority. In the greater number of cases elderly people are institutionalized because they have no family members left or because those members have exhausted their own emotional and physical resources and use institutionalization when they have no alternative. Often they are forced to accept that choice by the older person's degree of impairment and by the type and intensity of care required, for almost 80 per cent of all admissions are for medical conditions, most no longer manageable at home. Furthermore, about 82 per cent of the elderly admitted to nursing homes previously had no access to services, such as food delivery, housekeeping, home health care, and transportation. Given these factors, there is scant support for the assumption that large numbers of adults "dump" their aged parents into nursing homes simply to be rid of them. In fact, about two-thirds of the residents have visitors weekly and less than a tenth have none at all,[44] and visitation is so important that the majority of people cite location as the principal reason for selecting a particular institution.

Future Nursing Home Needs

The size of the elderly institutional population has been increasing rapidly, because both the numbers and proportions of older people have been growing, while the average number of younger relatives to care for each elderly family member has been declining. The increase in the institutional group will continue for a time, because the cohorts born in the Great Depression of the 1930s are relatively small compared with those of the preceding generation. Therefore, people who reach their 50s and 60s in the 1980s and 1990s will have a comparatively heavy burden of support for older people, many with only one adult child or even none to look after them. So a larger share of the elderly, especially as they reach very old age, will have to enter nursing homes and other institutions. Some will have needs that cannot be met at home; others will be only mildly impaired, but will have no one at home to help with daily tasks. Even now, however, there is a shortage of nursing homes, because their numbers and capacity are not growing and their waiting lists are long. Moreover, high interest rates and uncertainty about the future of Medicare and Medicaid funds have delayed needed construction.

As the small cohort of the Depression years enters the older ages, they will have the comparatively large baby-boom cohorts of 1945-1960 to help see to their needs, and each elderly person will have a larger average number of middle-aged children to help provide physical, emotional, and financial support. Therefore, other things being equal, it should be possible for a larger percentage of the elderly to remain at home and part of the community. In turn, it is likely that, briefly, the population admitted to nursing homes and other institutions will grow less rapidly that it has, though it will still grow. Presumably, in the future as now, it will be "the lack of a spouse, adult child, or other relative to help with routine daily tasks and not medical reasons per se that sends many slightly inform older persons to nursing homes."[45]

The longer term future, however, will produce another increase in the need for institutional care. In 2010 the first of the baby-boom people will reach age 65 but will have a comparatively small cohort of adult children to help provide for them, because the birth rate declined significantly after 1960 and reached an all-time low in the mid-1970s. Therefore, the two decades after 2010 will again see a sizable number of the elderly with one child or none to help with daily tasks and routine support. As a result, the population that will have to seek out institutions for care not available in the community will increase, perhaps dramatically.

Before that happens, however, there will be still another group of elderly people who will draw more heavily on resources, including institutions. They are the veterans of World War II and for whom the Veterans Administration already operates a huge, costly health care system. At present, there are about 3.3 million veterans aged 65 and older, but by 1990 there will be 7.6 million,[46] and they will be increasingly in need of medical and other care as they age. Moreover, since 1971, federal law has guaranteed free medical care to veterans 65 and over no matter what their financial condition and whether or not their health problems are service-related.[47] The coming task of caring for these veterans is further complicated by uncertainty about the areas in which they will be living and where the services should be concentrated, though the groups are likely to grow the fastest in the areas with large net in-migration in general. As a result of this impending growth, the needs related to it, and governmental financial commitments already made, the size of the veteran population using governmentally subsidized institutions will increase rapidly and soon, placing a much larger burden on Veterans Administration hospitals, out-patient clinics, nursing homes, and institutional residences. These places will be especially attractive because the quality of care is often superior to that available in other institutional settings.

By 2010, when the new crush of elderly begins, we may have learned that it is cheaper to keep all but the most severely impaired at home and will provide more public assistance to private caregivers — spouses and middle-aged offspring — in order to lessen their personal burdens and the need for expensive institutional care. At present, the large majority of elderly in families are cared for with no agency help, and much of their sustenance costs the public far less per person than does the process of institutionalization. Consequently, there is room for government at various levels to help families sustain the dependent elderly and to make the effort cost-effective. Without such help, more families will have to place the burden of support for their elderly upon public caregivers, and the costs to taxpayers will escalate accordingly.

The objectives of the Older Americans Act of 1965 certainly provide the basis for the necessary federal efforts. Perhaps those endeavors only require more versatile application, better coordination, less duplication, and greater simplicity. One problem now is that the older person must identify the various services needed, search them out in a maze of federal, state, and local agencies, and somehow put together a program that meets his/her needs, so it is hardly surprising that many impaired older people have no real access to the programs that do exist.[48] Some of those people enter nursing homes because it is a simpler, more comprehensible process, even though readily available public aid might allow them to remain in the community. Ideally, the institutional population would consist only of those impaired people who have no friends or others to help them, the ones whose families have too many disabilities or other problems to provide care, and those who are so severely disabled that the emotional and financial costs of care are less in an institution than at home. Such a population would consist even more heavily than it does now of the very old, the chronically ill, and the solitary.

Quality of Care

The growing nursing home population and large governmental subsidies have increased opportunities for promoters and exploiters to enter the business of looking after the elderly in an institutional setting, though the care provided in many homes run by churches, private operators, and others is quite decent. At present there are about 23,000 nursing homes in the United States to house over a million elderly people, most with substantial assistance from taxation of various kinds,[49] and some of the facilities are substandard. In certain cases, conscientious operators are forced to provide less than adequate care because of financial constraints, while others simply exploit the elderly for the highest possible income at the lowest possible cost. A large share of those older people have no one to look after their interests and are at the mercy of profiteering caregivers, which often means inadequate nutrition, poorly paid and incompetent employees, and various deals with physicians and others to maximize income at the expense of the elderly patients. Therefore, while many homes are scrupulously run, many others represent a national scandal that governmental agencies fail to stop.

Trends in Marital Status

During all of the last 100 years, elderly women have been far less likely than elderly men to be married but far more likely to be widowed. Therefore, the high incidence of widowhood is not solely a consequence of medical miracles performed in the last few decades, but a persistent feature in American history. In fact, as shown in Figure 4-2, the fluctuations in the percentages of men and women classified as married have been small since 1890, with only about half as many women as men reporting themselves as married, though the difference between the sexes is a little greater now than in most years since the turn of the century. Furthermore, the proportions of widows and widowers both generally have fallen, though the decline was much faster for the men than for the

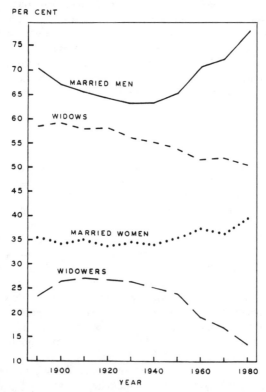

Figure 4-2. Percentages of People Aged 65 and Older Classified as Married or Widowed, by Sex, 1890-1980

Sources: U.S. Bureau of the Census, *U.S. Census of Population: 1960, Characteristics of the Population, U.S. Summary* (1964), table 177; *U.S. Census of Population: 1970, Detailed Characteristics, U.S. Summary* (1973), table 203; "Marital Status and Living Arrangements: March 1980," *Current Population Reports,* P-20, no. 365 (1981), table 1.

women. As a result, while the percentages of widowed people of both sexes are lower than ever, the superabundance of widows relative to the supply of widowers is also greater: In 1890 there were 2.5 widows for each widower, but in 1980 there were 3.8.

Some changes have also occurred in the percentages of elderly men and women classified as single and divorced, though taken together those categories have never accounted for more than 11 per cent of either sex. (See Figure 4-3.) After 1890 the proportions of elderly single people rose steadily until 1940 and then declined because of long-term increases in the marriage rate. It was more likely that those who reached age 65 around 1980 had married than was true of those who became 65 in the 1930s, 1940s, and 1950s. The proportions of elderly men and women classified as divorced (and not remarried) have risen steadily since 1890, and by 1980 the figure for men was more than nine times what it had been at the turn of the century, while that for women was 11 times greater. Those changes reflect radical alterations in the divorce rate in the twentieth century, and the proportions would be significantly higher if the remarriage rate were not much greater for divorced people than for widows and widowers. The incidence of remarriage is greater because divorce generally takes place

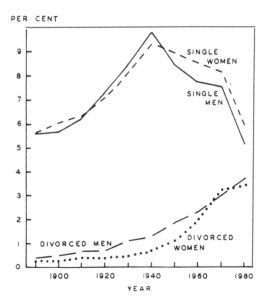

Figure 4-3. Percentages of People Aged 65 and Older Classified as Single or Divorced, by Sex, 1890-1980
Sources: U.S. Bureau of the Census, *U.S. Census of Population: 1960, Characteristics of the Population, U.S. Summary* (1964), table 177; *U.S. Census of Population: 1970, Detailed Characteristics, U.S. Summary* (1973), table 203; "Marital Status and Living Arrangements: March 1980," *Current Population Reports,* P-20, no. 365 (1981), table 1.

much younger than widowhood, and given the prejudice that aging men are more attractive than aging women, the younger divorced woman has a greater competitive advantage in finding a new mate. Furthermore, the many social and psychological barriers to remarriage, discussed earlier, either do not operate at all or are less formidable for many divorced women than for widows. No matter what the specific patterns, however, the steady increase in the percentages of divorced people reflects some of the basic changes in marriage and family during the last several decades, though the higher divorce rate is offset considerably by the relatively high remarriage rate among divorced persons.

Most of these trends apply to both white and black elderly people. Thus, since 1940 the proportions married have increased for both sexes and races, while the percentages widowed have decreased. Moreover, the percentages classified as divorced have risen markedly in all four groups, but especially among black men and women. In the category of single people, however, the races part company: The proportions of white men and women who have never married are considerably lower now than in 1940, while those of black men and women have increased somewhat. It is more significant, though, that the black and white populations are aging in many fundamentally similar ways, including the higher incidence of marriage now than in 1940, the widening mortality differential that produces many more widows than widowers, the higher rate of remarriage among people whose mates have died, and the greater tendency to be divorced. Most of the variations between elderly blacks and whites are a matter of degree rather than of kind, and the demographic similarities, in turn, suggest that the aging populations of both races have more in common socioeconomically than they did in the past.

Summary

Marital status, family relationships, and living arrangements help determine the content of the older years, so one highly significant fact for those reaching age 65 is the rapid decline in the proportion married and the concomitant increase in the percentage widowed, though the pattern varies greatly for men and women. Consequently, the large majority of elderly men are married and living with their wives, whereas the bulk of elderly women are widows with relatively poor statistical chances for remarriage, even when the social and psychological barriers are surmountable. As expected, these demographic realities become more exaggerated in the oldest age groups, though they also vary between blacks and whites, Hispanics and other ethnic groups, and rural and urban inhabitants.

Widowhood, which affects so many elderly women, is a social and psychological phenomenon that persists for most until they die, for remarriage is limited to a small minority. But even though the remarriage rate is far higher in the group of elderly widowers, there are still certain problems owing to the prevailing myths about love, mate selection, and the desirability of the elderly. Nevertheless, most elderly remarriages do seem to succeed, partly because they help people grapple with the experiences of death and isolation. Despite the incidence of widowhood, however, most couples have far more years of life together after the last child leaves home than did their parents and grandparents.

The functions of a family change with time and the older person comes to relate to them differently, but family ties remain significant for most elderly. Contrary to popular myth, the majority are neither isolated from a family context nor abandoned by family members, though it is not usual for an older person to reside with an adult offspring. That is true even for those whose mates have died and who face living alone, for the norm of independence in American society is a powerful one which, along with other factors, militates against the three- or four-generation family living in one household. But residential separation does not necessarily mean abandonment or emotional isolation, and various family bonds do help most elderly persons contend with the realities of the later years. So do sustained sexual interest and dating among some whose mates are gone.

Institutionalization, chiefly in nursing homes, involves no more than 6 per cent of the elderly population — a proportion that also belies the myth of widespread abandonment by adult children. In fact, the institutional population consists largely of people who are disabled to some degree and have no one to help them with daily tasks. They tend to be extremely old and female. Even the ones with children have not been wantonly abandoned to nursing homes, for most are institutionalized as a last resort after continuing their care at home becomes impossible. That often happens because the caregiver — usually a daughter or daughter-in-law — also is elderly and unable to provide what is necessary. For this and other reasons the institutional population can be expected to increase rapidly, at least for a few decades, although better governmental assistance for home care could slow that increase and help contain its costs.

108

NOTES

1. U.S. Bureau of the Census, "Demographic Aspects of Aging and the Older Population in the United States," *Current Population Reports,* P-23, no. 59 (1978): 45.

2. *Ibid.,* pp. 45; 47.

3. Paul C. Glick, "The Future of the American Family," in U.S. Bureau of the Census, *Current Population Reports,* P-23, no. 78 (1979): 1.

4. *Ibid.*

5. Matilda White Riley and Anne Foner, *Aging and Society,* v. 1, *An Inventory of Research Findings.* New York: Russell Sage Foundation, 1968, p. 158.

6. For the data, see United Nations, *Demographic Yearbook, 1980,* table 34.

7. Henry A. Sheldon, *The Older Population of the United States.* New York: Wiley, 1958, p. 90.

8. U.S. Bureau of the Census, "Demographic Aspects of Aging," *op. cit.,* p. 49.

9. Jacquelyne Johnson Jackson, *Minorities and Aging.* Belmont, CA: Wadsworth, 1980, p. 125.

10. *Ibid.,* p. 136.

11. *Ibid.,* p. 137.

12. National Center for Health Statistics, *Vital Statistics of the United States, 1977,* v. 3, *Marriage and Divorce* (1981), table 1-7.

13. U.S. Bureau of the Census, *op. cit.,* p. 47.

14. Helena Znaniecki Lopata, "The Widowed Family Member," in Nancy Datan and Nancy Lohman, eds., *Transitions of Aging.* New York: Academic Press, 1980, p. 107.

15. Lopata, *ibid.,* p. 108.

16. Lucile Duberman, *Marriage and Its Alternatives.* New York: Praeger, 1974, pp. 200-201.

17. Jessie Bernard, *Remarriage.* New York: Dryden Press, 1956, p. 64.

18. Helena Znaniecki Lopata, "Loneliness: Forms and Components," *Social Problems* 17 (1969): 249.

19. Lopata, "The Widowed Family Member," *op. cit.,* p. 95.

20. *Ibid.,* pp. 98-99. Cf. Richard A. Kalish, "Death and Survivorship: The Final Transition," *Annals of American Academy of Political and Social Science,* 464 (1982): 172-173.

21. Alfred P. Fengler and Nicholas Danigelis, "Residence, the Elderly Widow, and Life Satisfaction," *Research on Aging* 4 (1982): 113.

22. Richard A. Kalish, *Late Adulthood: Perspectives on Human Development.* Monterey, CA: Brooks/Cole, 1975, p. 76.

23. Herman J. Loether, *Problems of Aging.* 2nd ed. Belmont, CA: Dickenson, 1975, p. 16.

24. Elaine M. Brody, "The Aging of the Family," *Annals of American Academy of Political and Social Science,* 438 (1978): 23-24. Cf. Ethel Shanas and Marvin B. Sussman, eds., *Family, Bureaucracy, and the Elderly.* Durham, NC: Duke University Press, 1977.

25. See the work on this matter by Ethel Shanas and Gordon F. Streib, eds., *Social Structure and the Family: Generational Relations*. Englewood Cliffs, NJ: Prentice-Hall, 1965.

26. John E. Dono, Cecilia M. Falbe, Barbara L. Kail, Eugene Litwak, Roger H. Sherman and David Siegel, "Primary Groups in Old Age," *Research on Aging* 1 (1979): 405-406.

27. For studies of this matter, see Timothy H. Brubaker, ed., *Family Relationships in Later Life*. Beverly Hills, CA: Sage, 1983.

28. Mary Barberis, "America's Elderly: Policy Implications," *Population Bulletin* 35 (1981): 12. Cf. Fred C. Pampel, "Changes in the Propensity to Live Alone: Evidence from Consecutive Cross-Sectional Surveys," *Demography* 20 (1983): 433-447.

29. Beth J. Soldo, "America's Elderly in the 1980s," *Population Bulletin* 35 (1980): 26.

30. Elaine M. Brody, statement in House Select Committee on Aging, June 4, 1980, "Families: Aging and Changing," p. 56.

31. Riley and Foner, *op. cit.*, pp. 157 and 162.

32. Brody, "The Aging of the Family," *op. cit.*, p. 14.

33. Alfred Kinsey, Wardell Pomeroy and Clyde Martin, *Sexual Behavior in the Human Male*. Philadelphia: Saunders, 1953.

34. Erdman Palmore, *Social Patterns in Normal Aging: Findings from the Duke Longitudinal Study*. Durham, NC: Duke University Press, 1981, pp. 83-84.

35. For a treatment of this matter, see Mary S. Calderone, "Sex and the Aging," in Ronald Gross, Beatrice Gross and Sylvia Seidman, eds., *The New Old: Struggling for Decent Aging*. Garden City, NY: Doubleday, 1978, pp. 205-208.

36. *Ibid.*, p. 206.

37. Ardyth Stimson, Jane F. Wise and John Stimson, "Sexuality and Self-Esteem Among the Aged," *Research on Aging* 3 (1981): 235-236, 237.

38. Fred Cottrell, *Aging and the Aged*. Dubuque, IA: Wm. C. Brown, 1974, p. 47.

39. Palmore, *op. cit.*, pp. 93-94.

40. Soldo, *op. cit.*, pp. 26-27.

41. For the data, see U.S. Bureau of the Census, "1976 Survey of Institutionalized Persons: A Study of Persons Receiving Long-Term Care," *Current Population Reports*, P-23, no. 69 (1978), table II-6.

42. Al Sirroco, "An Overview of the 1980 National Master Facility Inventory Survey of Nursing and Related Care Homes," in National Center for Health Statistics, *Advance Data from Vital and Health Statistics*, no. 91 (1983).

43. Robert N. Butler, "Ageism," in Kurt Finsterbusch, ed., *Social Problems 82/83*. Guilford, CT: Dushkin, 1982, p. 130.

44. U.S. Bureau of the Census, "1976 Survey of Institutionalized Persons," *op. cit.*, p. 268.

45. Soldo, *op. cit.*, p. 27.

46. Paul R. Voss, "The Increasing Ranks of Elderly Veterans: Where They Will Be in 1990," paper presented to the Southern Regional Demographic Group, Greensboro, NC., October 6-8, 1982.

110

47. *Ibid.,* p. 4.

48. Soldo, *op. cit.,* p. 32.

49. Paul B. Horton and Gerald R. Leslie, *The Sociology of Social Problems.* 7th ed. Englewood Cliffs, NJ: Prentice-Hall, 1981, p. 179.

Chapter 5

The Educational Status of the Older Population

When today's elderly people were young, long years of schooling were a less compelling necessity than they are now and more people left school at an earlier age for a variety of reasons. A sizable part of the older population grew up on farms, where the informal apprenticeship system was a major element in one's education, and other people were diverted from additional schooling by World War I. Still others received inadequate formal education because strained family finances caused them to enter the labor force as soon as possible, especially during the Great Depression in the 1930s, or because the quality of teachers and education was comparatively low in many places, especially the rural areas. Consequently, each succeeding cohort has had more educational opportunities than the one preceding, corresponding to the rise in socioeconomic status of the American population, and each has aspired to and actually achieved higher levels of formal education. This has left the present elderly population with a significantly lower level of educational attainment than exists in the adult population as a whole,[1] and has imposed certain disadvantages on many older people.

Immigration also played a part in the relatively low educational standing of elderly people, though its effect is waning significantly. The huge populations of immigrants who came early in the century averaged less schooling than the native-born population and often didn't acquire much more after they arrived. Instead, they had to find unskilled and semiskilled jobs to support themselves and their families, though many did obtain some "night-school" training, mostly to learn English and achieve citizenship. A few even went farther up the educational ladder. As these large groups of foreign-born people became age 65, their higher rates of

111

illiteracy and lower educational attainment helped depress the average educational status of the elderly population, especially the group that is now 75 and over, while that of the younger population was rising rapidly. The disappearance of the old immigrants now, however, helps account for the rapid increase in the level of educational attainment among the elderly, as does the entry into that group of cohorts who are increasingly better schooled. Most of the latter are native born, but even many in the new groups of immigrants are better educated than their predecessors and tend to enter better jobs. Nonetheless, comparatively low levels of formal schooling are still a major characteristic of the nation's older population. In turn, those levels affect the older person's values, his/her views of the economy and the political system, and the way he/she interacts with intimates; it has much to do with one's ability to keep a job or find new work if necessary.[2]

Levels of Educational Attainment

There are several ways to report the educational accomplishments of a population, including the percentages who cannot read or write, the proportions who have acquired some schooling but too little to master basic skills, and the percentages who have completed various higher grades. Ordinarily, the national data on these matters are provided for people who presumably have completed their formal educations — usually those aged 25 and older — and for various groups beyond that age. If we were to study a whole population rather than merely the elderly, we would also be concerned with school enrollment, retention and dropout rates, and other matters applicable to children, teenagers, and traditional college-age people. But an assessment of the older population and how it compares with other adults needs to focus on outputs from the educational process several decades in the past, and requires that we emphasize educational attainment. Therefore, we will consider the proportions of people who have had no schooling and the ones who are illiterate, those who are functional illiterates, and the groups who are eighth-grade, high school, and college graduates. The median level of education also helps differentiate the various groups within the older population.

Median Years of Schooling Completed

The relatively poor educational showing that elderly people make in comparison with younger groups is illustrated in Table 5-1, which uses the amounts of formal schooling attained by men and women in several age categories. In 1982 the total population aged 25 and older had completed an average of 12.6 years of schooling, which made the average person a high school graduate with a few months of college work. But the average person aged 70-74 had finished only 10.9 years of formal education, and the level dropped progressively into the older years. This comparatively poor showing is the culmination of progressive decreases in formal education at each successive level in the age scale from 25 upward. The oldest people are at a particular disadvantage, however, for in 1982 even the average person 65-69 was a high school graduate.

These patterns apply to both major races, though the average educational levels of the black elderly are substantially below those of whites. There are differences between men and women, too, to be discussed later, but in the older years the gender differential within any one race is usually smaller than the variation between the races.

Table 5-1. Percentages of People with Specified Years of Schooling, by Sex and Age, 1982

Sex and Age	Per Cent Completing			Median Years Completed
	8 Years or Less	High School, 4 or More Years	College, 4 or More Years	
Male				
25+	15.7	71.7	21.9	12.6
55-59	18.6	64.4	19.7	12.4
60-64	24.0	59.9	13.7	12.3
65-69	30.9	51.7	13.2	12.1
70-74	40.1	43.0	12.0	10.9
75+	53.1	33.9	10.3	9.4
Female				
25+	15.6	70.3	14.0	12.5
55-59	16.3	67.1	9.5	12.4
60-64	22.6	61.5	8.3	12.3
65-69	27.8	54.2	8.0	12.1
70-74	36.7	46.0	7.9	10.9
75+	47.7	36.1	6.7	9.4

Source: U.S. Bureau of the Census, "America in Transition: An Aging Society," Current Population Reports, P-23, no. 128 (1983), table 10.

Literacy and Illiteracy

The percentages of people who cannot read or write in any language are supposedly so low in the industrialized countries, that data on illiteracy have not been collected in the decennial census of the United States since 1930. The estimates that do exist place about 0.5 per cent of all people aged 14 and older and 1.4 per cent of those aged 65 and older in the illiterate category, although the official data on the matter undoubtedly underestimate the actual magnitude of the problem among all age groups. At the turn of the century, however, about 17 per cent of the people 65 and over were illiterate, with significantly higher rates for women than for men. That compares with only about 11 per cent in the total population aged 15 and over, and indicates that the lower educational standing of the elderly is no recent phenomenon, though the data may also be distorted by deliberate misreporting of illiteracy by persons who are ashamed of their deficiencies,[3] and by assuming that all people who attend high school become literate. In fact, many do not.

Many of today's illiterate elderly have never attended school, but the illiterate population is not the same as the group that has completed no years of schooling. A considerable share of the latter have learned to read and write on their own or in various special programs that are not included in the reports on school grades completed. That is especially true of many foreign-born people, who did use means other than typical schooling to acquire the language skills necessary to function in jobs that facilitated their move up the social scale or at least provided a living. On the other hand, many illiterate people attended some years of school, but either did not learn to read and write or lost the ability they once had.[4] Therefore, while the percentage of elderly people with no formal schooling is similar to the percentage of illiterates, the two groups are not the same. In fact, among all elderly people who have completed no years of schooling, only about half are classified as illiterate.[5]

Functional Illiteracy

The concept of *functional illiteracy* was first used by the Civilian Conservation Corps in the 1930s and by the army during World War II, and now refers to people who have had less than five years of formal schooling.[6] The concept implies that a person has not had even the minimal formal training in basic language and conceptual skills necessary to manage well in a highly complex and sophisticated society, though in this case, too, some people with less than five years of formal schooling are adequately self-educated. Nonetheless, many functional illiterates of all ages appear near the bottom of the social scale, and they usually lack the ability to command even average incomes or occupy any but the most menial jobs.

Functional illiteracy still afflicts just under 10 per cent of the nation's elderly population, compared with less than a third of that percentage in the whole population aged 25 and older. Moreover, the percentage of functional illiterates rises with age, until it is one-eighth of the group aged 75 and older. In fact, the functionally illiterate population is so heavily concentrated among the elderly that nearly half of all people in that educational class are aged 65 and older, even though elderly people make up only 19 per cent of the population aged 25 and over. A substantial part of the functionally illiterate group has had no schooling at all, amounting to well over a half million older people, or nearly 3 per cent of the entire elderly population.

An Eighth-Grade Education

During the years when today's elderly people were young, an elementary school education was regarded much the same way a high school education is viewed now — the minimum amount of schooling necessary for a reasonably informed person. Therefore, in the face of urgent needs to enter the labor force, a very large proportion of the oldest people completed their formal schooling with graduation from the eighth grade, though that level of achievement is now seriously inadequate and very few young people stop their schooling there. (See Table 5-1.) When those eighth-grade graduates are added to the people who left school in even lower grades, it means that well over a third of the elderly population finished their schooling without ever having gone to high school, contrast-with less than 5 per cent of those aged 25-29. In fact, a high school education was so uncommon for today's oldest people, that half those past age 74 acquired only eighth-grade educations or less. The young-old fare better, but even in that group nearly a third did not go past the eighth grade.

High School and College Graduates

If a relatively small proportion of today's elderly entered high school as young people, even smaller shares graduated and only a tiny minority were able to obtain a college education. Thus, less than half the older population managed to graduate from high school, compared with almost nine-tenths of the 25-29 age group, for whom some college training is now the norm. Once again, the old-old are at the greatest disadvantage, for only a third of the group aged 75 and older graduated from high school. The proportion of the nation's oldest people who graduated from college is less than half the percentage among the total population aged 25 and

116

older, and little more than half that among people aged 55-59. The latter comparison shows how rapidly the educational status of the elderly is changing and illustrates the dramatic increases in the share of college graduates among even the young-old. Elderly people are especially unlikely to have post-graduate educations, although that situation also is changing rather quickly.

Summary

Irrespective of the index, the nation's elderly people have lower levels of schooling than cohorts just behind them, and much lower levels than young adults. The wide discrepancies reflect major changes in attitudes about education and the amount of formal training necessary for entry into the jobs that typify post-industrial America. The variations also mirror the nature of education in the United States, for it is seen largely as a tool to enter the labor force and to advance once in it, rather than as a means to intellectual development for its own sake. Therefore, many of today's elderly acquired only the schooling necessary to hold the semiskilled jobs that awaited them, and they could not afford to invest additional time in their educations. Consequently, many of our least educated elderly people have been by-passed by the knowledge explosion of the last few decades, and some are easily exploited because of their relatively unsophisticated formal educations. Quite a few scrape by on inadequate pensions because they lacked the education to obtain high salaried jobs that would have provided larger retirement incomes. Others are able to cope adequately with the realities of a complex society, but sometimes even they must struggle hard because of educational handicaps.

Educational Differentials

Though the elderly population of the United States ranks far below younger groups in their levels of education, it also has some variations internally, including that between men and women, but especially the discrepancy between blacks and whites. The variations reflect distinct differences in socioeconomic advantages and disadvantages, both in the past and at present, for the level of education is one major indicator of social status. They also reflect the historical definitions of social roles performed by the sexes and the races, because each group encountered differences in the expectations about the value of education, the degree of access to schooling, and the quality of the education provided.

Differences Between Men and Women

Elderly women have somewhat higher average levels of education than elderly men, particularly in the oldest ages. (See Table 5-1.) As a consequence, the men are more likely to be functional illiterates or to have finished their formal schooling with the eighth grade, whereas the women are more apt to have graduated from high school, though they are considerably less likely to be college graduates or to have post-graduate educations. On the average, therefore, elderly men are more heavily represented in the lowest and the highest levels of schooling, whereas women are more heavily concentrated among high school graduates. The net result is a somewhat higher average level of schooling for the women.

These patterns reflect several social conditions when today's elderly were in the traditional school ages. Males were more likely to leave school early or never to enter at all, because of the demands placed on many of them as youngsters to find jobs or to help with farm tasks. Girls were more likely to be excused from those necessities, though some were hurried through their educations to marry and fill the traditional roles of women. Moreover, given the social context in which they were reared, the girls often accepted the discipline of schooling more passively than did the boys and were less likely to drop out. The world wars also kept many young men from finishing their schooling, while more young women were able to continue, at least through high school. At the same time, a four-year college education was thought to be more crucial for men than for women, so a much higher proportion of the men who went to college actually graduated, many of them encouraged by governmental subsidies after World War II. The women, on the other hand, more often found husbands in the first few years of college and dropped out to help support their husbands and to start homes and families, partly because the professional opportunities for college-educated women were relatively limited.

Racial Differences

The educational variations between elderly men and women are far smaller than those between the two major races, because the education of today's elderly black people still bears the mark of "separate-but-equal" schools, in which the quality of education was vastly unequal for the races. (See Table 5-2.) The lower levels attained by blacks also show the results of discrimination in a broader sense, for education was available to fewer blacks than whites; it had less relevance to the immediate needs and future orientations of many enmeshed in Southern agriculture; and it required a large investment of time that many blacks could ill afford to let their children make, given the demands of survival. It is not surprising, therefore, that while the average elderly white person has obtained some high school training, the average elderly black was never able to complete the eighth grade, despite the premium that blacks have long placed on education.

The differential disabilities by race are so great that almost a third of the nation's elderly blacks are functional illiterates, compared with only 7 per cent of the whites. Moreover, while a third of the elderly whites never went beyond elementary school, that is true of two-thirds of the older blacks. Conversely, almost half of the whites but less than a fifth of the blacks are high school graduates. Among college graduates the black-white ratio is even more distorted, for 10 per cent of the whites but only 4 per cent of the blacks have finished at least four years.[7] No matter what the index, the black population suffers very profound disadvantages in its levels of schooling when compared with the white group, and the difference is closely tied to broad income differentials between the races and other components of socioeconomic status. The lower levels of education also make older blacks more vulnerable to exploiters and less able to deal with the social system in ways that are to their advantage. Their retirement years are more apt to be economically deprived, because as workers they lacked the education and the "right" skin color to get the better jobs and had to settle for those that paid low wages and accrued very small retirement benefits, if any. Therefore, many in the elderly black population still suffer the consequences of low educational levels, coupled with other results of the punitive racial discrimination of earlier times.

Most of the educational differences by sex appear in both the white and black populations in that elderly women in both groups have higher average levels of schooling than elderly men. But unlike the case among whites, the percentage of college graduates is higher for black women than for black men, though the latter are more likely to have obtained post-graduate degrees. The higher proportion of female college graduates is related to their use of an elementary or secondary teaching career to climb the social ladder, for that was one of the few channels of upward mobility open when today's elderly black women were young. Since that profession called for some higher education, almost always at a black college or university, black women were somewhat more likely than the men to continue their schooling past the secondary level. Many blacks of both sexes, however, have long felt education to be a way out of various social and economic disadvantages,[8] which helps explain the similar proportions of college graduates among black men and women aged 25-29, and the fact that black college enrollments have been rising faster than those of whites. Eventually the results will appear in the educational status of the elderly black population, and the sexes and both major races are likely to converge in average levels of education.

Education and Marital Status

Levels of education differ substantially by marital status and the patterns vary widely for men and women. Thus, among elderly men the lowest average amount of schooling was obtained by those who are widowed, though single and divorced men also have comparatively low levels. In all three groups the average man has completed only the ninth grade or less. Married men, on the other hand, have substantially greater average amounts of formal schooling, though educationally the men still rank significantly below the women in each marital status category. Among women, those who are single have substantially more schooling than any other marital status group, and the average single woman is a

Table 5-2. Percentages of People With Specified Years of Schooling, by Race and Age, 1982

Race and Age	Per Cent Completing			Median Years Completed
	8 Years or Less	High School, 4 or More Years	College, 4 or More Years	
White				
25+	14.7	72.8	18.5	12.6
55-59	14.9	69.1	15.2	12.5
60-64	20.9	63.6	11.4	12.3
65-69	25.9	56.5	10.8	12.2
70-74	35.2	47.6	10.3	11.3
75+	47.3	37.2	8.5	9.4
Black				
25+	24.8	54.9	8.8	12.2
55-59	38.8	35.9	4.9	10.3
60-64	45.4	33.2	3.8	9.7
65-69	59.0	21.0	4.7	8.4
70-74	65.9	18.9	3.0	7.9
75+	74.0	15.4	3.4	6.6

Source: U.S. Bureau of the Census, "America in Transition: An Aging Society," Current Population Reports, P-23, no. 128 (1983), table 10.

high school graduate with a few months of college study. Widows have the lowest levels of education, while married women and those who are divorced share the same level, intermediate between those who are single and those who are widowed.

What are some of the reasons for these differences, especially the relatively high educational levels of single women? When today's elderly people were young, marriage usually ended a woman's formal schooling as she assumed home duties and family roles on a full-time basis. Therefore, the woman who did not marry had a better chance to continue in school. At the same time, the wish for more education also caused some women to postpone marriage, and a share of them never married at all. In both cases, however, education and marriage proved mutually exclusive for many of today's elderly women, and schooling usually stopped in the same year that marriage took place. Men were not quite as likely to terminate their educations after marriage, so the highest levels of education are found not among single men, but those who are married and whose wives often worked to help them through college. Furthermore, the higher average age at first marriage among men allowed them about two additional years in which to continue with schooling before assuming domestic responsibilities. Not many people of either sex, though, seem to have been permanently deterred from marriage by having a particular level of schooling, for the percentages of men and women who eventually married vary only a little from one educational level to another.

The low levels of education in the elderly widowed populations of both sexes are closely associated with general socioeconomic status. The older people who are poor or who come from poor backgrounds generally received the smallest amounts of schooling when they were young, either because it seemed unrelated to their needs or because they had to seek jobs as soon as possible, though for some it simply was not available. In many cases, the quality of education was low anyway and did little to encourage continued attendance, particularly if families didn't see much value in it. Now many of those same people are still relatively poor and they have higher rates of widowhood at earlier ages than the more affluent members of the older population. Therefore, widows and widowers of both races are the most poorly educated of the marital status categories. In addition, the proportions of widowed people are much higher in the oldest ages than in those just past 65, and the older the group, the lower its average level of education.

Trends in Education

The educational attainment of elderly Americans is rising quite rapidly, just as it has been for the total population, because younger people with more schooling are aging into the 65-and-over group and the older ones with less education are dying.[9] Moreover, the various age groups will become more alike in educational achievement, for the rate of improvement among people under age 65 is slowing down and the more rapid advances among the elderly will allow the schooling gap to close, perhaps in 10 years or so. Graduation from high school and some college training is the median level of attainment now for people between age 65 and 69, and within a decade or so it will probably be so far those aged 70 and older as well. It is necessary to remember, though, that the median figure divides the population in half and that many in the lower half will still be poorly educated, some of them in the ranks of functional illiterates, premature dropouts, and unlearned victims of "social promotion." In that sense, there will still be ample challenge to educate many adults.

The progress that is occurring represents dramatic reductions in illiteracy among the elderly population, from 17 per cent in 1900 to 1.4 per cent now. This seems to portend its virtual elimination, because those unable to read and write are more heavily concentrated than ever before among the oldest people, who will soon die. But there are still substantial numbers of illiterates to replace them, despite educational improvements in the population as a whole, and significant numbers if not percentages of the future elderly population will be illiterate if there are not improvements in educational achievement among younger people.

The rapid rise in educational standing among older people is also reflected in all of the other indexes that are used to measure attainment. For example, the median years of schooling of the population aged 65-69 rose from 8.2 in 1940 to 12.1 at present as a result of substantial increases among blacks and whites and men and women, though the four groups improved at different rates. Furthermore, people aged 65-69 experienced greater improvement than their elders, especially between 1970 and 1982. (See Table 5-3.) Much of that rapid change is due to better-educated younger people entering the 65-69 age range and to losses of the more poorly schooled old immigrants, people with farm backgrounds, and unskilled and semiskilled workers in early twentieth-century industries. The improvements are showing up in the age groups above 70 as well, basically for the same reasons, though the rate of change is slower than among people aged 65-69. The trends suggest that all groups of older people will soon have far higher average levels of schooling than their predecessors, but also that the rate of improvement will slow down considerably, because that has already happened in much of the population under age 65.

122

Trends by Sex

The rates of educational improvement during much of the 1940-1982 period were greater for women than for men, but by the latter year the only significant difference in median years of schooling was that between the oldest men and women. In the ages 65-69 there was no variation, and as the present oldest groups disappear, so will the sex discrepancy in levels of education. (See Table 5-3.) Nevertheless, women are still less likely than men to be functional illiterates or merely eighth-grade graduates, while they are more likely to be high school graduates or to have attained one to three years of college. Older men are still significantly

Table 5-3. Changes in the Median Years of School Completed, by Sex and Age, 1940-1982

Sex and Age	1940	1950	1960	1970	1982
Male					
25+	8.6	9.0	10.3	12.1	12.6
55-59	8.2	8.4	8.7	10.7	12.4
60-64	8.2	8.3	8.5	9.6	12.3
65-69	8.1	8.1	8.3	8.8	12.1
70-74	8.0	8.0	8.1	8.6	10.5
75+	7.7	7.9	8.0	8.3	8.9
Female					
25+	8.7	9.6	10.7	12.1	12.5
55-59	8.4	8.6	9.0	11.1	12.4
60-64	8.3	8.4	8.7	10.4	12.3
65-69	8.2	8.3	8.5	9.1	12.1
70-74	8.2	8.3	8.4	8.8	10.9
75+	8.1	8.2	8.3	8.6	9.4

Sources: U.S. Bureau of the Census, U.S. Census of Population: 1950, Detailed Characteristics, U.S. Summary (1953), table 115; U.S. Census of Population: 1960, Detailed Characteristics, U.S. Summary (1964), table 173; U.S. Census of Population: 1970, Detailed Characteristics, U.S. Summary (1973), table 199; "America in Transition: An Aging Society," Current Population Reports, P-23, no. 128 (1983), table 10.

more likely to be college graduates, but that gap between the sexes is diminishing. It will widen again, however, at least for awhile, because the proportion of women aged 40-59 with four or more years of college is scarcely more than half that of men. In the age group under 40 the proportions of college graduates in both sexes are more nearly alike, and in the ages 25-29 about a quarter of the men and a fifth of the women have completed four or more years of college. Therefore, when those people eventually reach 65, the male-female gap at the highest level of schooling will narrow again, though men will still have some advantage. By that time the average man and woman aged 65-69 will be a high school graduate with at least one year of college.

Trends by Race

The huge educational disadvantage experienced by elderly black people in the United States has been diminishing rapidly and their average levels of education are more like those of whites than they were in 1940. In that year, for example, the median years of schooling completed by blacks aged 65-69 was far less than half that for whites, but by 1982 the difference had been reduced to less than a third. (See Table 5-4.) Black women experienced an especially rapid rate of improvement, making their pace of increase in median years of schooling the greatest of the four race and sex categories. Elderly black people were not able to overcome functional illiteracy at the same rate as white people, however, owing to the great educational disadvantages when the former were young. Moreover, while the percentage of older whites who completed their eductions with the eighth grade dropped between 1940 and 1982, that of blacks rose, because even that modest level of educational attainment represents an improvement over the high rates of illiteracy and functional illiteracy that prevailed in 1940. Beyond the eighth-grade level, older blacks have also moved ahead rapidly, for the percentage of high school graduates has increased faster for blacks than for whites, as has that of college graduates, including people who go on to post-graduate education. Thus, every index shows that the elderly black population has progressed faster than the white segment in raising the level of education, though blacks had a far greater initial disadvantage to overcome.

As a result of these improvements, the older members of both races have converged some in educational standing, though the blacks still rank substantially below the whites on every measure. Furthermore, black women have been making faster progress than black men, thereby adding to their initial educational advantage over the men. Thus, at each census since 1940, elderly black women have been less represented than black men in the group of functional illiterates and they are rising out of that low

124

status at a faster rate. The women are more likely to have gone to college and to have finished four years than are the men; the women are even enjoying more rapid increases in the percentages who obtain college and post-graduate degrees. Therefore, given these changes, elderly black men remain the least well-educated group in American society, and while their levels are rising faster than those of whites, who are already much better educated on the average, they are not keeping pace with the improvements among black women.

Table 5-4. Changes in the Median Years of School
            Completed, by Race and Age, 1940-1982

Race and Age	1940	1950	1960	1970	1982
White					
25+	8.8	9.6	10.8	12.1	12.6
55-59	8.4	8.6	9.0	11.3	12.5
60-64	8.3	8.4	8.7	10.4	12.3
65-69	8.2	8.3	8.5	9.3	12.2
70-74	8.2	8.3	8.4	8.9	11.3
75+	8.1	8.2	8.3	8.6	9.4
Black					
25+	5.8	6.9	8.3	9.8	12.2
55-59	4.7	5.5	6.5	8.1	10.3
60-64	4.4	5.1	6.0	7.5	9.7
65-69	3.8	4.3	5.2	6.6	8.4
70-74	2.8	4.1	5.2	6.0	7.9
75+	1.2	3.3	4.9	5.7	6.6

Sources: U.S. Bureau of the Census, U.S. Census of Population: 1950, Detailed Characteristics, U.S. Summary (1953), table 115; U.S. Census of Population: 1960, Detailed Characteristics, U.S. Summary (1964), table 173; U.S. Census of Population: 1970, Detailed Characteristics, U.S. Summary (1973), table 199; "America in Transition: An Aging Society," Current Population Reports, P-23, no. 128 (1983), table 10.

Some Projections

As each younger cohort with its higher level of education moves into the elderly group, the overall average in the older population will continue to rise dramatically, though not indefinitely. At the same time, the rise in educational attainment will slow considerably among people under age 65, because some age groups are already getting about all the formal schooling it is practical to obtain, and that fact will help narrow the educational gap between older and younger Americans.

All of the people who will reach age 65 in the first several decades of the twenty-first century are now alive, and most of those 25 and over have obtained the bulk of formal education they will ever receive. Therefore, as each cohort enters the older category in the future, the average levels of education in that older group will be approximately the one which exists now in the several younger cohorts. In fact, it will even be a little higher, because the people with the poorest educations also tend to have the highest death rates and are least likely to seek more schooling as adults. These realities make it possible to project the median years of schooling among elderly people until 2020, when the group aged 25-29 in 1980 will have reached the ages 65-69. Table 5-5 provides the data on this matter.

The deficiencies in education among older people will continue to decrease through the period and the medians will rise, but not at the rates that prevailed between 1960 and 1980. Therefore, by 1990 the educational gap between people aged 65-69 and all those who are younger will have narrowed very significantly, though the elderly will still remain somewhat behind the younger population and the oldest groups will lag most severely. Moreover, the educational differential between the sexes will decrease and men may even hold a slight advantage, largely because they are still more likely than women to complete college and to seek postgraduate educations. By 2020, however, the average person aged 65-69 of each sex will be a high school graduate with a year or so of college education.

Black and white elderly people also will grow more alike in levels of schooling, as the oldest blacks with the severest educational handicaps are replaced by younger ones whose formal schooling has increased greatly in the past couple of decades. It will be at least 2000, though, before the average black person aged 65-69 will be a high school graduate. White men and women will become more similar in average levels of schooling, as will blacks of both sexes, though white men are apt to hold a slight lead over white women, while black women will probably retain a slight edge over black men.

All of the trends and projections suggest that the huge educational disadvantage of elderly people relative to younger ones will diminish sharply and that the large proportions of poorly schooled older Americans will not be duplicated in future generations. Nonetheless, even though serious educational deficiences among the elderly may not be permanent, they will still affect a sizable share of that group, especially people 75 and over, for several years, while some in all of the elderly ages will continue to need additional education. But even if better continuing education were provided for those people, it would come too late for many because their ability to contend with reality was shaped long ago, and some will be unable to overcome many of the educational deficiences of that time. Many also lack the self-confidence that would enable them to capitalize on additional education, tending instead to accept current constraints as inevitable. But there is a significant population of older people who can stretch their intellects, learn new skills and ideas, and expand their ability to manipulate their immediate environments. For them, adult education is a large-scale need not being fully met, and it remains for colleges and universities to compensate for the decling pool of traditional-age students by providing more useful and attractive services to older adults. That will long be so.

Table 5-5. Projections of Median Years of School Completed by Cohorts Reaching Age 65-69 in Specified Years, by Race and Sex

Race and Sex	1990	2000	2010	2020
All Races				
Male	12.4	12.5	12.8	13.0
Female	12.3	12.4	12.6	12.8
White				
Male	12.5	12.6	12.8	13.2
Female	12.4	12.5	12.6	12.9
Black				
Male	8.9	11.8	12.5	12.5
Female	9.7	11.7	12.3	12.6

Source: U.S. Bureau of the Census, "Educational Attainment in the United States: March 1979 and 1978," Current Population Reports, P-20, no. 356 (1980), table 1.

Educational Needs of the Elderly

The relationship betwen aging and education really involves three aspects: (1) education of people at all ages about the process of aging; (2) education of specialists who will work closely with the elderly and their needs; and (3) education of older people themselves, especially continuing education through all of the later years.[10] Important as the first two are, in this section we will focus on the educational needs of the elderly themselves.

Why Educate the Elderly?

It is too easy to regard the progress in educational levels among older people as an excuse to write off the present group of poorly schooled elderly. In fact, many of those inadequately educated people will be around for a decade or more and some will be replaced by other elderly with educational deficiences, for not all younger people are receiving adequate educations. Consequently, insufficient schooling will continue to work to the disadvantage of many older *individuals* even in the time when *average* levels come to resemble those of the total population. Those for whom levels of education remain low are heir to various social problems, because they are the most likely to suffer from poor health, improper nutrition, inadequate housing, fear of crime, exploitation, and loneliness, though the cause-and-effect relationships of these factors are very complex. Moreover, the deficient educational standing of many elderly persons originally forced them into unskilled and semiskilled jobs that later produced very small or even no retirement benefits, and there is every reason to re-educate at least some of them for jobs that will supplement incomes and diminish that initial handicap. Low levels of education even reduce the ability of older people to seek help with their problems, because it is difficult for the least educated to find out about assistance and to contend with the agencies that supply it.[11] In short, the social, technical, and financial resources of many older people are insufficient to meet the demands of a complex society,[12] and education is one fundamental way to enhance those resources. Moreover, as the proportion of workers in their 50s and beyond increases, the society will need to modernize their skills if those people are to maintain their productivity or switch to new jobs in order to help maintain a healthy economy.[13]

Low levels of education also contribute to inadequate self-confidence for many older people, whereas the better-educated ones tend to be more positive about themselves and to have greater confidence in their mental and physical abilities.[14] Many of the poorly educated have little faith in their ability to make decisions and they become cautious and even withdrawn, partly because they lack the information and skills necessary to function in a contemporary culture that requires many sophisticated decisions. In fact, a substantial part of the aging process for many elderly people is progressive social disengagement,[15] in which a lack of confidence in one's ability to interact productively plays a large part, though not all older people succumb to it. Considering that more than a third of today's elderly never got past the eighth grade, it isn't surprising that many lack confidence in their own abilities, despite decades of experience and productivity.

Few of the learning problems that elderly people encounter seem to result from decreases in the level of intelligence, for the ability to learn declines less with aging than was formerly thought and fewer specific areas are subject to such reductions.[16] The declines that do occur tend to come very late in life and often as a result of illness, such as Alzheimer's Disease. Therefore, the limited skill level of many elderly people, which reduces their ability to make productive use of their innate intelligence, is largely a consequence of the social rather than the physiological process of aging.

Some older people with those limitations need new skills to cope with life, while others require more satisfactory ways to use the skills they have, along with additional opportunities to be useful. The potential in this area is so great that some of the gradual wasting that often accompanies aging could be reduced or even largely undone if adequate education were available for the elderly.[17] Even the physiological declines associated with aging, such as those involving sensory abilities and physical mobility, need not reduce the motivation or ability to learn new things, to remember, and to respond intelligently, for those are the real keys to educational success among older people.[18] Consequently, education for the elderly can provide better skills to cope with daily living, create new ways to employ the skills one has, and overcome some of the psychological constraints that may accompany the aging process. Additional education is particularly useful to the individual if he/she believes it will improve status or ability, whereas those who feel they can achieve no higher level generally lose much of the incentive for additional learning as they age.[19] Thus, the prospect of a tangible payoff is strategic if the older person is to seek additional education.

Education is also one way to deal with the personal tragedies that come to most elderly people. When a spouse is seriously ill or dies, new activities may produce some relief and solace, and the very involvement in an educational program can be one of those new activities, regardless of the precise things one learns. But some educational experiences also provide coping skills directly, and can be far more than just a way to stay busy.

Responses to the Need for Education

To deal with some of these needs, there is a relatively new movement in education that has impelled one of every five colleges and universities toward education for older adults.[20] Most of the programs, which are free of grades and formal degrees as credentials to enter the labor force, involve learning for its own sake. In that respect, the adult programs have a basic component that has been uncommon in American education,[21] for they encourage learning as a process rather than as the expedient accumulation of information.[22] They also help older adults overcome the obsolescence of some of their early education, obtained when the content of schooling differed markedly from what it is now. In fact, not only are older adults poorly educated relative to younger groups, but some aspects of their educations are so remote in time as to be irrelevant.[23] Moreover, not all of what one needs for a lifetime can possibly be learned in 12 or 16 years of schooling, recent or not. Therefore, adult education programs can also streamline the knowledge that elderly people are using, thereby supplementing rich experiences that facilitate interpretation and adaptation, and encouraging the concept of lifetime learning. The growth of such programs also tends to accelerate as the average level of schooling of the elderly rises, because the more education a person has, the more likely he/she is to seek additional training,[24] whether in formal schooling, self-education, or other endeavors. Thus, because each successive cohort has more education than the one just before it, each is also more apt to get involved in adult education programs, and there is every prospect the latter will grow substantially.

In order to provide a rationale for the emerging programs and especially to articulate specific needs, in 1980 the National Council on the Aging formulated several recommendations for educators and governments, based on the assumption that the elderly will become increasingly interested in educational opportunities.[25] They are intended to do the following:

1. Promote the concept of lifelong learning.

2. Create opportunities specifically suited to older people that educate them not merely in tangible skills, but in "the arts and humanities, self-development, retirement-related skills and knowledge, civic issues and advocacy techniques, and career education in human services (particularly services to the elderly)."[26]

3. Provide education for the elderly at little or no cost in order to compensate for the fixed incomes on which many live.

4. Use settings apart from the normal classroom in order to bring education to the places where elderly people congregate, such as churches and senior centers.

5. Encourage school systems to use specialists in education for older people.

6. Promote research on the variable educational needs of older people in different ethnic groups and classes.

7. Introduce into high school and college curricula, courses on the aging of persons and the whole population.

If these recommendations are followed, many of the needs and interests of the elderly will be met by offerings that help overcome their educational liabilities, and knowledge of the aging process will become a sufficiently pervasive part of the whole educational system for the community to grow more aware of the needs of elderly people.[27] Both accomplishments would reduce substantially the educational gap that now separates much of the older population from many younger groups. The formal educational levels among younger people might still remain higher than those among the elderly, but the absolute deficiencies of many older people would diminish significantly and the two groups would have a better basis for communication to minimize the age clash that may well accompany the rising burden of support for the growing elderly population. Comprehensive adult education has a role to play in these areas, especially in a rapidly changing society where time renders the formal education of any generation partly obsolete long before that generation dies, no matter how effective the schooling may have been initially. In that sense, adult education will be necessary not just for the present group of elderly who were relatively poorly educated as youth, but for upcoming generations of older people who received much better schooling but who will need to remain current. That will be especially important for older workers who wish to stay in the labor force, though timeliness is a significant social skill for others as well.[28]

For the elderly or any other group, education needs to be continuous in order to hone intellectual skills. Given the tendency to perceive schooling only as a tool one acquires to enter the labor force, education is often viewed as something to be "done with," and many elderly see themselves beyond the time when education can be "useful." Therefore, education for them needs to be a lifelong process that provides not employment primarily, but insight into the aging process itself and the equipment necessary to carry on a range of activities in the older years. Moreover, if older people are to seek and use continuing education, they need a high chance of success in those endeavors, partly because failure would further shake the self-confidence of many and discourage them from additional educational efforts.[29]

They must also perceive a need for the education. That is more common among better-educated older people than among the poorly educated who actually have the greatest need. The latter often feel useless and unwanted, and while education might help restore their sense of personal worth, they are the ones least motivated to return to school. Therefore, continuing education should provide not just classes, but also a way to catch the interest and imagination of the elderly and to give them a clear picture of the benefits to be obtained from re-entry into the educational process. Once that is accomplished, continuing education can teach the skills and insights to help make the elderly feel more needed, useful, and positive about themselves, and can improve the chances that their new skills and interests actually will produce suitable rewards.[30] The elderly are too valuable a resource to be wasted because of inadequate education and the disabilities it imposes, and much of that waste can be reduced with appropriate motivation, educational programs that meet real needs, and satisfying rewards for educational pursuits.[31]

Summary

Elderly people have significantly lower average levels of education than younger ones, because they bear the imprint of a time when education was less available, less valued, and less important than the need to earn wages. In addition, the large immigrant population of the early twentieth century usually had little schooling, and they still affect the educational standing of the oldest people. In turn, deficient education tends to aggravate other problems, and many elderly lack the basic skills to cope successfully with a complex society and even the aging process itself. Consequently, even though the level of education is rising rapidly as better-educated cohorts age into the elderly category, there are still large numbers of older Americans whose lives are seriously constrained by their poor educational levels.

The elderly make a relatively poor showing on all of the measures of educational status: They average fewer years of schooling completed than do younger people; they are more likely to be illiterates or functional illiterates; they are less likely to have completed the eighth grade or to have graduated from high school or college. As a result, the vast expansion of knowledge, computerization, and robotics has by-passed many, while others have educations that are too obsolete to allow them useful access to these changes. Some are disengaged from all but the narrowest of social interaction and lack even the social, psychological, and technical skills to resist exploiters, understand available services, or plan meaningful activities. That group is at once most in need of continuing education and least likely to obtain it, partly because the better-educated elderly are the ones who seek even more training.

Within the older population, women have somewhat higher average levels of education than men because fewer women have eighth-grade educations or less, while more are high school graduates and have attended college. The men, however, are more likely to have finished college. Blacks have far lower educational levels than whites, owing largely to the old segregated, low-quality school systems and to the lesser relevance that education had for blacks in the rural South.

The level of formal schooling among America's elderly is rising very rapidly as younger, better-educated cohorts reach age 65. Consequently, the gap between the various age groups has narrowed substantially and will nearly disappear within a decade or so. This progress represents major reductions of illiteracy, a dramatic decline in functional illiteracy, and a significant increase in the proportions of older people with high school and college educations. The improvements were especially marked after 1960 as younger people became 65 and the oldest groups, containing many with immigrant or farm backgrounds, lost members. Furthermore, the rate of improvement has been greater for blacks than for whites, which is gradually decreasing the educational gap between these races. In the first two decades of the next century, most of the great educational differences between them may well become minor, though elderly whites will still have a slight advantage.

Despite the improvements, many older persons still have important needs that can be met by continuing education, provided it is geared to those needs and the elderly can be motivated to use it. If so, education can help older people overcome various social problems that often accompany aging and can contribute to a stronger self-image. In fact, part of the presumed process of aging itself, including indecisiveness, caution, withdrawal, and a feeling of uselessness, can be moderated by meaningful education that provides new skills and helps the older person understand the aging process. Too many older people have wasted away intellectually, not because of declines in their native intelligence, but because they have become obsolete. In a society that deplores obsolescence and readily affixes that label, continuing education has a high mission to save many of the elderly for a better fate.

NOTES

1. U.S. Bureau of the Census, "America in Transition: An Aging Society," *Current Population Reports,* P-23, no. 128 (1983): 21.

2. Lowell Eklund, "Aging and the Field of Education," in Matilda White Riley, John W. Riley, Jr. and Marilyn E. Johnson, eds., *Aging and Society,* v. 2, *Aging and the Professions.* New York: Russell Sage Foundation, 1969, p. 325.

3. John K. Folger and Charles B. Nam, *Education of the American Population.* Washington, DC: U.S. Government Printing Office, 1967, p. 122.

4. *Ibid.,* pp. 125-126.

5. U.S. Bureau of the Census, "Illiteracy in the United States: November 1969," *Current Population Reports,* P-20, no. 217 (1971): 9.

133

6. Folger and Nam, *op. cit.*, p. 126.

7. U.S. Bureau of the Census, "America in Transition...," *op. cit.*, pp. 21-22.

8. Paul E. Zopf, Jr., *Population: An Introduction to Social Demography.* Palo Alto, CA: Mayfield, 1984, p. 376.

9. U.S. Bureau of the Census, "America in Transition...," *loc. cit.*

10. Irving L. Webber, "The Educable Aged," in J.C. Dixon, ed., *Continuing Education in the Later Years.* Gainesville, FL: University of Florida Press, 1963, p. 14.

11. Beth J. Soldo, "America's Elderly in the 1980s," *Population Bulletin* 35 (1980): 19.

12. Webber, *op. cit.*, p. 15.

13. Robert L. Clark, Juanita Kreps and Joseph J. Spengler, "Aging Population: United States," in John A. Ross, ed., *International Encyclopedia of Population.* v. 1. New York: Free Press, 1982, p. 38.

14. Louis Harris & Associates, "Myths About Life for Older Americans," in Ronald Gross, Beatrice Gross and Sylvia Seidman, eds., *The New Old: Struggling for Decent Aging.* Garden City, NY: Doubleday, 1978, p. 103.

15. Kurt W. Back and Kenneth J. Gergen, "Cognitive Constriction in Aging and Attitudes Toward International Issues," in Ida Harper Simpson and John C. McKinney, eds., *Social Aspects of Aging.* Durham, NC: Duke University Press, 1966, p. 323. Cf. Elaine Cumming and William E. Henry, *Growing Old: The Process of Disengagement.* New York: Basic Books, 1961.

16. Robert N. Butler, "Ageism," in Kurt Finsterbusch, ed., *Social Problems 82/83.* Guilford, CT: Dushkin, 1982, p. 128.

17. Eklund, *op. cit.*, p. 324.

18. *Ibid.*, pp. 331; 333.

19. Matilda White Riley and Anne Foner, *Aging and Society.* v. 1, *An Inventory of Research Findings.* New York: Russell Sage Foundation, 1968, p. 440.

20. Ronald Gross, "I Am Still Learning," in Gross, Gross and Seidman, *op. cit.*, p. 364.

21. *Ibid.*

22. Eklund, *op. cit.*, p. 327.

23. Riley and Foner, *op. cit.*, p. 116.

24. *Ibid.*, p. 117.

25. The recommendations are adapted from National Council on the Aging, "NCOA Public Policy Agenda," *Perspective on Aging* 9 (1980): 28-29.

26. *Ibid.*, p. 29.

27. Joseph Drake, *The Aged in American Society.* New York: Ronald Press, 1958, p. 397.

28. Joseph J. Spengler, "Some Economic and Related Determinants Affecting the Older Worker's Occupational Role," in Simpson and McKinney, *op. cit.*, p. 13.

29. Eklund, *op. cit.*, pp. 335-336.

30. *Ibid.*, pp. 338-339.

31. One approach to education for older people is Patricia Harper Apt and Roger Heimstra, ''A Model for Learning Resource Networks for Senior Adults,'' *Educational Gerontology* 5 (1980): 163-173.

Chapter 6

Work Characteristics
Of the Elderly

The work roles of elderly people, especially men, have changed substantially in the twentieth century, and the large majority have become a non-working population. In 1900, for example, more than two-thirds of the men aged 65 and older were still in the labor force, because both the economic system and their families needed them to be producers and there were few alternatives, while at present less than one-fifth are in the work force. Moreover, older people make up a steadily declining proportion of the whole working population and now account for less than 4 per cent of all employed. At the same time, the opportunity and pressure to retire have both increased, and large numbers leave the labor force because they want and can afford more leisure, while others are forced out by mandatory retirement provisions.[1] Some others suffer health problems that cause them to stop working. Furthermore, there is some pressure from younger workers for older ones to make way and it contributes to the substantial increase in the retired population; that pressure is often a factor in the mandatory retirement provisions negotiated by industries and unions. Despite various negative consequences and the need to make adjustments, however, the elderly generally have positive attitudes about retirement, unless income is a significant problem, and a sense of job deprivation seems less common than popular myth would have it.[2]

As a result of the rapidly growing retired population, including many who have not yet reached age 65, there is a heavy financial load on pension systems and the people who must underwrite them now and in the future, sometimes creating crises in those systems, including Social

Security.[3] It is a burden the society imposes on itself because of forced retirement policies, but one we may be unable to afford much longer as a financial constraint, a waste of skills and experience, and a form of discrimination against those elderly persons who need jobs to earn adequate incomes.

This situation is currently under close scrutiny, partly in light of the limited job opportunities for young workers who also need to be accommodated in the labor force, and partly as a result of the Social Security crisis. Certainly a more rational sorting process is needed in which those older people who are able and wish to work can continue without stigma, penalty, or pressure to retire; change in the mandatory retirement age is a step in that direction. At the same time, larger proportions of workers are choosing to retire early, mostly at age 62 but sometimes earlier, although that trend was slowed by the recession and inflation of the late 1970s and early 1980s. If the trend picks up again, however, it may precipitate substantial increases in the minimum age to receive Social Security benefits in order to keep the older worker on the job, perhaps until age 68 or 70, not just 67 as now projected for 2027. But such a change would be contrary to the preferences of workers who wish to retire earlier and would reduce the job opportunities for younger people, especially first-time entrants into the work force and those whose lack of seniority makes them the first fired during layoffs. Some of these dilemmas have come about because the work ethic has relaxed for many people and because retirement programs make it financially attractive to retire early, while changes in birth and death rates have enlarged the numbers and proportions of older workers available to claim retirement benefits.

Thus, even though work roles no longer have the same meaning they had when today's elderly entered the labor force, a large share of older people must survive on significantly lower incomes than the wages they earned, many because they have been cut off involuntarily from the opportunity to work. For some that severance causes feelings of uselessness, a decline in self-confidence, and uncertainty as they are converted from producers to pensioners. Their problems also tend to be reinforced by the larger society, which assumes that the aging process makes a person an ineffective or a hazardous employee, even though the older worker is usually able to meet existing occupational demands and adapt to new ones, provided he/she is appropriately rewarded. Furthermore, there is a tendency to overestimate the problems of retired people and to underestimate their successful adjustments, and to ignore the large proportions who prefer retirement to employment, including many who were forced out of their jobs.

Older People in the Labor Force

Participation Rates

A nation's potential labor force, or economically active population, includes all people who are available by age or other criteria to be employed in organized economic endeavors,[4] whether or not they are actually working. The actual labor force is the proportion of that group who are employed and the ones who are unemployed but actively seeking work. In the United States the labor force consists of all people aged 16 and over who are employed in civilian jobs, those who are unemployed but available for work, and members of the armed services,[5] though we will focus on civilians. Within that group, the elderly labor force consists of people aged 65 and older who meet the other criteria, though part of our analysis will also refer to people aged 55-64, because changes in work roles often take place during those years.

Moreover, the *labor force participation rate* of the elderly is a ratio of the number actually in the labor force to the total population aged 65 and over. In 1981, for example, 3 million of the 25 million noninstitutionalized elderly were still in the labor force, producing a rate of 12 per cent. That figure represents a steady decline from the younger ages. Among men, labor force participation reaches a peak of 95 per cent in the ages 35-44 and then drops steadily, while among women in those ages it rises to 70 per cent and then declines, though the patterns do differ by race. (See Figure 6-1.) Until the mid-1970s, women's participation fell during the childrearing years and then rose to another peak in the late 30s and early 40s,[6] but those fluctuations have now diminished and the rate remains relatively steady in the ages 20-44 and then begins to decline. For men, the participation rate remains relatively high through their 50s and then begins its downward plunge, largely because of voluntary retirements, though some men are unable to work for various reasons. (See Table 6-1.) For women, the participation rate falls significantly by age 60. In 1981 these changes left 1.8 million elderly men and 1.2 elderly women in the labor force, but the participation rates of both sexes were quite low compared with those of younger people. Many elderly of both sexes who are still working are employed in low-paying, low-status jobs, mostly because they need the income,[7] though some are also self-employed or high-salaried people of considerable value to their employers, and who work beyond the age when most others retire.

The official participation rates actually underestimate the numbers and proportions of older people who work for wages during the year. The data on labor force involvement reflect the number of jobs filled at the time the surveys are taken, but they leave out the people who are not working then

138

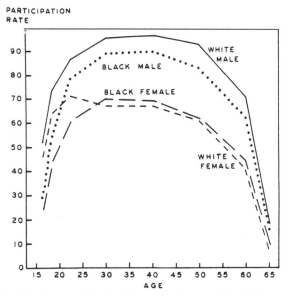

Figure 6-1. Labor Force Participation Rate, by Age, Race, and Sex, 1981
Source: U.S. Bureau of Labor Statistics, *Labor Force Statistics Derived from the Current Population Survey: A Databook*, v. 1 (1982), tables A-3; A-4.

but who have worked at some time during the 12-month period. That is a particularly significant omission among older people, because sizable numbers are employed on a part-time or part-year basis, often to earn the maximum amount before Social Security benefits are reduced, and those workers do not usually figure in the data.[*8*] Therefore, perhaps as many as a quarter or more of the older people who have worked during a year are not represented in the official participation rates. Moreover, the rates would be higher if all older people who wanted jobs could get them.[*9*]

Leaving the Labor Force

The age variations in labor force participation rates reflect the complex social process by which elderly people vacate work roles, whether or not by choice, and assume others. In certain respects, the older person now separates from the role of worker more abruptly than in the past, when larger proportions were self-employed in agriculture and other fields and could remain partially productive longer. Now more workers are employed in large corporations that specify a uniform retirement age that makes the change from worker to pensioner relatively abrupt and, for some, traumatic.[*10*]

The process of removal from the labor force has subtle dynamics that actually begin in the 40s and 50s and push the worker toward retirement in the early to mid-60s. For example, the worker may find that after a certain age promotions are less likely, either because he/she has attained the maximum level or is passed over in favor of a younger person. In addition, the revolutionary technological changes in some industries make it difficult for some older workers to keep pace and thus make retirement a welcome relief from a frustrating struggle. The aging employee's salary also may not rise as rapidly as those of younger workers, often because supervisors accept the stereotype of lower performance levels among older workers.

Whatever the specific reasons, however, retirement is frequently preceded by a certain amount of disengagement for the worker in his/her 50s and early 60s, when the rewards go to younger people who can be hired more cheaply. Then, actual retirement simply culminates several antecedent events.[11] Many of them are unrelated to the older worker's actual performance or capacity, but reflect the beliefs and attitudes in America's occupational structure, though many people approaching retirement welcome progressive separation from work roles. Moreover, the mass exodus of older workers from the labor force occurs in the early to mid-60s, despite the Age Discrimination in Employment Act of 1967 and other legal

Table 6-1. Labor Force Participation Rates, by Age, Race, and Sex, 1981

Race and Sex	55-59	60-64	65+
All Races			
Male	81.2	58.5	18.4
Female	49.3	32.6	8.0
White			
Male	82.3	59.1	18.5
Female	49.1	32.0	7.9
Other Races			
Male	72.0	52.6	16.7
Female	50.7	37.8	9.1

Source: U.S. Bureau of the Census, "America in Transition: An Aging Society," Current Population Reports, P-23, no. 128 (1983), table 12.

protections, because the separation process is often too subtle to be detected or thwarted by the law, well-intentioned employers, or the workers themselves. The process is also a reciprocal one, however, because people are not merely ejected from the work force, but are attracted into retirement by adequate pensions, useful alternative roles, persuasive family members and previous retirees, and other influences. Moreover, some workers have no choice but to retire because of health problems.

In considering the situation of the older worker who is retired involuntarily, it is easy to overestimate the pervasiveness and the negative effects of the disengagement process, and even to see virtually the whole retired population as a tragic mass expelled from useful social activity and plagued by numerous problems. In fact, a large majority of workers look forward to retirement, hasten the process if they can afford it, and adapt well when they actually do retire, though the proportions who can retire vary as inflation and other problems change in intensity. Nor do most former workers slow down very significantly, withdraw into solitude, or sever major social contacts with family, friends, or even former co-workers,[12] though many experience these consequences in a mild form and a minority suffer them acutely. People whose incomes, educations, and health are good incur few or none of the negative results attributed to disengagement from the labor force, and they remain full social participants during retirement; for a time they may even increase their social activity.[13] Almost all elderly people, however, do tend to disengage gradually from social interaction as they age, partly because friends and spouses die, health deteriorates, and other changes occur as one moves toward the oldest years. Therefore, some degree of disengagement is a reality for most even beyond the question of employment, but its intensity varies greatly and it only creates serious difficulties for a fairly small number.

Once the older person has left the labor force it is relatively difficult to return because of hiring practices, the lower levels of formal education that many older workers have, the periodic recessions that reduce the demand for elderly job seekers, and the frequent glut of applicants for those jobs. Consequently, some of the 65-and-over group outside the labor force simply give up trying to return and settle for whatever retirement income they can get. Even labor unions, as they negotiate pension plans with employers, accept age limits that help push older workers out of the work force and hamper their return. The age requirements of the Social Security system and other governmental programs for the elderly have much the same effect. Therefore, to a certain degree the pension is "a formal reward for waiving the right to work,"[14] in order that the elderly can be removed from the labor force. But no matter how one assesses these various elements, they do reduce labor force participation rates rapidly after age 55 or 60.

Perhaps the major problem is a categorical view of the elderly that doesn't account for individual variations. Productivity does decline among some older workers, but many compete successfully with younger ones, and others substitute accuracy and dependability for high rates of productivity.[15] Furthermore, experience is often a strong compensation for certain decrements of aging, especially in sensory abilities; experience helps the older worker produce more consistently than many younger counterparts and still maintain as high a quality of work. Despite some chronic absentees, the average attendance record of elderly workers also is as good as that of younger ones, even when the older employees are bothered by certain health problems. Thus, removing workers from jobs at a uniform age is inconsistent with variations in their skills and performance, though the raising of the mandatory retirement age to 70 and the trend toward earlier voluntary retirement are modifying this artificial uniformity.

Some International Comparisons

Older people in most societies tend to withdraw from the labor force, but they are much more likely to do so in the industrialized nations than in the so-called developing countries, where poverty and subsistence labors are part of the way of life of many people. Moreover, even though longer life expectancy in the developed countries increases the average number of working years, those years represent a smaller percentage of life than is true in the developing nations, especially the more agrarian ones. Thus, Table 6-2 shows lower participation rates among elderly men in the representative developed countries than in the developing ones, though Japan is something of an exception because of its unique industrial situation. But it is rare in most developed countries for more than a quarter of the older men to be in the labor force, whereas the proportions are half, two-thirds, or more in the less developed ones.

The participation rates of elderly women also tend to be somewhat greater in many of the developing nations, though the pattern is less consistent than it is for men, because religion, the status of women, and other factors influence the proportions. In Pakistan, for example, only 3 per cent of the older women are in the labor force, partly because of restrictions imposed by Islam, which also helps account for women's low participation rates in Iran and some countries not listed in Table 6-2, including Bangladesh. Moreover, the work that women do in many developing countries, especially in agriculture, is substantially underreported in the official statistics on the economically active population. In fact, the ways of conceptualizing who is and is not in the work force in the developing countries differ considerably from the procedures used in the developed ones.[16]

142

The countries with the lowest participation rates for men and women
are those with comprehensive services for elderly workers who retire, for
they make retirement attractive and mandatory for large percentages of
the work force. Most are European countries. Some provide better benefits for the elderly than does the United States, which helps account for
our relatively high participation rates among older people, both men and
women.[17] But retirement benefits are only one of the factors that affect
labor force participation rates of the elderly. In Japan, for example, early
in the twentieth century industries introduced the concept of lifetime
employment with one firm, along with increases in income according to

Table 6-2. Percentages of People 65 and Over
Classified as Economically Active in
Selected Countries, by Sex

Country	Year	Per Cent	
		Male	Female
Japan	1978	41.5	15.8
Denmark	1978	20.9	5.6
UNITED STATES	1978	19.7	7.8
Spain	1978	17.1	6.1
Australia	1976	16.8	5.1
New Zealand	1976	16.2	2.8
Italy	1978	13.4	3.7
Finland	1976	10.8	3.1
West Germany	1978	8.4	3.4
Netherlands	1977	6.3	1.4
Bolivia	1976	80.5	14.1
Ethiopia	1977	68.1	14.2
Honduras	1977	67.2	6.5
Jamaica	1978	65.6	30.7
Cameroon	1976	62.8	31.2
Zambia	1977	61.3	30.2
Mexico	1979	60.3	8.9
Pakistan	1978	59.7	3.2
Iran	1976	56.6	4.2
Venezuela	1977	53.1	8.3

Source: International Labour Office, Year Book of
Labour Statistics, 1979 (1979), table 1.

length of service. But because that tenure system is expensive, most firms require retirement at age 55 but begin paying benefits at age 60. In addition, the governmental social security plan is a recent one and its benefits are relatively small, even after age 60. Therefore, the older Japanese worker is often forced to seek employment after forced retirement, often in a poorly paid, low-status, part-time job, though the government, industries, and unions are now promoting measures to make older workers more employable. These several circumstances account for a considerable part of the high labor force participation rates of the elderly in Japan.[18]

Labor Force Participation Differentials in the United States

Participation Differences by Sex

Labor force participation has changed dramatically for American men and women under age 65, especially since 1970, because women are much more likely to be in the work force than they were previously, whereas the participation rates of men have declined. Despite the job and wage discrimination they still encounter, women have been increasingly available and motivated to work outside the home, partly because their child-care responsibilities have been diminished by more childlessness and smaller family size. Other significant factors include expanded job opportunities, higher levels of education that qualify women to work at better jobs, the wish for a level of living that only two salaries can provide,[19] the increase in one-parent families supported by women, and especially the high inflation rates of recent years. As a result, the proportions of men and women working for wages have grown much more alike.

In the elderly group, however, only some of this change has occurred, for although older men are now far less likely to be in the labor force than were those in 1900, the participation rate for women has dropped very little. Thus, while the rates of the nation's elderly men and women differed by 59 percentage points in 1900, in 1981 the two groups were separated by only 10 percentage points. During the period, the participation rate of elderly women has fluctuated a little, but now, at 8 per cent, it is not much below the 9 per cent of 1900 or even the 10 per cent of the 1950s and 1960s. Older men, on the other hand, are less than a third as likely to be in the labor force as they were in 1900. The factors chiefly responsible are pension plans that encourage voluntary retirement, age restrictions imposed by industries and unions, reductions in the rate of self-employment,[20] and the difficulty of finding work after age 65. For both sexes, however, older people are far less likely than younger ones to remain in the labor force, and the rates for men and women aged 65 and over are far below those of the group aged 60-64. (See Table 6-1 and Figure 6-1.)

The tendency for participation rates of older women to change relatively little since 1900 doesn't mean that the women are immune to the forces that reduced the rates among older men. Many elderly female workers are also motivated to leave the labor force because of improved retirement benefits and other incentives, or are forced to withdraw because of formal age limits, subtle age discrimination, stationary salaries, stereotypes about physical attractiveness, and other disincentives that favor younger women over older ones. Their separation from work roles may be concealed, however, by the greatly increased flow of women of all ages into the labor force, especially during the 1970s,[21] and the aging of many into the elderly category where they replace most who retire.

Like the men, women workers also tend to remain in the labor force in large numbers until age 62 or 65, especially if they are single or divorced and self-supporting, though many widows also must seek employment for financial reasons, sometimes at relatively old ages. That group is particularly likely to end up in low-paying service and white-collar jobs, partly because the widow whose income is so low that she must work is also apt to have a relatively poor education and limited job skills. Often she has spent much of her life engaged in housework, which has little negotiating value when she seeks paid employment, unfair though that may be.

The variable work force particpation rates of elderly men and women also reflect the different ways in which the sexes have viewed work historically. When today's elderly were young adults, paid work was far more central to a man's overall role than to a woman's, because it tied him to the larger social system and provided a major part of his self-concept.[22] Typically, the man was judged less as a husband and father than as a worker, and it was often difficult for him to relinquish the work role. That was true even for many who had no serious financial constraints, though pension plans were much poorer then than now. When elderly women were young adults, on the other hand, a woman's role was bound up with housekeeping and childrearing; she was identified chiefly as a wife and mother and part of her status simply reflected that of her husband. Paid employment was pursued by a comparatively small minority. Therefore, the present low labor force participation rates of elderly women and the higher ones of men are partly a residue of those earlier social realities.

The ways in which the sexes related to work are changing markedly, however, for the labor force participation rates of women in all age groups under 65 have risen sharply, while those of men have fallen somewhat. Therefore, paid work has become an important if not central feature in the lives of at least half the nation's women aged 18-54, and for a sizable minority it is just as basic as it has been for men. When these women reach age 65, many will carry with them the same attitudes about work and retirement held by many men, and future populations of older women will have far more versatile work experience than housekeeping and childrearing. In fact, a sizable share of women now reaching age 65 already have had long careers and face the same questions about role definitions, retirement and its meaning, and use of time that many men have had to resolve when their working years were over. That change is part of the fundamental convergence in the work histories of more and more elderly men and women, and is another of the dynamics involved in the aging of America's population.

Participation Differences by Race

Labor force participation rates among older people do not vary tremendously by race, though they are slightly higher for white men than for blacks and somewhat higher for black women than for whites.[23] (See Table 6-1 and Figure 6-1.) These patterns represent some changes, however, for as recently as 1950 the participation rates of elderly black men were significantly higher than those of white men; older black women, though, have long had higher rates than white women. In recent decades, the labor force involvement of older black men has declined somewhat more rapidly than that of any other elderly group,[24] but even at all of the ages under 65 the participation rates of black men have dropped substantially below those of white men. If the pattern doesn't change for those reaching age 65, blacks will continue to be less represented than whites in the elderly work force.

The labor force participation rate of elderly women of both races has been more nearly constant than that of men, owing to the sizable number of younger women who enter the work force, reach age 65, and replace the ones able to retire. White women of all ages have been entering the labor force at an especially rapid pace, but at age 65 and older their participation rates are still below those of black women, partly because larger proportions of the latter hold low-paying service jobs from which they cannot afford to retire. On the other hand, the percentage of elderly black women unable to work because of physical disability and other problems is more than twice that of white women; the same proportion holds among men.

Participation Differences by Other Characteristics

Rural-urban residence. Elderly men in the rural-farm population are more likely to remain in the labor force than are men in the urban and rural-nonfarm groups. Many of the farm men continue working in agriculture, either for themselves or for an adult child who has taken over principal responsibility for the business, or they are employed in other enterprises related to agriculture. Elderly women, on the other hand, are most likely to continue in the labor force if they reside in cities, where there are higher proportions of unmarried women who must support themselves.

Marital status. The labor force participation rates are highest for elderly married men (20% in 1981) and a little lower for those who are divorced (19%). The rates are still lower for single men (14%) and lowest of all for widowers (12%). Most of the married men still help support an aging spouse, which would be more difficult on a small retirement income, and they also tend to have better average health than widowers and are more able to work. In addition, widowers tend to be considerably older than 65 and less able to get or hold jobs because of advanced age. Elderly women are far less likely to be in the labor force if they are married than if they are single or divorced. Many in the last two groups are essentially on their own financially and must work to survive, particularly if their jobs are at the low end of the status scale and promise only small retirement incomes. Widows have participation rates nearly as low as those of married women, for while some must work to support themselves, many others have adequate incomes because of their late husbands' pension plans, survivor benefits, and other advantages. Moreover, considering that the soaring increase in the divorce rate is relatively recent, divorced and separated women tend to cluster closer to age 65 than do widows, so the former are often better able to work.

Educational attainment. Labor force participation rates are generally lowest for elderly people with the poorest educational attainment, highest for those who have the most schooling, because many of the latter hold jobs or practice professions that are less susceptible to mandatory retirement, and frequently they are doing things they enjoy and prefer to continue. Furthermore, the best-educated people have better average levels of health than the poorly educated and are more able to hold jobs, and they also have an advantage should they wish to return to work. At the same time, older workers as a group have less schooling than younger ones, are less likely to have the occupational training that equips them with valued skills, and are found less often in government-sponsored retraining programs.[25] Some of those discrepancies are diminishing, however, as better-educated younger workers age into the older labor force and as some elderly workers recognize the need to hone old job skills or learn new ones. But well-educated people also generally have attractive pension options that favor early retirement and keep their labor force participation rates from being higher than they are.

Part-Time and Part-Year Work

Elderly workers are especially likely to be employed part time, and the older one becomes, the greater the likelihood.[26] Thus, in 1981 about 48 per cent of the men aged 65 and older who were still working and 60 per cent of the working women were employed on a part-time basis. These figures compare with 30 per cent and 42 per cent, respectively, in 1960. Consequently, as the participation rate has declined among the elderly, part-time work has become an increasingly important source of employment for the minority who remain in the labor force.[27] In addition, elderly workers are far more likely than younger ones to work only part of each year, though more than half put in at least some hours during 50-52 weeks a year. Elderly women are slightly more likely than elderly men to be part-year workers, but the difference is small. Therefore, when older men and women do work, somewhat over half of each group are employed on a 50-52 week basis, but the women are significantly more likely to work less than 35 hours per week.

Although some elderly people work part-time because they cannot get more regular jobs, most prefer part-time work as a way to supplement their retirement incomes. Some, especially at the higher educational levels, get pleasure from the work itself but prefer to avoid the demands and commitments of full-time employment. Thus, the less regular employment of many elderly persons reflects the mix of activities with which they fill their older years, and while work supplements income and adds variety to life, it is not usually demanding enough to interfere seriously with other things that people want to do. In that sense, part-time and part-year work represents a tapering off in economic activity to avoid abrupt or even traumatic separation from the working world. Therefore, given the choice to work, many elderly people prefer to do so on a less rigorous schedule than their regular jobs previously required, though the limitation on earnings for Social Security recipients also plays a major role in the amount of work the older person chooses to do. In addition, many of the part-time jobs available to older people pay poorly and provide only a meager supplement to Social Security income. Thus, while fairly large numbers of older people hold part-time jobs, most do so out of economic necessity and most of the jobs pay only modest wages.[28]

The reasons for part-time rather than full-time employment also vary by sex. The most frequent reason women workers remain on a part-time basis is because of housekeeping responsibilities, whereas two-thirds of the men give retirement as their principal reason. Ill health or disability is an equally important reason for both sexes and is fairly minor, though it is, of course, a much more significant factor among the elderly who do not work at all.

Occupations of Older Workers

Older workers are concentrated rather heavily in the occupations that are declining in proportional importance in the economy, such as farm work, certain service jobs, and some types of manufacturing, though they are also heavily represented in occupations that require long years of experience. Young workers, on the other hand, are more likely to appear in the newer occupations, the ones that are expanding in importance, those that are physically demanding, the professions, and the jobs that are stepping stones to better positions.[29]

Occupational Differences by Sex

Reflecting these differences between age groups, the data in Table 6-3 on occupations show that elderly men are far more likely than younger ones to be employed in farming, especially as private operators, and in nonhousehold service jobs of various kinds, such as guards or janitors. Moreover, the older men are somewhat overrepresented in white-collar jobs, chiefly as managers and administrators, sales workers, and clerical employees; they are underrepresented in professional and technical occupations and greatly so in blue-collar jobs with mandatory retirement. In large companies particularly, persons who reach age 65 as blue-collar workers are more likely to retire than are older workers in small companies. Far more elderly men are employed in white-collar jobs than in any other category, whereas blue-collar occupations account for 45 per cent of all jobs held by men aged 16-64.

Elderly women workers are very heavily concentrated in white-collar positions and service jobs. In 1981 those two job categories accounted for 87 per cent of the female work force aged 65 and older. Even so, elderly women are less represented in many specific white-collar jobs than are younger ones, including professional and technical work, managerial positions, and sales and clerical jobs, partly because prejudices still favor young women in some of those categories. The unusually large share of elderly women in service jobs includes a significant number of household workers and baby-sitters, for many of the older women, especially those past age 70, still have to work for whatever wages they can get in the only positions they can get. Many of their situations represent an accumulation of low levels of education, limited job skills, modest or no retirement income from private pensions, and subsistence wages that help stave off the more serious deprivation they would suffer if they depended on Social Security or Supplemental Security Income (SSI) alone. Not all women in those jobs are poor, however, and some do the work because they enjoy the activity and the contacts it provides.

Older women have lower rates of participation than younger ones in all of the blue-collar jobs, but much higher rates in farm work, especially as operators. Some of these women are the widows of farmers and are still working to hold onto a family farm, though nearly half of them are laborers working for wages or other remuneration. The group of farm laborers, however, is limited largely to women under age 70, for very few past that age could meet the physical demands of such work.

It is clear that older workers of both sexes appear disproportionately in the more menial and poorly paid occupations and those that demand lesser skills, while they are underrepresented in the jobs that provide relatively high income and status. Consequently, many of the nation's older workers hold the least coveted white-collar positions and service jobs,[30] laboring as janitors, guards, household employees, and similar workers. Job status does not decline much for some after they reach age

Table 6-3. Percentages of Workers Employed in Various Occupation Groups, by Age and Sex, 1981

Occupation Group	Male		Female	
	16-64	65+	16-64	65+
White-Collar Workers	42.7	47.3	66.2	56.7
Professional & Technical	15.9	13.7	17.2	11.1
Managers & Administrators	14.5	17.5	7.3	9.3
Sales	6.0	9.3	6.7	11.5
Clerical	6.3	6.8	35.0	24.8
Blue-Collar Workers	45.0	25.7	13.6	10.2
Crafts	21.0	11.8	1.9	1.1
Nontransport Operatives	11.3	4.5	9.8	7.9
Transport Operatives	5.6	3.4	0.7	0.2
Nonfarm Laborers	7.1	6.0	1.2	1.0
Service Workers	8.7	13.2	19.1	30.5
Farm Workers	3.6	13.8	1.1	2.6

Source: U.S. Bureau of Labor Statistics, Labor Force Statistics Derived from the Current Population Survey: A Databook, vol. 1 (1982), p. 648.

65, however, and they simply continue in the relatively menial positions they held before age 65,[31] while for others the low-level jobs are a tolerable way to supplement income.

But education, not age, is the variable that determines occupational placement for most older workers. For example, the large majority of elderly working men with college educations are white-collar employees in the professions, technical fields, administrative positions, and other situations with relatively high status, whereas the men with less than eighth-grade educations are heavily represented in farm jobs and service occupations.[32] Moreover, the proportions of older and younger workers engaged in most occupations do not vary a great deal if the level of education is held constant. Therefore, poor educational attainment tends to dog elderly people throughout their lives and to diminish their chances of high-status employment in the older years, just as it did when they were younger. It can also reduce the elderly person's confidence to be able to do a job and can erode his/her self-concept after retirement.[33]

Inadequate education also prevents older workers from having much occupational mobility, either upward in the social scale or from one job to another at the same level, although job security, pension investments, and other factors also reduce mobility. Many are reluctant to attempt a move because they know the prospects to find a better position diminish sharply after age 45 or 50, and unless forced out, older workers rarely leave one position to find another. Even when they do, relatively large shares remain unemployed for long periods or even permanently, or they end up taking part-time work. In addition, with the relocation of many plants to other parts of the country in the last few decades, often from the Snowbelt to the Sunbelt, many older workers were left behind by their companies or were unwilling to move. The least skilled have often been unable to find new jobs, particularly if the economy of an area is in general decline and its unemployment rate for all ages is relatively high. On the other hand, older people with the highest levels of education and job status continue working the longest, particularly if they are self-employed,[34] and though they often choose not to move to new jobs, many could do so if they wished.

Occupational Difference by Race

Many of the occupational variations between elderly men and women apply to both blacks and whites, but there are some differences between the sexes by race and major ones between the races for each sex. Thus, elderly white women are more likely than men to be white-collar workers, whereas the proportions are about the same in the older black group, partly because the percentage of female professional and technical workers, many of them teachers, is higher than that of men; so is that of clerical workers. (See Table 6-4.) But in the blue-collar and farm categories, men predominate in both racial groups, whereas higher proportions of women of both races are service workers.

There are large variations between the races, however, that reflect long-term advantages and disadvantages in employment status. Thus, black men are far less likely than white men to be white-collar workers in all of the sub-categories but much more apt to be blue-collar workers, especially laborers. Black men are also more than twice as likely to be service workers, but somewhat less apt to be farm workers. Elderly black

Table 6-4. Percentages of Workers 65 and Over
            Employed in Various Occupation Groups,
            by Race and Sex, 1981

Occupation Group	White		Other Races	
	Male	Female	Male	Female
White-Collar Workers	49.6	60.8	22.1	22.3
Professional & Technical	14.5	11.6	5.4	7.4
Managers & Administrators	18.4	9.9	8.6	5.0
Sales	9.8	12.5	2.7	2.5
Clerical	6.9	26.8	5.4	7.4
Blue-Collar Workers	24.5	10.6	38.3	6.6
Crafts	12.0	1.1	8.9	0.8
Nontransport Operatives	4.3	8.4	6.9	5.0
Transport Operatives	3.3	0.2	4.8	a
Nonfarm Laborers	4.9	0.9	17.7	0.8
Service Workers	12.0	26.0	26.8	68.6
Farm Workers	13.9	2.6	12.8	2.5

Source: U.S. Bureau of Labor Statistics, Labor Force Statistics Derived from the Current Population Survey: A Databook, vol. 1 (1982), p. 649.

aLess than 0.1 per cent.

women who work are heavily concentrated in service occupations, which employ more than two-thirds of them. They are proportionately less abundant than white women in all of the white-collar and blue-collar categories, though they are about equally likely to be farm workers. It is clear, though, that the status profile of jobs held by elderly blacks is significantly poorer than that of older whites, and that the occupational choices of the elderly black woman are especially limited.

Industries of Older Workers

Because of these occupational patterns among older workers, the largest proportions of them are employed in service industries, especially education, personal services, business and repair services, and various kinds of welfare, religious, and medical services. Trade also employs a large share of older workers, particularly as retail store clerks. Together, service industries and trade provide the jobs for about two-thirds of all elderly workers, and for a much larger percentage of the women than of the men.

Manufacturing is the third most important industrial category employing older workers, but after age 65 the percentage engaged in it drops substantially. Part of the decrease is due to the pension plans and mandatory retirement provisions enacted as the labor movement gained strength and wrested concessions from factory owners and managers, though the physical demands of some jobs and the routine nature of others also help reduce the employment of the elderly in manufacturing. For some, health problems play a major part, but often the worker on the assembly line or in other forms of manufacturing has had enough of the factory and simply wants to retire as soon as possible. The job prospects for older people in manufacturing and other industries are also reduced by product competition from abroad, robotics and other rapid advances in computer technology, and increases in the educational sophistication expected of many employees. Those changes have forced out some who would like to work after age 65 and have reduced new employment opportunities for many people who have reached that age or are even in the 40s and 50s. The changes also help concentrate older workers in the service industries and trade, because they are the only areas in which many elderly can hope to find jobs. And whenever the economy slides into a recession, their prospects are poor even in those industries, especially with younger people and undocumented alien immigrants competing for the same jobs. Many manufacturing industries also have no provisions for part-time or part-year employment, which many older workers must have if they are to maintain a tolerable level of living; the service industries and trade are the most likely to provide those opportunities.

The only other industry in which there is a heavier proportional concentration of workers age 65 and over than of those 55-64 is finance, insurance, and real estate, though that is true only for men. Within that category of industries older workers are especially drawn to real estate, and many continue in that field after "normal" retirement age, while others enter it for the first time. Even there, however, when high interest rates and other conditions inhibit the real estate market, the older worker is apt to have fewer opportunies than the younger one.

Older workers are relatively scarce in mining, transportation and public utilities, construction, and public administration. Moreover, all but the last category represent "male" occupations that provide jobs for very few elderly women. The latter are at a disadvantage even in public administration, though the discrepancy is not as great.

Employment and Unemployment

In one sense, the elderly are less susceptible to unemployment than are younger people, especially teenages, because the labor force participation rates of older people are so much lower.[35] Thus, in 1981 the unemployment rates for workers generally declined with age, until only 2.9 per cent of the men and 3.6 per cent of the women aged 65 and older were reported as seeking work but unable to find it. (See Table 6-5.) Elderly whites were especially unlikely to be classified as unemployed, while members of other races, chiefly blacks, had substantially higher rates. Nonetheless, the unemployment figures for the elderly, whether male or female, black or white, are less than half those of workers aged 16 and over, except for black women. It might seem, therefore, that the employment situation of elderly job-seekers is a relatively favorable one and that the youngest people in the labor force are far worse off.

But the situation of the elderly is actually poorer than it appears, for the data refer to unemployment among people classified as being *in the labor force*. Very sizable numbers of the elderly population, especially men, are classified as retired and thus not in the work force, even though a significant share of that group would take work if they could get it.[36] In fact, when economic growth slows and general unemployment rates rise, the elderly are especially unlikely to find the work they would like and often need. Many abandon the search, accept the designation "retired," and are not reported in the unemployment figures. A person out of work must be actively seeking a job to be considered officially unemployed, and for some elderly people it is less degrading to be retired than unemployed, and they report themselves accordingly.[37] People aged 65-69 are especially affected, because they are the large majority of older people who do work or would like to, and men are still more affected than women, because the majority of today's elderly women never worked for wages outside the home. That, of course, may change dramatically with future generations of elderly women who held paying jobs in their younger years.

Competition with younger workers is a key factor in the unemployment patterns of older workers, for even though the older person offers more experience than the younger one, the job is more likely to go to the latter, especially if it calls for a type and level of training the older worker lacks. Frequently, the younger worker is also thought to need the job more in order to support a growing family, whereas the older worker is felt to have at least some retirement income, fewer financial responsibilities, and more governmental protection from the costs of illness and accident. Older workers have been particularly hard pressed by this competition during the 1970s and 1980s, because their numbers and proportions have been increasing rapidly at the same time the large baby-boom generation has entered the labor force and worked its way into the industrial structure. Complicated by periodic recessions, this means there are more younger applicants for the jobs that older people might have been able to get or retain in the past.

Table 6-5. Percentages of the Labor Force Unemployed, by Age, Race, and Sex, 1981

Age	All Races		White		Other Races	
	Male	Female	Male	Female	Male	Female
16+	7.4	7.9	6.5	6.9	14.1	14.3
16-17	22.0	20.7	19.9	18.4	40.1	41.4
18-19	18.8	17.9	16.4	15.3	36.0	36.5
20-24	13.2	11.2	11.6	9.1	24.4	24.2
25-34	6.9	7.7	6.1	6.6	12.6	13.9
35-44	4.5	5.7	4.0	5.1	8.3	8.9
45-54	4.0	4.6	3.6	4.2	7.1	6.7
55-64	3.6	3.8	3.4	3.7	6.2	4.6
65+	2.9	3.6	2.4	3.4	7.0	8.0

Source: U.S. Bureau of Labor Statistics, Labor Force Statistics Derived from the Current Population Survey: A Databook, vol. 1 (1982), table A-28.

Thus, incentives and pressures for elderly people to leave the labor force have pushed their actual unemployment rates substantially above the official rates. Furthermore, when older job-seekers do find employment, much of it offers less prestige and income than the jobs people held before they were aged 60 or 65. Even the exceptions among professional, technical, and other highly skilled workers do not negate the general pattern. And when the older worker does look for a job, the search takes much longer than it does for the average younger worker,[38] increasing the likelihood the elderly job-seeker will become discouraged and retire. Sometimes the problems of the search are worsened by employers who choose younger workers even when they are compelled by law to interview older ones, because employers often expect to train younger people more cheaply and to get a longer period of productivity.[39] Perhaps the prospects of older workers will improve when the low birth rates since the late 1960s reduce the proportions of very young job-seekers, but at present the prospects are limited and will grow worse as the baby-boom people reach age 65. In addition, the indebtedness and reduced purchasing power of many developing countries, such as Mexico and Brazil, have reduced the demand for American products, eliminated jobs, and made the elderly job-seeker's quest even more difficult. So has product competition from other nations.

Finally, the unemployment situation of older people is no longer ameliorated as it once was by a relatively high incidence of self-employment. In particular, farming has declined as an employer of older people who could continue working as long as they were able and then reduce their activity gradually rather than abruptly. Much of the same is true of small shopkeepers, grocers, and others who could not compete with chain and discount stores, and self-employment has also decreased in those businesses, especially among the elderly.

Some Trends and Projections

Labor Force Participation Trends

The labor force participation rates of older people have declined substantially over the past several decades, principally because of very significant decreases in the proportions of older men who work, though the employment rate of older women is also declining slowly. At the turn of the present century, nearly two-thirds of the men aged 65 and older were "gainful workers" (participants in the labor force),[40] but by 1950 fewer than half were so classified. The proportion declined steadily up to the present and promises to drop even more in the 1990s.[41] (See Table 6-6.) Moreover, while the participation rates of men aged 65 and older have fallen the most rapidly, those of men aged 55-64 have also dropped since 1970. As a consequence, although the whole labor force aged 16 and over will probably increase from 105 million in 1980 to 128 million by 1995, the group 65 and over is likely to remain at about 3 million throughout the period.[42] That will make elderly workers an even smaller percentage of the total work force and of the whole elderly population, unless significant changes take place in employment policies and opportunities, economic pressures on the elderly, or other conditions that affect labor force participation.

The reasons why the labor force participation rates of older men have declined so dramatically are complex, but five factors help to explain this drop:[43]

1. As work has shifted away from agriculture and self-employment and toward bureaucratized forms, more men have come under mandatory retirement rules designed by industries to enhance efficiency and favor younger workers, who can often be hired at lower wages than people with long seniority. This has forced out many workers at various ages from 55 to 75, though especially at 65, and in the future it will eject many at age 70. But status also enters the picture, because people in menial jobs are more likely than those in prestigious ones to retire, even on fairly low incomes if they must, though the retirement rates of various status groups are converging.

2. The increase in pension plans, both public and private, has made retirement more attractive to many workers, and to others the plans represent welcome relief from an unhappy work situation. The private plans are often part of a system that mandates retirement at a given age, so the worker is both drawn and pushed out of the work force. Moreover, the maximum-earnings test in the Social Security system and the prospect to receive some benefits as early as age 62 help to reduce labor force participation, while the meaning of retirement has also changed so much that some people prefer leisure to full-time work even if they must get it at considerable sacrifice of income. Therefore, some persons retire even under relatively poor pension plans or with Social Security alone, though many must then resort to part-time employment. Even for them, however, the pension does prevent the late-life destitution that many unemployed elderly experienced in earlier generations.[44] Retirement has also come to be defined as appropriate for older Americans, while non-work has lost its stigma and is even reinforced, both financially and normatively.[45]

3. When jobs are difficult to find because general unemployment rates are high, the older unemployed male is apt to become discouraged in his search for work and to stop looking. Furthermore, once unemployed he is more likely than the younger worker to remain out of the labor force, partly because he can qualify for retirement benefits the younger man cannot yet claim, but also because of barriers to re-employment. Those

circumstances have helped lower the labor force participation rates of older men, including those aged 55-64.

4. Ill health and disability also drive some older men from the labor force, while improved disability benefits enable them to survive financially if they must stop working. The proportion who claim disability as a reason for leaving the work force is a small fraction of those who credit retirement, however, though the latter may be an excuse for the former. The percentage of older men who claim poor health or disability is also smaller than in the past, so more could work if they wished and if suitable jobs were available.

Table 6-6. Labor Force Participation Rates in Two Major Age Groups, by Sex, 1890-1995

Year	Male		Female	
	55-64	65+	55-64	65+
1890	89.0	68.3	11.4	7.6
1920	86.3	55.6	14.3	7.3
1950	87.0	45.8	27.0	9.7
1955	86.4	38.5	32.2	10.3
1960	86.8	33.1	37.2	10.8
1965	84.6	27.9	41.1	10.0
1970	83.0	26.8	43.0	9.7
1975	75.8	21.7	41.0	8.3
1980	72.3	19.1	41.5	8.1
1985	69.7	17.5	41.6	7.7
1990	67.5	15.8	41.7	7.3
1995	66.5	14.3	42.3	6.8

Sources: U.S. Bureau of the Census, Statistical Abstract of the United States: 1960, tables 16, 262, and 264; 1981, table 636; Kingsley Davis and Pietronella van den Oever, "Age Relations and Public Policy in Advanced Industrial Societies," Population and Development Review, vol. 7 (1981), table 1; Howard N. Fullerton, "The 1995 Labor Force: A First Look," in U.S. Bureau of Labor Statistics, Economic Projections to 1990, Bulletin 2121 (1982), p. 52.

5. Employers still discriminate covertly against the older job-seeker, despite protective legislation. Often relying on stereotypes, many employers assume that older workers are less efficient than younger ones, less capable physically and even mentally, and less adaptable, though obsolete skills in a time of rapid technological change are a genuine problem. Moreover, many employers fear that hiring or even retaining older workers would increase insurance and pension costs. Newly hired older workers would also be unable to work long enough to participate in existing pension plans, and employers often assume they are less trainable than young ones and more likely to fall ill.

As noted earlier, the labor force participation rates of elderly women have fluctuated far less than those of men, basically because the larger proportion of younger women who entered the labor force in recent decades and then aged into the 65-and-over group tends to compensate for the growing number of those aged 65 and older who retire. Therefore, the participation rates of women are declining only slowly and will probably continue to fall gradually into the 1990s. The factors that have reduced the labor force involvement of older men are increasingly at play for women as well, however, although other forces encourage many women to enter or remain in the labor force during middle age and to stay in it past age 65.

As a consequence of various socioeconomic changes in the twentieth century, including improvements in retirement income, the falling labor force participation rates of the elderly have caused older workers to become a smaller share of the total work force. Their proportions have risen at times because of national emergencies that kept them at their jobs after age 65, but those were only temporary reversals in the long-term trend. Moreover, the tendency for the elderly to be less and less represented in the work force seems likely to continue, although new crises in the Social Security system and other financial problems could alter that trend and cause more older people to seek work or keep the jobs they have. That likelihood should decrease for awhile, however, because from 1985 to 2000 the baby-boom people will be in their prime working years, whereas the small group born during the Depression will be retiring; the pressure on retirement systems should ease, though only until the baby-boom group itself reaches retirement age.

Occupational Trends

Employed men aged 65 and older. Since 1950 the male labor force of all ages has grown most rapidly in the service occupations, followed by white-collar positions and blue-collar categories. (See Table 6-7.) Their participation in farming has been cut by nearly two-thirds. Within the broad occupational groups, professional and technical workers have increased at the greatest rate, followed by nonhousehold service workers, managers and administrators, craft workers, clerical people, sales workers, nonfarm laborers, and operatives. The number of private household workers has fallen substantially.

Elderly employed men show some of these same patterns, though others differ markedly. Most significant is the 19 per cent decline in the older employed labor force between 1950 and 1981, compared with an increase of 48 per cent in the male labor force aged 16-64. Moreover, the numbers of older men have decreased significantly in all of the blue-collar categories, in the group of private household workers, and in the class of farm workers. On the other hand, the older white-collar group grew,

Table 6-7. Percentage Change in Major Occupation Groups, by Age and Sex, 1950-1981

Occupation Group	Male		Female	
	16-64	65+	16-64	65+
All Groups	48.3	-19.3	182.1	148.3
White-Collar Workers	101.7	29.8	244.2	265.2
Professional & Technical	213.6	70.6	282.8	116.1
Managers & Administrators	98.5	37.2	380.0	173.4
Sales	39.1	29.1	116.8	267.2
Clerical	40.5	17.4	245.3	543.0
Blue-Collar Workers	37.2	-35.2	73.1	49.1
Crafts	61.2	-35.8	246.5	64.4
Operatives	18.8	-34.9	49.4	37.3
Nonfarm Laborers	27.2	-34.9	320.2	214.3
Service Workers	122.0	1.8	163.5	103.2
Farm Workers	-62.6	-60.4	-10.0	-7.4

Sources: U.S. Bureau of the Census, U.S. Census of Population: 1950, Detailed Characteristics, U.S. Summary (1953), table 127; U.S. Bureau of Labor Statistics, Labor Force Statistics Derived from the Current Population Survey: A Databook, vol. 1 (1982), p. 648.

particularly because of a large increase in the number of professional and technical workers and a smaller one among managers and administrators, whose jobs are often attractive enough for them to continue working and who are less subject to mandatory retirement than are blue-collar workers. Sales and clerical workers, who are usually farther down the social scale, also registered increases, as did nonhousehold service workers.

These changes suggest that the older men who do remain in the labor force have become more concentrated in a small number of occupations, largely white collar, though they are also getting out of farming at a slower pace than younger men. At the same time, the proportion of older workers in the blue-collar jobs has declined while that of younger ones has risen, though rather slowly. The percentage of workers aged 16-64 engaged in service occupations has risen significantly since 1950, while that of elderly men has scarcely changed. That is the net result, however, of a two-thirds reduction of elderly workers in private households and a 23 per cent increase in other service jobs. In no occupational category has the male labor force aged 65 and older increased nearly as fast as that aged 16-64, so the former continue to fall as a proportion in each category.

Employed women aged 65 and older. Since 1950 the female labor force of all ages has grown much faster than the male group in every occupational category except farm labor, and even there the number of women declined more slowly than that of men. These changes reflect the large influx of women workers into the work force in the past three decades and the tendency for some younger women to replace older men in the jobs that can be done by either sex.[46] Moreover, white-collar occupations as a whole attracted women faster than any other large category, followed by service jobs outside private households and blue-collar positions, particularly as laborers and craft workers. The growth in specific occupations in the white-collar category shows women rapidly becoming professional and technical workers and managers and administrators, though the more traditional clerical jobs have also attracted large numbers. Nonhousehold service jobs have also shown very substantial growth.

The number of elderly women employed has grown somewhat slower than that of all women, but the large increase in the elderly group contrasts dramatically with the decrease among older men. Given the rapid growth of the female population aged 65 and older, however, even this large increase in labor force participants has not raised the participation rate of elderly women.

The numbers of elderly women have grown faster than those of younger ones in the white-collar category, but only because of extremely large increases in the sales and clerical subgroups. In the blue-collar category and service occupations the numbers of older women grew more slowly than those of younger ones in every subgroup; the number of older women in farming fell, but more slowly than that of younger ones.

By 1990 women will probably be about 40 per cent of the elderly work force, up from 17 per cent in 1950, because some of the many employed women aged 55-64 will keep their jobs after age 65 and the number of older male workers will probably continue to shrink.[47] Older workers of both sexes will tend to concentrate even more heavily in nonhousehold service jobs and clerical and sales positions, though growth in the higher status professional and technical occupations also will be important. At least for a time, older women will increase quite substantially in the blue-collar jobs that elderly men are leaving in large numbers. These trends also suggest that while the percentage of older women who work probably won't rise or fall much, the *number* who work will be substantially greater, largely because of inadequate retirement incomes. Heavily represented in that group will be single and divorced women and widows.

The nation will also need more occupational opportunities for the elderly, because some who are retired or unemployed would like to work. In addition, the financial difficulties of the Social Security system are not over and may cause other cutbacks that will make Social Security alone a less adequate source of income, while inflation, even at a decreasing rate, will reduce buying power, and periodic high unemployment will make jobs especially scarce for the elderly. Mandatory retirement policies also are being challenged in the courts as discrimination, and may either fall or undergo additional change. Older people are also increasingly well educated and healthy and are able to hold more sophisticated occupations longer, while the self-images of some are changing to include continued work as a viable option. Finally, the social services needed by older people, especially in the advanced ages, have grown so costly that the elderly and their families are having to bear more of those costs. Work for wages over a longer period is one way to help solve this problem.[48] and may prove a necessity for people aged 65-70 who are caring for even older parents.

Summary

The proportion of elderly people who work has declined sharply in recent decades, and those who do hold jobs tend to be concentrated in relatively low-status, low-paying occupations. Older men have been particularly likely to leave the labor force, though the participation rates of older women also are declining gradually. Perhaps as many as half the elderly workers who leave the work force are pushed out by mandatory retirement policies, and while pension plans and Social Security make that practice palatable financially, it is still discriminatory and expels some older persons who would like to work. Moreover, most who do retire,

162

whether voluntarily or involuntarily, find their incomes cut substantially. Many poorer ones are forced to seek re-employment, usually part time at the lower end of the status scale.

Despite these problems, more workers than ever choose early retirement, often several years before age 65. Thus, the aging work force consists of some workers who will have to retire but prefer to continue working and others who want to leave their jobs as early as possible. Income is the critical factor for many, though the nature of the work, the satisfaction it provides, the types of post-retirement activities available, the worker's self-image, and many other factors influence the complex process of leaving the labor force. Once out, however, it is relatively difficult for the older person to find another job, and the low official unemployment rates among the elderly fail to account for those who get discouraged and stop seeking work and for the long periods of unemployment faced by many of those who do eventually find jobs.

The labor force participation rates of older people will probably continue to decline, despite the increase to 70 of the mandatory retirement age. Yet each cohort that enters the older population is better educated than its predecessors and more able to do the sophisticated work in the evolving occupational-industrial system. Employers are also increasingly likely to look at individual abilities and preferences, and the nation may be moving slowly toward a job pattern that is more responsive to those older persons who want to work, as well as to those under age 65 who want to retire. Court challenges to mandatory retirement are partly responsible, as is the tendency for the elderly to consolidate their voices in opposition to age discrimination in the work-place and other parts of the American social system. Genuine cohesion in any age cohort is difficult to foster, for while people remain male or female, white or black, all their lives, they soon pass from one age group to another and common interests are diluted by that passage and by individual variations.[49] Even now, however, it is clear that older people as a group are not really expected to provide for themselves by working and that large numbers do prefer retirement, while they are also becoming an increasing financial burden for the employed population. That paradox may well become a major intergenerational crisis.

NOTES

1. Fred C. Pampel, *Social Change and the Aged.* Lexington, Ma: Heath, (1981), p. 61.

2. Beth J. Soldo, "America's Elderly in the 1980s," *Population Bulletin* 35 (1981): 21.

3. Robert N. Butler, "Ageism," in Kurt Finsterbusch, ed., *Social Problems 82/83.* Guilford, CT: Dushkin, 1982, p. 127.

4. Judah Matras, *Introduction to Population.* Englewood Cliffs, NJ: Prentice-Hall, 1977, p. 301.

5. For the detailed definition, see U.S. Bureau of the Census, *Statistical Abstract of the United States: 1982-83.* Washington, DC: U.S. Government Printing Office, 1982, p. 372.

6. Herman J. Loether, *Problems of Aging.* 2nd ed. Belmont, CA: Dickenson, 1975, pp. 61-62.

7. Soldo, *op. cit.,* p. 19.

8. Harold L. Sheppard, "Aging and Manpower Development," in Matilda White Riley, John W. Riley, Jr. and Marilyn E. Johnson, eds., *Aging and Society.* v. 2, *Aging and the Professions.* New York: Russell Sage Foundation, 1969, pp. 186-187.

9. Charles S. Harris, *Fact Book on Aging: A Profile of America's Older Population.* Washington, DC: National Council on the Aging, 1978, p. 74.

10. Matilda White Riley, Marilyn E. Johnson and Anne Foner, eds., *Aging and Society.* v. 3, *A Sociology of Age Stratification.* New York: Russell Sage Foundation, 1972, pp. 165-166.

11. *Ibid.,* pp. 173-174.

12. Erdman Palmore, *Social Patterns in Normal Aging: Findings from the Duke Longitudinal Study.* Durham, NC: Duke University Press, 1981, pp. 3-4; 108-109.

13. *Ibid.,* pp. 52; 61.

14. Riley, Johnson and Foner, *op. cit.,* p. 179.

15. Matilda White Riley and Anne Foner, *Aging and Society,* v. 1, *An Inventory of Research Findings.* New York: Russell Sage Foundation, 1968, pp. 427-428.

16. Henry S. Shryock and Jacob S. Siegel, *The Methods and Materials of Demography.* v. 1. Washington, DC: U.S. Government Printing Office, 1973, p. 353.

17. United States data are for 1978 in order to keep the countries in Table 6-2 as close together in time as possible.

18. Organisation for Economic Co-operation and Development, *Socio-economic Policies for the Elderly.* Paris: OECD, 1979, pp. 57-58.

19. Harold L. Sheppard, "Work and Retirement," in Robert N. Binstock and Ethel Shanas, eds., *Handbook of Aging and the Social Sciences.* New York: Van Nostrand, 1976, p. 291.

20. U.S. Bureau of the Census, "Some Demographic Aspects of Aging in the United States," *Current Population Reports,* P-23, no. 43 (1973): 27.

21. Riley and Foner, *op. cit.,* p. 44.

22. Loether, *op. cit.,* p. 51. Cf. Kurt W. Back and Carleton S. Guptill, "Retirement and Self Ratings," in Ida Harper Simpson and John C. McKinney, eds., *Social Aspects of Aging.* Durham, NC: Duke University Press, 1966, p. 120.

23. Riley and Foner, *op. cit.,* p. 51. Cf. Harris, *op. cit.,* p. 75.

24. U.S. Bureau of the Census, "The Social and Economic Status of the Black Population in the United States: An Historical View, 1790-1978," *Current Population Reports,* P-23, no. 80 (1979): 60.

25. Riley and Foner, *op. cit.,* pp. 58-59.

26. Harris, *op. cit.,* p. 80.

164

27. U.S. Bureau of the Census, "America in Transition: An Aging Society," *Current Population Reports*, P-23, no. 128 (1983): 23.

28. Harris, *loc. cit.*

29. John A. Priebe, "Occupation," in U.S. Bureau of the Census, "Population of the United States, Trends and Prospects: 1950-1990," *Current Population Reports*, P-23, no. 49 (1974): 155. See also Ida Harper Simpson, Richard L. Simpson, Mark Evers and Sharon Sandomirsky Poss, "Occupational Recruitment, Retention, and Labor Force Cohort Representation," *American Journal of Sociology* 87 (1982): 1305.

30. Mary Barberis, "America's Elderly: Policy Implications," *Population Bulletin* 35 (1981): 7.

31. Palmore, *op. cit.*, p. 15.

32. Sheppard, *op. cit.*, p. 197.

33. Ida Harper Simpson, Kurt W. Back and John C. McKinney, "Work and Retirement," in Simpson and McKinney, *op. cit.*, p. 59.

34. Riley and Foner, *op. cit.*, p. 50.

35. Juanita M. Kreps, "The Economy and the Aged," in Binstock and Shanas, *op. cit.*, p. 272.

36. *Ibid.*, p. 278.

37. Loether, *op. cit.*, pp. 65-66.

38. Soldo, *op. cit.*, p. 20.

39. Fred Cottrell, *Aging and the Aged*. Dubuque, IA: Wm. C. Brown, 1974, p. 31.

40. Riley, Johnson and Foner, *op. cit.*, p. 164. Cf. Harris, *op. cit.*, p. 75.

41. The projections assume moderate rather than high or low growth in the labor force as a whole. See Howard N. Fullerton, Jr., "The 1995 Labor Force: A First Look," in U.S. Bureau of Labor Statistics, *Economic Projections to 1990*, Bulletin 2121 (1982): 48-58.

42. Congressional Budget Office, *Work and Retirement: Options for Continued Employment for Older Workers*. Washington, DC: U.S. Government Printing Office, 1982, p. 10.

43. Parts of the first three reasons are adapted from Pampel, *op. cit.*, pp. 24-25; 60-61.

44. Judith Treas and Vern L. Bengston, "The Demography of Mid- and Late-Life Transitions," *Annals of American Academy of Political and Social Science*, 464 (1982): 17-18.

45. Melissa A. Hardy, "Social Policy and Determinants of Retirement: A Longitudinal Analysis of Older White Males," *Social Forces* 60 (1982): 1119.

46. Paula J. Schneider and Thomas J. Palumbo, "Social and Demographic Characteristics of the Labor Force," in U.S. Bureau of the Census, "Population of the United States....," *op. cit.*, p. 144.

47. Sheppard, *op. cit.*, p. 292.

48. For a summary of these factors, see Harris, *op. cit.*, p. 774.

49. Kingsley Davis and Pietronella van den Oever, "Age Relations and Public Policy in Advanced Industrial Societies," *Population and Development Review* 7 (1981): 2.

Chapter 7

Retirement

The vast majority of America's elderly are retired, and the amount, sources, and adequacy of their incomes have caused much popular debate and misunderstanding. The perceptions range from masses of older people huddled in rundown tenements and rural shacks and eating dog food, to a huge group of nonproducers who generally live very comfortably because of the heavy financial support burden that falls on the producing population. There are questions, too, about why people retire, what meaning retirement has for them, and how well they adjust to it. Do most desire retirement because it is an attractive alternative life style, or because they are thrown out of their jobs by uncaring employers obsessed with derogatory stereotypes about the abilities and productivity of older workers? Would most retired people rather work or not? Are most of them poor or aren't they? This chapter addresses these and other related questions.

Views of Retirement

Much has been written about the retirement patterns of older people, especially men, the reasons why they leave the labor force, and what they do afterwards.[1] Chapter 6 has already alluded to several aspects of the subject, and in this section it is possible only to summarize some significant findings about retirement — voluntary or involuntary — as a reality in the lives of older people, though the reader needs to know that some of the literature on the retired population is characterized by stereotyping, over-generalizing, and contradictory findings. Too often retired people have been pictured as poorly adjusted and desperate to return to jobs they never wanted to leave in the first place. Some of the apparent contradictions, however, also reflect changes in attitudes among retired people over the past couple of decades, especially as financial opportunities to retire have improved.

Analytically, retirement is simply the withdrawal of a person from the work force and entitlement to an income based on previous employment,[2] and is a process that has many forms and effects. One of the most strategic characteristics of retirement is that it need not be destructive or the beginning of a meaningless existence, any more than it is forced on all those who do leave the labor force. At the same time, negative images of retirement abound among people of all ages, and for some elderly it does symbolize the end of youth, vigor, usefulness, and social involvement, particularly if ill health forces them to retire.

In part, these views exist because some older persons are not prepared to retire *to* something rather than just *from* something, and because retirement often does connote "old age,"[3] even though most people who are forced to retire make reasonably good adjustments after a time. It is easy to miss the tremendous individual variability among retired people, including their different levels of satisfaction, the many ways they use their time, the highly variable amounts of money they have available, their diffences in health, the degrees of satisfaction and happiness they expect, and other variations that keep the retired population from being homogeneous. Thus, one of the complex issues that a discussion of retirement must address is the extent to which the event really is a crisis for retired persons and their spouses. Another issue is why they retire in the first place, for while many leave the labor force involuntarily because of illness or mandatory provisions, many others choose to retire, often before age 65. That trend toward early retirement began in the 1950s and was accelerated by a 1961 Social Security provision that granted reduced benefits at age 62.[4] In the late 1970s, however, inflationary pressures tended to slow this trend, and many people who would have retired early actually had to postpone moving into that phase of the life cycle. Even so, for many retired people the adjustments are successful, and finances, physical and mental health, and outlook seem adequate for the bulk of the retired population to adjust satisfactorily.[5]

The Retired Population

The retired group is more difficult to identify than it might seem, for there are various ways to classify them. Some do not work at all in a given year; others are not at work or in the labor force during the week they are surveyed; some hold only part-time or part-year jobs, though they may have retired from full-time positions. The last group experiences a certain degree of retirement, but not complete disengagement from the workplace. One can define retired people as those who receive retirement benefits, even though some of them also work, many up to the earnings-limit allowed by the Social Security system. Perhaps the most inclusive definition involves that group who hold less than full-time, year-round jobs, for under that designation about 90 per cent of the men and 95 per cent of the women aged 65 and older are retired.[6]

If the receipt of Social Security retirement benefits is used as a criterion, in 1980 almost 20 million Americans aged 62 and older were drawing such benefits, but only about a third that number received full benefits, which begin at age 65. Thus, 4.6 million men and 2.8 million women fell into the latter category, which means that about 64 per cent of the men and 31 per cent of the women were full beneficiaries. But women often do not receive full benefits because of their work histories and the way the Social Security system has classified them relative to their husbands. Many people of both sexes still work at part-time jobs while they receive benefits, so these data do not really reflect the retired population either.

If retirement is gauged by the proportions not in the labor force, then in 1980 about 81 per cent of the men and 92 per cent of the women 65 and over were classified as retired. (See Table 7-1.) But these data are strongly influenced by what people were doing during the survey week, the number of hours worked by those who were employed, whether or not unemployed people were seeking work, and other factors that prevent non-involvement in the work force from being a perfect measure of the nation's retired population. Nonetheless, the materials available do show that between the ages of 55 and 64 the retirement rate rises significantly, that at age 65 the vast majority of workers of both sexes are retired, and that in the 10 years after age 65 virtually all remaining workers retire from the labor force. For the society at large those proportions represent two opposing trends: (1) reductions in the death rate and increases in life expectancy raise the number of years the average person could work; while (2) the tendency for virtually all elderly people to retire and for many to do so before age 65 reduces the number of years one actually works and increases the time he/she is a dependent.[7] Those trends have basic implications for the productivity of the older population and for the financial costs borne by the younger group.

Men and Women

The patterns of retirement have changed quite dramatically over the past few decades, and have done so differently for men and women. For example, even among men aged 45-54 the retirement rate appears to have increased since 1950, though more than 90 per cent of that age group is still in the labor force. A sizable share of those who do retire in their 40s or early 50s are military personnel and people who worked in police and fire departments or were otherwise occupied as civil servants;[8] others are forced to stop working because of poor health. In the 55-64 age group the retirement rate doubled between 1950 and 1980, largely because retirement at age 62 or even earlier has caught on with a quarter or more of the men in the 55-64 age range. The proportion of men aged 65 and older who are retired is also much higher than in any past decade, largely due to improvements in benefits that allow an older couple sufficient money to live on, though the income is usually considerably lower than their last pre-retirement wage.

Mandatory retirement provisions have also helped push the proportion of retired men aged 65 and older to more than 80 per cent of the total. But even with the mandatory retirement age now at 70, the trends suggest that other forces favoring early retirement are far more powerful than the legal right to work until that age. One of those forces is the recent relatively high unemployment rates which have caused large groups of workers to be laid off despite seniority, and which make it difficult for elderly workers to find new jobs.

At the same time, continued inflation has forced some older workers to

Table 7-1. Percentages of People Not in the Labor Force, by Sex and Age, 1900-1990

Year	Male			Female		
	45-54	55-64	65+	45-54	55-64	65+
1900	4.5	10.0	31.6	85.3	86.8	91.9
1930	3.5	9.8	41.7	79.6	83.9	92.0
1940	7.9	16.2	58.5	87.9	83.6	94.1
1950	4.2	13.0	54.2	62.0	73.0	90.3
1960	4.3	13.2	66.9	50.2	62.8	89.2
1970	5.8	17.0	73.2	45.6	57.0	90.3
1980	8.8	27.7	80.9	40.1	58.5	91.9
1990	9.2	32.5	84.2	35.7	58.3	92.7

Sources: U.S. Bureau of the Census, Sixteenth Census of the United States: 1940, The Labor Force, U.S. Summary (1943), table 8; Statistical Abstract of the United States: 1981, table 636; U.S. Bureau of Labor Statistics, Handbook of Labor Statistics: 1980, table 2; Howard N. Fullerton, "The 1995 Labor Force," in U.S. Bureau of Labor Statistics, Economic Projections to 1990, Bulletin 2121 (1982), table 4.

continue until age 70 and caused others who did retire to seek part-time employment. But it probably isn't realistic to expect that any large number of older people can return to the work force during times of relatively high unemployment.[9] The jobs are simply too scarce and younger people have too much of an edge in obtaining and holding the ones that are available. Moreover, each new recession tends to start with a higher unemployment rate than did the previous one, and that reduces the older person's job prospects.

As we have seen, the involvement of women in the labor force has increased substantially since 1950, and the percentages of participants aged 45-64 are now much higher. For those aged 65 and older, however, there has been little change, and women seem more likely than men to retire. The Duke Longitudinal Study suggests that even when the women who list themselves as "housewife" and who are not in the official labor force are omitted from consideration, women workers are still more likely than men to retire early, having a substantially higher retirement rate in their 50s and beyond.[10] In part, this difference comes about because the work role is still more important to today's older men than it is to older women, given their earlier socialization, their lower average wages, persistent negative stereotypes about elderly women, and other disincentives to remain in the labor force after age 62 or 65. Furthermore, married women have far higher retirement rates than single women and somewhat higher ones than divorced women, partly because the married ones are less compelled by economic necessity to continue in the work force.

But the sex differences in retirement patterns are diminishing because of the gradual shift toward equality of men and women in the work-place. More women than ever are in the labor force and more are working full time without long interruptions for childrearing or other reasons. In addition, men's attitudes toward working women have been changing, as have those of the women themselves, and they are now less likely to end up in the relatively few categories of "female" jobs available to earlier generations. Therefore, women are apt to work for wages longer and more continuously than their mothers did, and to do so in better jobs and at higher wages, though the income differential between the sexes remains a persistent problem. Given these conditions, more women tend to have longer tenure in the work force than did earlier cohorts, and their retirement patterns by age are becoming more like those of men.[11 At the same time, more men are retiring earlier and their retirement rate is pushing toward that of women.[12]

Reasons for Retirement

People retire from the work force for many reasons, some of which were discussed in Chapter 6, but as the data in Table 7-1 suggest, advancing age is the principal one; the older one gets, the more likely one is to retire. Therefore, the general aging of the population will create a growing retired segment to be supported by a proportionately smaller working group, unless the basic trends reverse and larger percentages of older workers remain in or return to the labor force. That seems unlikely in the near future, though over a longer period the economic system may have to be fundamentally restructured so they can, because older workers will still need jobs, some employers will need their services, and they will be too large a population to be supported adequately if they are all retired. Of course, other things go along with advancing age, such as discrimination, the general expectation that older people should retire, increased financial benefits, and, for some, disability.[13]

Therefore, retirement is not just an individual matter, for it serves many purposes and has many motivations. For the person it may represent relief from a difficult, unpleasant, or boring job, and it is now a socially accepted way to stop working in a work-oriented society and do other things. In that sense, the person usually feels he/she has earned the right to live as much on his/her own terms as allowed by health, finances, family considerations, and other realities. Retirement also allows flexibility in the work force, so that employers can replace people they deem undesirable and can reduce the number of employees in tight economic times, often by not filling jobs vacated by retirees. Retirement helps lower the rate of unemployment and admits more young people to the labor force, while it also protects those elderly covered by pensions from the abject poverty that the loss of a job would otherwise impose. This is especially significant in times of high unemployment when labor is abundant. Even unions agree to mandatory retirement in order to extract concessions from employers, including pensions.[14]

Given these forces and factors, involuntary and voluntary retirement need to be considered separately, though they overlap substantially in many actual cases, especially when the worker who is pushed out of the labor force is also provided advantages that pull him/her out.

Involuntary Retirement

Given the impact of aging and other forces on retirement, it is clear that involuntary reasons loom large in causing people to retire after age 65, and that mandatory provisions adopted by industries are the most important cause of involuntary retirement. Thus, the Duke Longitudinal Study, whose findings agree with a 1963 survey done by the Social Security Administration, found that about 40 per cent of the older retired male workers and 35 per cent of the females left the work force because of mandatory retirement or layoffs, while another significant share cited poor health or disability.[15] Therefore, considerably more than half the retired workers of both sexes left their jobs involuntarily, although much mandatory retirement does allow sufficient benefits for the retirees to live reasonably comfortably, and thereby merges an incentive with the necessity to retire. In fact, that combination raises serious questions for the future, when the number of older workers forced to retire and the strains on public and private pension plans both will increase.

The issue of discrimination is also inherent in forcing people out of work at any age no matter what income is provided, for mandatory retirement does fail to account for individual differences in productivity, ambition, and occupational usefulness. Moreover, about half the working population is not covered by private pension plans, and the financial problems many face after forced retirement do discriminate against the group that must rely only on Social Security and other governmental programs, savings,[16] help from family members, and other sources that are sometimes insufficient or unpredictable.

But given the sizable proportions who live reasonably comfortable, well-adjusted lives after retirement and the benefits still needed by those whose incomes are inadequate, the most basic question is this: Can the economic system afford to force more workers out because of age and still provide the income that makes retirement humane?[17] Mandatory retirement at a uniform age well below average life expectancy of the elderly is a rite of passage that the society may be unable to subsidize in the future, especially if the cost of maintaining the average retired worker continues to escalate beyond his/her contributions to the Social Security system, and if the ratio of workers to retirees continues to drop.

Despite its problems, mandatory retirement is a more humane alternative than dismissing older workers for inadequate performance, although the latter practice would better reflect individual variations. Moreover, mandatory retirement gives workers a "target" date toward which they must plan, while younger workers know when certain positions will open up. As those younger workers move up, presumably more entry-level jobs also become available for people just completing their educations. This is especially critical in times of high unemployment, such as the early 1980s, though some of those jobs are also being eliminated by more sophisticated technology. Finally, given the tendency for white men to dominate the ranks of upper-level senior employees in most industries, mandatory retirement gives employers the opportunity to recruit additional women, blacks, Hispanics, and others whose chances would otherwise be more limited.[18]

Mandatory retirement is certainly a complex issue, but it does appear that moving the age limit from 65 to 70 will solve some problems while it intensifies others. If the change keeps more older workers in the labor force, it will shorten the time during which they receive benefits from the hard-pressed Social Security system and from private pension plans, most of which are not growing and provide no cost-of-living increases, and many of which are also under severe financial strains. Furthermore, a few extra years in the labor force will make the worker a continuing contributor to Social Security and might provide some additional private savings for retirement, though high rates of inflation and interest on purchases would erode some of those gains. Finally, longer years in the labor force would partially offset the fact that the elderly population is growing faster than the group aged 20-64, and would relieve some of the burden on the latter.

But because the forces that result in retirement are so complex, even if all people were allowed to work longer, it is uncertain how many would choose to do so. The average age of retirement is already substantially below the old mandatory age of 65, and many people still find retirement so attractive that they are willing to take substantial cuts in income to achieve it, though the relative adequacy of that income after retirement is often better than the dollar losses might imply. If many people continue to want retirement in their early 60s or at age 65, it seems useful to encourage the wider development of private pension plans that will allow earlier voluntary retirement and help relieve unemployment and other problems, while they also help the Social Security system preserve the long-term solvency intended by the 1983 reforms, one of which is a gradual increase in the minimum age at which workers can claim full benefits. The system was never meant to be the sole source of income for retired persons anyway.

Voluntary Retirement

Though about 40 per cent of all retired workers leave the labor force involuntarily because of compulsory provisions and another 15 per cent quit because of disability, the other 45 per cent are not subject to mandatory retirement, are in good health, and yet choose to leave the work force for a variety of reasons. For men, the wish to enjoy more leisure and recreation is a major incentive, as is the availability of an adequate pension or other financial resources that allow a decent retirement income. For women, family considerations seem the most important, because they either wish to spend more time at home or are needed to do so. In many cases, the woman worker in her late 50s or her 60s becomes the chief caregiver for an aged parent, usually a mother or mother-in-law, and that role takes precedence over her job.

In addition, a substantial number of women prefer more leisure and recreational opportunities, often with husbands who have also retired.

This helps account for the higher retirement rates among women who are married than among those who are not, as does the availability and adequacy of the husband's retirement income. It is also significant, therefore, that the proportion of women who choose to retire because they personally have good pensions is far lower than the percentage of men who cite that reason.[19] Many of the older women who continue to work are sole wage-earners in a household; not a few live alone, and some have had long work experiences that encourage them to continue working. Thus, given the tendency for fewer women to be covered by adequate pension plans and the lower wages on which their retirement benefits are computed, it is not surprising that financial incentives are a less attractive reason for women to choose retirement than they are for men.

The level of education and type of job also affect voluntary retirement rates, for people with the highest levels of schooling tend to retire relatively late and at a lower rate. Many of them are doing work that demands little physical exertion and are not as overwhelmed by the energy demands of their jobs as a laborer might be, though some may be too sedentary. In addition, well-educated people are more likely to hold interesting and rewarding occupations they are reluctant to leave, and are more apt to have skills that make them less easy to replace or power that makes them difficult to expel. They are also more likely to be self-employed and unaffected by mandatory retirement, and some are able to scale down their activities gradually while partners or heirs take on more responsibility, such as in a law or medical practice. The well-educated are also less subject to the age discrimination that often forces the poorly educated out of their low-status jobs.

Conversely, people whose educations and opportunities have caused them to be laborers all of their working lives are apt to retire as soon as they can afford to do so, thus escaping the arduous physical demands of their jobs. Other blue-collar workers, especially in manufacturing, must depart at the mandatory age and their retirement rate is relatively high, though many are also glad to leave the work force. At the same time, older people in service positions have a fairly low rate of retirement, basically because they cannot afford to leave their jobs, but also because those jobs don't make impossible physical demands on the elderly worker. In fact, many older workers who do retire from other occupations take service jobs as a way to supplement their incomes, which might otherwise come exclusively from Social Security, though the jobs tend to be relatively low in the status hierarchy. Finally, workers in middle management also tend to have relatively high retirement rates, often because their chances for promotion decline sharply after age 45 or 50 and they tend to be "stuck" at the same level for many years,[20] some because of obsolete skills and educations.

In general, then, the retirement rates are lowest at the extremes of the income and job-status range: Professional and technical workers and senior management personnel tend to work past age 65 because of high rewards and their value as workers or because they are self-employed. Service workers tend to hold on to jobs which pay relatively little and which they may even dislike, but which supply small supplements to Social Security payments and are not too difficult physically for the older person to perform. Workers between these extremes tend to have higher retirement rates because of adequate pensions, mandatory provisions, or "dead-end" jobs that are not an inspiring alternative to leisure; the rates are also comparatively high for laborers.

In the retired population of all ages, voluntary reasons seem responsible for the fact that the average worker now has a 30 per cent greater chance of retirement than one with the same job and nonwork income had in 1950. Much of this increase is due to early retirement that is unaffected by mandatory provisions, and that helps account for the rapid growth in the total retired population. And most of the people who are subject to mandatory retirement appear to leave willingly at the specified age, or at least to adjust eventually to the nonwork role. Therefore, the workers who have been forced out of jobs they really wanted to keep are only a minority, whereas those who have chosen or adjusted readily to retirement are the majority. The former group is enlarged some by the people who must retire because of disability, the latter by the increasing numbers who can count on reasonable pensions after they retire, though certain numbers choose to retire on low incomes because retirement has significant attractions for many people even when it creates financial strains; the retirement choice is at least partly independent of income and the effects of inflation.[21]

Nevertheless, there remains a sizable number of retirement resisters, perhaps 4 million or more retired people age 65 and older who do not like their situations and want to work for wages. Once again, however, the state of health and the adequacy of income play major roles in whether or not a person resists or accepts retirement, as do the nature of the job, the strains it imposes, how the person perceives his/her degree of autonomy in the job, and other factors that may be quite subjective.[22]

Adjusting to Retirement

Retirement calls for more adjustment by some people than others, but as in most phases of the life cycle, the large majority deal with it as smoothly as possible and go on with their lives. In fact, most who retire find the event and subsequent accommodations far less traumatic than the popular wisdom suggests. The process does not appear to create unbearable poverty, serious mental or physical problems, idle boredom, or grim unhappiness for the great majority; for many people it has the opposite effects. It is crucial, however, for retirement to allow people continued self-respect, no matter how they may construe it, and a reasonable measure of social responsibility and usefulness, partly to offset the negative status that Americans still tend to assign persons who are retired.[23] In a society that is strongly youth-oriented and where one's worth is still tied partly to work, retirement signifies the loss of two socially desirable traits and the concomitant acquisition of two less desirable ones. Therefore, even though retirement doesn't shatter many lives unless it plunges people into extreme poverty, it does necessitate adjustments and redefinitions, some of them painful, others easy and pleasurable. On the whole, however, retirement doesn't seem to reduce life satisfaction for most people, and "very few suffer severe poverty, illness, inactivity, or depression as a result."[24]

In contrast to some earlier studies, the recent ones cited herein show that people's attitudes toward impending retirement are generally favorable, and that the number of years a person has to go before retirement or the years already spent in it have little relationship to how he/she assesses retirement. The two factors that do strongly affect attitudes are health and projected or actual income, because they influence the person's options during retirement.[25] Both of these factors have improved markedly for the older population in the past few decades, so that many who might have feared retirement in the 1950s and 1960s do not do so now. Therefore, while the findings of some earlier studies on the matter are inconsistent with those of later investigations, the apparent contradictions actually reflect significant shifts in the attitudes of the elderly themselves,[26] and those, in turn, mirror important financial improvements for the elderly population as a whole.

Some caution is necessary, however, as one interprets the results of surveys that attempt to gauge the life satisfaction of older people, especially those who are retired. Some may report that they are genuinely satisfied with conditions that other age groups would reject or which the elderly themselves would have deplored when they were younger, whereas their favorable responses may represent an ego-defense. Even if elderly respondents truly believe they are deprived and less happy than other groups, they may still report themselves in more optimistic terms as a way to deny the feeling that they have failed, are poor, and are otherwise unable to live up to the life-satisfaction norms they think prevail.[27] Such a phenomenon is closely related to the tendency for the elderly to see themselves as a more homogeneous group than they are, as discussed in Chapter 2.[28]

Income

When most persons retire, income does go down substantially and they must get by on the much-discussed smaller "fixed income," though cost-of-living increases in Social Security benefits have provided some flexibility. But lingering fears about income insufficiency are often exaggerated, for despite the inflationary spiral the proportion of elderly people living in families below the official poverty line declined from 27 per cent in 1959 to 8 per cent in 1981, while the proportion among unrelated individuals (essentially the people living alone) fell from 62 per cent to 29 per cent. Moreover, most of the elderly who live in poverty did so when they were younger, though it is noteworthy that even the lower percentage of elderly poor in 1981 meant there were still 4 million people, or 15 per cent of the entire older population, below the official poverty line. Obviously, those people need more of the help an affluent society can provide, whether privately or publicly.

The decrease that retired people experience in *actual* income is generally far more than the decrease in the *adequacy* of income, because most retired people no longer pay home mortgages, while they have small or no responsibilities to rear and educate children and are less burdened by certain other expenses carried by younger adults, including the bulk of Social Security taxes. Retired people also have the protection of medical care that is partly publicly financed, increases in Social Security benefits to counter cost-of-living changes, discounts on many purchases, and other offsetting advantages,[29] though some of these were reduced as the federal government attempted to restore the financial health of the Social Security system. In general, the spectacle of a class of elderly persons forced into poverty by mandatory retirement is a myth for all but a relatively small minority, though they do need attention and some are truly destitute. In addition, retirees report they miss money more than any other aspects of the job, while comparatively few miss the work itself,[30] which means that older people's assumption of widespread poverty in their age group may be a problem no matter what the realities.

Chapter 8 to follow deals more fully with the elderly who are truly poor and with the larger matter of income received by various groups of older people.

Health

Almost everyone seems to know at least one older person who retired and died soon afterward, appearing to languish and waste away in the interim. Such cases have created the assumption that retirement causes a decline in health, both physical and mental. It may do so for those whose lives were consumed by a job and who became totally inactive after retirement. But the principal reasons retired people have higher rates of illness and death than other groups is because existing health problems forced more of them to retire, and because advancing age increases the likelihood of illness irrespective of employment status.

Moreover, while some retirees report poorer health after retirement, equal numbers experience improvements, especially those who worked in hazardous or unusually stressful jobs, and the ones who became more active physically after retirement.[31] As expected, most of those whose health is poor tend to be less satisfied with retirement than people who have few disabilities, largely because illness keeps the former from living life as they please, including the choice to keep on working. But retirement also allows the unhealthy person to lay down the burden of a job, and his/her level of satisfaction with life may rise as a result. Nonetheless, health and income are the two most strategic predictors of how well a person adapts to retirement, though the decision to retire in the first place seems to be influenced much more strongly by the availability of retirement income than by the level of health, unless the latter is severely incapacitating.[32]

Personal Adaptation

Retirement does not cause depression or unhappiness for the great majority of elderly people, though a small minority with limited interests and the compulsion to continue working do suffer such problems. Furthermore, some of those who resist retirement are often able to keep their jobs, at least in certain occupations, while others can sometimes find new ones to offset forced retirement. Altogether, therefore, perhaps 80 or 90 per cent of the retired population seem no less happy than when they worked, and the great majority do not slip into extreme loneliness, depression, isolation, and inactivity.[33] although those difficulties were probably more severe in the 1950s and 1960s than they are now. Nevertheless, there is a tendency toward greater solitude among many retirees, for not all of the hours one formerly worked are necessarily filled with other social activity, and one's productivity in the conventional sense does decrease; nor does the person have a work role around which to orient other activities.

Retirement also has some unfavorable social meanings the person must confront, and status may fall because the society still assigns rather negative meanings to a person's departure from work, and because his/her income will probably decrease.[34] Even worse, the drop in income does force some retirees to experience poverty or near poverty for the first time in their lives.[35] Nearly all retirees tend to be labeled "old," which also has negative connotations despite individual differences in chronological and physiological age, mental and physical states, and levels of activity. Therefore, some retired workers must struggle to preserve a decent level of living, self-respect, and a sense of usefulness in the face of these realities and their meanings, especially if significant associates believe that retirement is "the end of things." The task is particularly difficult for those who lack an adequate network of integrative relationships to replace the work role.

But new retirees begin to give more effort to activities for which they once had little time, such as recreation with a spouse or friends who have also left the labor force. Many people who had hobbies spend more time on them and obtain a feeling of productivity from those efforts or from part-time employment, volunteer work, home maintenance, religious involvement, new educational experiences, and other activities. Consequently, most of the negative effects of retirement that do occur, including disengagement from full-time work, lower incomes, and the change from "middle aged" to "old," seem to be temporary and manageable for most retired persons. Their successes, however, should not belittle the adjustments that virtually all retirees must make, or the substantial strains experienced by a minority who do not progress smoothly into that phase of the life cycle and who suffer once in it. Some of them are too poor to afford activities that would enhance social integration. But no matter what the cause, social activity for the elderly can be improved by public and private efforts to create centers for the elderly, group dining arrangements, and other activities that enhance social integration and adaptation.[36]

Changes in the Nature of Retirement

A New Institution

In assessing the ways people adapt to retirement, it is useful to recognize that it is a relatively new institution in American society, other industrialized societies, and the socialist countries, while it scarcely exists for the great majority of people in most of the developing nations. As suggested by the data in Table 7-1, only in the last few decades has any group but a wealthy minority been able to afford retirement, while the majority either died while still employed or were forced out by disability or employment policies, usually without pensions or much other financial security. Many didn't have to retire at all because they were self-employed, mainly in farming, and in those farm households that did include three generations the elderly continued to contribute what they could, being neither forced by age alone to give up productive work nor protected by pensions from sharing any deprivations experienced by the rest of the family. As noted in Chapter 4, however, the three-generation family was never as common as often assumed; nor are most modern families indifferent to elderly members and their needs, though the task of caring for very old retired members may fall on offspring who are retired themselves.[37]

The newness of the retirement process means, therefore, that American society is just now developing mechanisms and attitudes to smooth the transition from work to nonwork and to make retirement a fully respectable and satisfying stage in the life cycle. Moreover, the great variation in the post-retirement incomes received by individuals means that financial comfort for some people in the older years contrasts sharply with deprivation for others. Consequently, before older people can adapt more easily and productively to retirement, the society must complete the process of creating institutions that provide adequate incomes, medical care, housing, and other aspects of retirement that are still not as thoroughly incorporated into the American system as is work. Only then will retirement become a fully acceptable status in a reasonably ordered period of life for virtually all individuals, rather than the last struggle after an earlier ordered period of life is over.[38]

Supporting the Retired Population

There is another side to this matter. It involves the increasing burden of support for the elderly that falls on the working population, for that situation has also changed significantly. Chapter 2 dealt with the statistical relationship between producers and the elderly and pointed out that the *combined* youth and elderly dependency ratio is no greater now than it has been, but that the relative importance of the two components has changed significantly. This section considers the financial implications of a growing, non-producing elderly population, including the degree to which the working population will continue to accept the rising costs of supporting that group.

The burden of support for the elderly has passed increasingly from the family to public responsibility, though the working population still carries the burden. Several factors, including rapid social change, geographic movement, vertical social mobility, and high divorce rates, have broadened the social distance between many elderly persons and their children, and in many cases they have reduced the direct care that offspring provide their elderly parents. Simultaneously, these and other factors have increased the dependence of the elderly on pension plans, Social Security, Medicare, community agencies, and other formal public programs and agencies.

Moreover, despite the family relationships that still pervade the care that large numbers of older people receive, the elderly have come to expect less from children directly and more from the society, which is to say more from the working population indirectly through taxation and various transfer payments. And because this expectation has been institutionalized, the small population of wealthy elderly whose family resources allowed them to retire in earlier generations has been joined by the large majority of all people aged 65 and older, for they can now call on the resources of the whole society. In the process, the cost for support of the retired population has risen astronomically.[39] As a result, the older person who retires now recoups his/her total Social Security investment in a few years and then draws from funds paid by current workers, whereas young people may never receive the full amount they will contribute during their working lives.

This situation raises several questions: How high can taxation for support of the elderly go before it is counterproductive? How long will the working population be willing to pay for such support, balancing costs against genuine benevolence for older people and the knowledge that they, the younger people, will eventually become recipients rather than contributors? What additional reforms are needed in the Social Security and Medicare systems to keep them solvent indefinitely and yet allow us to meet the costs of other necessary services? How can the elderly come to rely more heavily on wages generated by their own efforts, and how can attitudes be changed to encourage work as a way to reduce the strains on public finances? Can the economy accommodate a larger population of working elderly and still provide "full employment" for younger people, including teenagers? Can we head off a serious intergenerational conflict over these matters?

American society is struggling with these questions now and will need to deal with them more intensively in the future. In the meantime, it is undeniable that the elderly whose support derives from nonwork income, use but do not produce goods and services, no matter how much they may have earned that privilege and no matter what other useful things they may do. In turn, the burden on those who do produce grows, because the numbers and proportions of retired people have increased rapidly, the ratio of workers to retired people has fallen sharply, and the relative incomes of the elderly have risen.[40] All of this represents an unprecedented burden on producing adults, no matter how much the support burden for children may have declined, and is a major social change that has made care for the elderly much more a public matter with major political implications. There is no escaping the fact that fertility fluctuations in the twentieth century, along with mortality reductions, have greatly increased the elderly population, and that the retirement of the great majority of older people has made them a dependent group for an increasingly long period.[41] With the average age of retirement falling and life expectancy increasing, more elderly are drawing more heavily from both public and private pension plans financed by a working population that is growing at a slower rate than is the older group. That is another basic feature in the aging of America's population, and is a major dilemma.

Summary

Most Americans aged 65 and older are retired, though numerous misperceptions stereotype them as poor or as an overwhelming burden on the working population; as with most stereotypes, there is *some* truth in both views. The "retired" population is actually very diverse, because some people work part-time or part-year; others retire on comfortable pensions but have difficulty in adjusting to income reductions; still others continue to be just as poor as they always were or become even poorer. Therefore, it is difficult to identify who is retired and the nature of their circumstances.

People retire for many reasons, but one large group is forced to do so by mandatory provisions or poor health, while the other large segment chooses retirement willingly, usually because they can afford it and look forward to a financially tolerable future. Moreover, much voluntary retirement is accompanied by a package of Social Security benefits and private pension income, so that many people are simultaneously forced and attracted out of the labor force. Those who must retire early because of serious disabilities, however, often have limited resources and large expenses. Those who retire voluntarily because they can afford to and want more leisure account for the bulk of early retirees, and they have helped lower the average age at retirement significantly.

How well people accept and adjust to retirement is subject to conflicting findings, but largely because adjustment seems to have been more difficult in the recent past than it is now. The critical factors in adjustment are the adequacy of one's income, the state of one's health, and the kinds of activities that one experiences in the older years. But most retirees appear to adjust well and relatively easily and to go on with their lives fairly smoothly. Those who really miss work itself are a comparatively small and declining minority, though most people do miss the higher income that work provided. Large-scale retirement is a relatively new phenomenon, however, confined to the industrialized countries and the socialist nations, and many questions remain about its impact on the retired population and the support burden that the working population must carry for the rapidly growing retired group.

182

NOTES

1. See, for example, Gordon F. Streib and Clement J. Schneider, *Retirement and American Society*. Ithaca, NY: Cornell University Press, 1971; Frances M. Carp, ed., *Retirement*. New York: Behavioral Publications, 1972; Robert C. Atchley, *The Sociology of Retirement*. Cambridge, MA: Schenkman, 1976; Anne Foner and Karen Schwab, *Aging and Retirement*. Monterey, CA: Brooks/Cole, 1981; Neil G. McCluskey and Edgar F. Borgatta, eds., *Aging and Retirement: Prospects, Planning, and Policy*. Beverly Hills, CA: Sage, 1981; Erdman Palmore, *Social Patterns in Normal Aging: Findings from the Duke Longitudinal Study*. Durham, NC: Duke University Press, 1981, chapter 3; and Robert C. Atchley, "Retirement: Leaving the World of Work," *Annals of American Academy of Political and Social Science* 464 (1982): 120-131.

2. Atchley, *op. cit.*, p. 120.

3. Marvin B. Sussman, "An Analytical Model for the Sociological Study of Retirement," in Carp, *op. cit.*, pp. 32; 36.

4. Judith Treas and Vern L. Bengston, "The Demography of Mid- and Late-Life Transitions," *Annals*, p. 19.

5. Palmore, *op. cit.*, p. 36.

6. For the various definitions, see *ibid.*, p. 32.

7. Trudy B. Anderson, "The Dependent Elderly Population: A Function of Retirement," *Research on Aging* 3 (1981): 314.

8. Richard A. Kalish, *Late Adulthood: Perspectives on Human Development*. Monterey, CA: Brooks/Cole, 1975, p. 111.

9. Juanita M. Kreps, "The Economy and the Aged," in Robert H. Binstock and Ethel Shanas, eds., *Handbook of Aging and the Social Sciences*. New York: Van Nostrand, 1976, p. 282.

10. Palmore, *op. cit.*, p. 34. Cf. Fred C. Pampel, *Social Change and the Aged*. Lexington, MA: Heath, 1981, p. 69.

11. Jacob S. Siegel, "On the Demography of Aging," *Demography* 17 (1980): 358.

12. For a treatment of this matter, see Robert C. Atchley, "The Process of Retirement: Comparing Women and Men," in Maximiliane Szinovacz, ed., *Women's Retirement*. Beverly Hills, CA: Sage, 1982, chapter 10.

13. Palmore, *op. cit.*, pp. 34-35.

14. For several of these points, see Atchley, "Retirement," *op. cit.*, p. 121.

15. Palmore, *op. cit.*, pp. 37-39.

16. Harrison Givens, Jr., "An Evaluation of Mandatory Retirement," *Annals of American Academy of Political and Social Science*, 438 (1978): 51-52.

17. Harold L. Sheppard, "The Issue of Mandatory Retirement," *Annals* 438 (1978): 48-49.

18. Givens, *op. cit.*, p. 51.

19. Palmore, *op. cit.*, pp. 37-38.

20. Organisation for Economic Co-operation and Development, *Socio-economic Policies for the Elderly*. Paris: OECD, 1979, pp. 82-83.

183

21. Pampel, *op. cit.,* pp. 60-61.

22. Harold L. Sheppard, "Work and Retirement," in Binstock and Shanas, *op. cit.,* p. 302. Cf. National Council on the Aging, *The Myth and Reality of Aging in America.* Washington, DC: NCOA, 1975.

23. Carp, *op. cit.,* pp. 40-41.

24. Palmore, *op. cit.,* pp. 45-46.

25. Robert C. Atchley and Judith L. Robinson, "Attitudes Toward Retirement and Distance from the Event," *Research on Aging* 4 (1982): 311.

26. On this matter, see Nancy Lohman, "Life Satisfaction Research in Aging: Implications for Policy Development," in Nancy Datan and Nancy Lohman, eds., *Transitions of Aging.* New York: Academic Press, 1980, chapter 2, especially pp. 31-32; 35.

27. For a treatment of this methodological problem, see Frances M. Carp and Abraham Carp, "It May Not Be the Answer, It May Be the Question," *Research on Aging* 3 (1981): 85-100, especially pp. 97-98.

28. Hubert J. O'Gorman, "False Consciousness of Kind," *Research on Aging* 2 (1980): 105-128.

29. Palmore, *op. cit.,* p. 40.

30. Kalish, *op. cit.,* pp. 108; 109.

31. Palmore, *op. cit.,* pp. 40-41.

32. Willis J. Goudy, "Antecedent Factors Related to Changing Work Expectations," *Research on Aging* 4 (1982): 153-154.

33. Palmore, *op. cit.,* p 41. Cf. Atchley and Robinson, *op. cit.,* pp. 301-303.

34. Sussman, *op. cit.,* pp. 40-41.

35. Beth J. Soldo, "America's Elderly in the 1980s," *Population Bulletin* 35 (1980): 21.

36. Lohman, *op. cit.,* pp. 34-35.

37. Elaine M. Brody, "The Aging of the Family," *Annals* 438 (1978): 17.

38. Sussman, *op. cit.,* p. 34.

39. Kingsley Davis and Pietronella van den Oever, "Age Relations and Public Policy in Advanced Industrial Societies," *Population and Development Review* 7 (1981): 4-6.

40. *Ibid.,* pp. 8-9.

41. Anderson, *op. cit.,* pp. 311; 314.

Chapter 8

Income and Poverty Status
Of the Elderly

Popular attitudes and literature tend to portray older people as poor or close to it, because most of the elderly experience such large cuts in their money incomes when they retire. Since 1960 their incomes have averaged only about half to two-thirds those of younger people,[1] and that drop is a severe blow to many, even those whose reduced resources are still adequate.[2] In addition, many people now reaching retirement age have worked at low-paying jobs, and the base on which their retirement benefits are computed is small, their incomes even less adequate when they do retire. Therefore, it would be cruel to minimize the plight of those older persons who encounter poverty for the first time when they leave work and of those who can't afford a decent level of living. Such groups include many sick and disabled people, widows, members of minority groups, and persons covered only by minimum Social Security benefits.

Despite these real problems, however, governmental programs and other forces have helped protect increasing proportions of the elderly from severe deprivation. Those forces include transfer payments, Medicare and other governmental health programs, the smaller number of dependents supported by older than by younger people, double tax exemptions, discounts on certain purchases, help from family members, and other advantages that partly offset the smaller cash incomes received by many elderly. These things are difficult to measure and rarely show up in the reports on financial resources, but even a few refinements in assessing the data on income show most older persons to be better off relative to younger ones than we often assume.

Income

Indexes of Income

This study relies principally on two indexes of income and focuses on the large majority of elderly who are not in the labor force or receiving full wages. The indexes are *family income* and *personal income*.

Family Income. The U.S. Census Bureau, through its Current Population Survey, regularly provides data on family income and household income, but unless those materials are used as carefully as they are recorded, they can support the impression of pervasive poverty among the elderly.[3] In 1980, for example, the mean income for all American families, unweighted by the number of family members or by age, was $23,974, while the unweighted mean for families with householders aged 65 and older was only $16,918, or about 71 per cent of the figure for all families.[4] But if family incomes are calculated on a per capita basis, the situation of older people seems far less dire, because most elderly householders need use the income only for themselves and a spouse; they are no longer responsible for high childrearing costs. Consequently, Table 8-1 shows how differently the elderly fare when per capita family income is substituted for overall family income, and that in 1980 the per capita income of families with a householder aged 65 or older was 99 per cent of the per capita amount received by all families.

Clearly, elderly families are about as well off on the average by this index as is the population as a whole, and they fare better than the families with a householder aged 15-24, 25-34, or 35-44. The last two groups are likely to have dependent children who impose a financial strain that most elderly no longer have to endure. In 1980, for example, while the average family with a householder aged 35-44 had 1.86 children and that with a householder aged 25-34 had 1.52, elderly families averaged a mere 0.10, while those with householders aged 15-24 averaged 0.87. Even the ones with householders aged 55-64 were down to an average of 0.28. Thus, while the elderly family had a smaller number of earners and less total income than most other age groups, it also had the fewest dependents.

If the per capita income data are further refined to reflect income before and after taxes, the elderly make an especially good showing. In 1980, for instance, all households collectively had a per capita income after taxes of $5,964, but those with an elderly householder had one of $6,299, so the elderly actually fared better on this index. All households paid nearly 23 per cent of their total money income in taxes, but the elderly paid only 13 per cent, which significantly improves their financial situation. In fact, the per cent of income that people aged 65 and older lost to taxes was only half that paid by households with a head aged 55-59, because of the progressive nature of the income tax, "bracket creep" created by inflation, and increases in Social Security taxes. Clearly, an assessment of the relative income situation of older people depends heavily on the type of index used.[5]

The usefulness of the per capita income index is also demonstrated by the wide variations in elderly household income according to the number of members. Thus, in 1980 one-person units with a householder aged 65 or over had a median income of $5,134, while two-person units received $12,134, three-person households obtained $17,436, and those with four persons had an average income of $20,485. But these figures also show how drastically the position of the elderly householder can change if one income receiver is lost, particularly if a spouse in a two-person household dies.[6]

Income of persons. The Census Bureau also reports personal income by age, cross-classified by sex and race, which allows an analysis of how well elderly individuals fare relative to younger ones in those categories. This index allows us to compute *relative income* for each age group, males and females, and blacks and whites. But more so than in the case of family income, the use of personal income as an index does support the conclusion that the elderly income receiver is at a substantial disadvantage

Table 8-1. Mean, Per Capita, and Relative Family Income, by Age of Householder, 1980

Age	Mean Family Income (Dollars)		Per Cent of Mean	
	Total	Per Capita	Total	Per Capita
15+	23,974	7,341	100.0	100.0
15-24	14,696	5,376	61.3	73.2
25-34	21,394	6,291	89.2	85.7
35-44	26,927	6,719	112.3	91.5
45-54	30,279	8,287	126.3	112.9
55-64	27,319	9,874	114.0	134.5
65+	16,918	7,275	70.6	99.1

Source: U.S. Bureau of the Census, "Money Income of Households, Families, and Persons in the United States: 1980," Current Population Reports, P-60, no. 132 (1982), table 21.

relative to most other groups, because personal income data include many older people living alone. In 1980, for example, persons aged 65-69 received a median income of $6,150, which was 77 per cent of that for all ages, while people aged 70 and over received $4,872, or only 61 per cent of the figure for all ages.

Recall, however, that elderly income receivers have fewer dependents than most other age groups, which improves the adequacy of their income. Moreover, the data on personal income do not account separately for people who have no income of their own but who live with relatives who do have income, and the census data tend to underestimate the overall resources available to the elderly.[7] That still does not justify the situation of those who really do live in or near poverty and whose lives are unreasonably constrained by inadequate incomes. Their cases provide ample room for improvement, though the degree of income inequality between the elderly and other groups has diminished because of changes in income distribution techniques. For those who no longer work, income generally comes from Social Security, earlier savings and investments, public and private pension plans, and private charity, and the mix of those things has changed in recent years so that income discrimination against the elderly as a whole has declined, though there are still wide discrepancies among individuals. Nor do the income indexes include indirect or non-money income, which can be quite significant for many people of all ages, including the elderly.[8] That group benefits from government programs; from the fact that mortgages are paid off, although property taxes continue to rise; and from shifts of money from younger people to older ones.[9]

Many types of income constitute the data from which the family and personal income indexes are computed. They include wages and salaries, net receipts from farm and nonfarm self-employment, Social Security (but not Medicare reimbursement), and Supplemental Security Income (SSI) from various levels of government for low-income people who are aged, blind, or disabled. Also included are welfare payments; dividends, interest, rents, royalties, and related payments; unemployment compensation, veterans' payments, and worker's compensation; and private and government pensions. Incomes also include annuities, alimony, and regular contributions from persons outside the household, as well as government transfer payments.[10] Thus, official "income" is a very broad category, and yet because not everything that people actually receive gets reported any place, the dollar amounts that are officially recorded still underrepresent total income. Moreover, the data omit money from the sale of property (e.g., stocks or a house), withdrawals of bank deposits, money borrowed, tax refunds, gifts, and lump-sum inheritances or insurance payments. These sources contribute to actual financial well-being and their omission also helps underestimate the real incomes of many elderly people. Nevertheless, the available data do facilitate various comparisons of the elderly with other age groups and among different groups within the older category.[11]

Incomes of Older and Younger People

The percentages of elderly people who have some income are greater than those for every other age group in the population. As a result, in the 1980 population of 25 million elderly people in the United States, only 333,000 had no income at all. Nevertheless, the median income received by persons aged 65 and older is significantly below that in all but the 15-19 age group and is especially low compared with those of middle-aged persons in their peak earning years. (See Table 8-2.)

People aged 65 and older are also very heavily concentrated in the $2,000-$4,999 category, and only somewhat less so in the $5,000-$9,999 range; even most of the latter cluster near the lower end. In fact, 63 per

Table 8-2. Median and Relative Income of Persons, by Age and Sex, 1980

Age	Median Income (Dollars)			Per Cent of Median		
	Both Sexes	Male	Female	Both Sexes	Male	Female
15+	7,944	12,530	4,920	100.0	100.0	100.0
15-19	1,736	1,801	1,673	21.9	14.4	34.0
20-24	6,612	7,923	5,286	83.2	63.2	107.4
25-34	11,173	15,580	6,973	140.6	124.3	141.7
35-44	12,254	20,037	6,465	154.3	159.9	131.4
45-54	11,927	19,974	6,403	150.1	159.4	130.1
55-64	9,420	15,914	4,926	118.6	127.0	100.1
65-69	6,150	8,953	4,379	77.4	71.5	89.0
70+	4,872	6,545	4,168	61.3	52.2	84.7

Source: U.S. Bureau of the Census, "Money Income of Households, Families, and Persons in the United States: 1980," Current Population Reports, P-60, no. 132 (1982), table 50.

cent of the persons aged 65-69 and 76 per cent of those aged 70 and older had incomes between $2,000 and $10,000 in 1980, compared with only 38 per cent of those aged 55-64 and even smaller proportions of people in their 30s and 40s. In addition, almost half the people 65 and over had incomes below $5,000. That amount scarcely provides survival for those living alone, though couples in which each member has an income fare better.

These concentrations of older people at the lower end of the scale reflect the abrupt income shifts most incur when they retire, for the proportion receiving more than $10,000 falls significantly, while the percentage receiving over $15,000 drops to a third or less of the proportion among middle-aged groups. Part of this age discrepancy occurs not just because of retirement, but also because any age group tends to have a lower average income than younger ones who move into that group, for each new cohort joins the labor force with higher entry salaries. Moreover, younger cohorts often receive larger salary increases than older ones, despite the escalating rewards of seniority, and the younger people have higher average levels of education that produce higher incomes. The younger workers also appear more frequently in high-paying growth industries, whereas many older people retire from low-paying industries on the decline.[12] Nonetheless, income inequality has been decreasing and the elderly as a group are in an improved position relative to other age groups, although the incomes of the oldest people have not risen as rapidly as those for people nearer 65, so that gap has widened some.[13]

For these and other reasons, including discrimination, the income of the average older person is lower than that in all other age groups, except for young people still in school or who have just entered the labor force. The elderly seem especially poor relative to people aged 35-44, but the latter also have the largest average child support burdens, because most have already produced as many children as they will have while they are still paying the high costs of rearing those children through adolescence and college. Thus, like people aged 15-19, the incomes of the elderly can be devoted almost entirely to supporting themselves, and the relative income position of many is better than dollar comparisons might suggest.

This is why it is important to study per capita income, discussed in connection with the data in Table 8-1. That index shows that the income situation of the elderly is often better than we assume, but it also allows us to pinpoint those older people, often solitary individuals, who really are desperately poor. That approach helps explain why families with a householder aged 55-64 are better off on a per capita basis than those with one aged 45-54, even though the latter group has the highest dollar income. By the time the householder reaches 55-64, most or all of the children have left home and the smaller income goes further. At the same time, however, costs for food, fuel, rents and property taxes, and health have risen rapidly and older people tend to spend a larger percentage of their incomes on those items than do younger ones.[*14*]

This may diminish the amounts available for things that make life more pleasant. Therefore, there are limits to the advantages older people gain by having fewer dependents to support, and some can hardly support themselves. For them, "the greatest destroyer of old-age security is inflation,"[*15*] because it erodes the income for which the elderly have planned and compromises the efforts society has made to improve pension plans, health care, and other supports. Therefore, many of the elderly may hold their own because of cost-of-living adjustments in Social Security and other increases in income, but most do not improve their positions measurably; many even have to draw principal from savings accounts, sell property, and otherwise diminish the assets from which they derive part of their income.[*16*]

Finally, the decline in income that most elderly persons experience when they retire has different meanings to different individuals, and many people whom a demographer might place below an arbitrary poverty line do not feel their status has fallen. Conversely, a middle-class wage earner plunged into poverty because a pension didn't materialize or was smaller than expected might experience an acute sense of deprivation and severe adjustment problems. So might a pensioner whose savings and fixed income are reduced by inflation, which has actually happened to many people on pensions that don't provide cost-of-living increases.[*17*] Similarly, a relatively wealthy person whose retirement income drops below previous earnings may feel deprived, even though he/she has a fully adequate income by less subjective standards.[*18*] Therefore, while the data on income provide a reasonably objective view of how the resources of different age groups compare, they cannot tell much about how people perceive those resources.

Elderly full-time workers. So far the discussion of income by age has dealt with the entire group of elderly people, the large majority of them retired and living on reduced incomes. But some people 65 and over still work full-time and their incomes are relatively high. Thus, in 1980 the group of workers aged 65-69 had a median personal income of $15,647, compared to that of $15,836 for full-time workers of all ages; and even working people aged 70 and older earned $14,963. The *mean* incomes of both elderly groups were actually above the national average because the older contingent includes a relatively large share of high-salaried persons who choose to continue working. The elderly group working full time is relatively small, however, for in 1980 it included only 15 per cent of all men aged 65-69 and 4 per cent of those 70 and over. The female contingent was even smaller. Therefore, this group has comparatively little statistical impact on the income situation of the whole elderly population.

Income Differences by Sex

At all ages the percentage of women receiving any income at all is smaller than that of men, though the difference declines in the 65-and-over group, especially for whites. Moreover, no matter what the age bracket, the median personal income of women is still significantly below that of men, though the discrepancy is less in the ages past 65 than it is for people between 25 and 64. (See Table 8-2.) Even so, in 1980 the median personal income of women aged 65-69 was only 49 per cent of that received by the men, and the income of women 70 and over was 64 per cent of that obtained by men. But the sex discrepancy for the elderly is less than it is for younger people, because women of all ages had a median personal income that was only 39 per cent of that received by men. That wide variation reflects the fact that the incomes of women are more likely to be based on part-time work, but it also shows that large numbers of women are still confined to typical "female" jobs that pay relatively poorly.

Furthermore, the persistent wage discrimination against women, even in the same jobs or in different jobs that ought to provide comparable rewards, is still a serious problem. For retired women, these circumstances mean that the lower earnings on which their pensions are based extend the discrimination into the older years as well. As a result, women aged 65 and older who reported themselves as retired in 1980 had a median personal income of $6,393, whereas the retired men had a median of $8,620.[19] However, the *relative income* of elderly women is fairly close to that of all women, while the relative income of elderly men is far below that of all men. With much higher pre-retirement incomes than women, the men experience a larger proportional drop when they leave the labor force, though the reduced incomes they do receive are still higher than those of elderly women.

When the personal incomes of the average elderly woman and man are combined into a family income that must support only two people, the elderly do not fare badly. When people live alone or with nonrelatives, however, their incomes are apt to be quite small compared with those of elderly families, and elderly women are at a considerable disadvantage relative to older men. A comparison of their circumstances uses the concept of *unrelated individuals,* who are people not living with any relative and who either reside alone, in group quarters, such as a rooming house, or with other nonrelatives. A large number of elderly women fall into this category, and in 1980 women accounted for 79 per cent of all unrelated individuals aged 65 and older.

Table 8-3 shows that the incomes of women classified as unrelated individuals fall below those of men in every age group, except in the case of blacks aged 25-34; but the sex discrepancy is also lower for whites in those ages than in any other bracket up to age 65. The reduced sex inequality among people aged 25-34 reflects the changes that are finally occurring for young women who have not been in the labor force very long, and who may be pursuing serious and rewarding careers in addition to or instead of marriage. As those people age and if new labor force entrants come close to income equitability, the present income discrepancy between men and women aged 35-64 may diminish significantly, though thus far that has been a slow process.

The sex disparity in the incomes of unrelated individuals aged 65 and older is still less than that of any other age group, not because women's retirement incomes are so high, but because those of men plunge more dramatically after age 65. Thus, in 1980 women aged 65 and older received 67 per cent of the income of women aged 55-64, whereas the figure for men was only 58 per cent. In fact, the sex disparity decreases after 55, when men begin to retire early, and it declines even more after age 62.

No matter what the index, elderly women have smaller average incomes than elderly men. Their personal incomes are lower, as are those of female householders (family heads), widows, and other women living alone. The

Table 8-3. Median Income of Unrelated Individuals, by Age, Race, and Sex, 1980

Age	Median Income (Dollars)					
	All Races		White		Black	
	Male	Female	Male	Female	Male	Female
15+	10,929	6,668	11,679	6,932	7,196	4,011
15-24	8,444	6,599	8,767	6,824	6,099	4,623
23-34	14,082	11,884	15,040	12,060	9,432	9,958
35-44	15,505	12,300	17,584	13,246	10,067	8,391
45-54	13,131	9,046	15,828	9,534	8,092	5,044
55-64	9,913	7,376	11,167	8,137	4,848	3,618
65+	5,746	4,957	6,161	5,186	4,219	3,558

Source: U.S. Bureau of the Census, "Money Income of Households, Families, and Persons in the United States: 1980," Current Population Reports, P-60, no. 132 (1982), table 27.

women without husbands but still supporting dependents who have little or no income, such as abandoned grandchildren or disabled parents, are especially badly off, even though they may have certain governmental assistance available. Despite the income inequality by sex among the elderly, however, the gap is narrowing gradually, for in 1970 women aged 65-69 had only 43 per cent of the personal income received by the men, whereas by 1980 women were receiving 49 per cent. In the 70-and-over group, the change was from 57 to 64 per cent. Therefore, elderly women are a little less disadvantaged relative to elderly men than they were, and all elderly are moving a bit closer to parity with other age groups. The latter change is facilitated by the movement of better-educated cohorts into the elderly group, for lifetime and retirement incomes both rise dramatically as the level of education improves.[20]

Until recently, women have suffered at least one other injustice because of their greater life expectancy. Almost all pension plans have paid women lower monthly benefits because they are expected to outlive men and to receive the payments over a longer period. Thus, even in those cases where their total benefits during the retirement years were comparable to those of men, their average monthly benefits were significantly less. In 1983, however, the Justice Department won a test case involving 3,400 colleges and universities and 650,000 employees that should eliminate the disparity, though the impact of the Supreme Court's findings of sex discrimination will take some time to accommodate.

Income Differences by Race

By every index, elderly black people have far lower average incomes than elderly whites, and Hispanic people also trail whites significantly. For example, in 1980 the per capita income in families headed by blacks aged 65 and older was only 47 per cent of that in elderly white families, while Hispanic families received 57 per cent of the white figure. (See Table 8-4.) Elderly white families also have per capita incomes that are virtually the same as those for all white families, whereas the ones headed by elderly blacks have significantly lower per capita incomes than do all black families collectively.

Irrespective of race, however, nearly all elderly people do receive *some* income, small though it may be for most minority elderly and for many whites as well. Important, too, is the greater tendency for elderly blacks to live with adult children, for while black per capita household income is low relative to that of whites, the black elderly person, especially a widow, is more apt to be accepted within a younger household, which helps in the struggle against a higher poverty rate. Moreover, a black grandmother is often useful in caring for children while one or both parents work, and she often enjoys greater family respect than her white counterpart, sharing more fully in whatever resources the family has and contributing more work.[21]

Poverty is also more evenly distributed among age groups in the black population, which means it may come as a considerably greater shock for elderly whites than for blacks,[22] though we do need to be careful not to assume that either group is homogeneous. Nonetheless, the data on family and household income imply that the black elderly population contains an abnormally large percentage of poorly educated people who were the victims of blatant job discrimination that forced them into menial jobs at low wages. As a result, those jobs provided minimal retirement incomes, savings, home ownership, and job skills with which to seek part-time work after age 65. That set of problems will not disappear quickly, for more middle-aged blacks than whites still suffer from them and will have higher rates of poverty in their older years.[23]

Table 8-4. Mean and Relative Per Capita Family Income, by Age of Householder, Race, and Spanish Origin, 1980

Age	Mean Per Capita Family Income (Dollars)			Per Cent of Mean Per Capita Family Income		
	White	Black	Spanish Origin	White	Black	Spanish Origin
15+	7,787	4,321	4,549	100.0	100.0	100.0
15-24	5,764	3,503	3,960	74.0	81.1	87.1
25-34	6,608	4,204	4,247	84.9	97.3	93.4
35-44	7,029	4,444	4,158	90.3	102.8	91.4
45-54	8,834	4,649	5,339	113.4	107.6	117.4
55-64	10,573	4,845	5,731	135.8	112.1	126.0
65+	7,745	3,639	4,382	99.5	84.0	96.3

Source: U.S. Bureau of the Census, "Money Income of Households, Families, and Persons in the United States: 1980," Current Population Reports, P-60, no. 132 (1982), table 21.

These realities also pertain when personal income is used as an index, and at every age level the incomes of blacks are below those of whites, while women of both races fare considerably worse than men. The least favorable comparison, therefore, is between black women and white men, for in the ages 65-69 the former receive only 35 per cent as much income as the latter; at age 70 they receive 45 per cent as much. But unfair as they are, these great disparities are softened somewhat by the greater proportional loss of income experienced by the more affluent groups in the population when they retire, either fully or partially. Thus, white men, with the highest incomes of all, sustain a drop of 44 per cent between the age groups 55-64 and 65-69, whereas black men, with the second highest average incomes in the 55-64 ages, experience a 36 per cent decline. The incomes of white women fall 10 per cent and those of black women decrease 15 per cent. Similar changes are also apparent in the incomes of unrelated individuals. In a limited sense, therefore, some status differences tend to level a bit after age 65, and the older people get, the more leveling takes place.[24] Even so, while the leveling phenomenon may someday reduce the income inequality that results from being black and female, it is still a long way from producing black-white or male-female equality in the older ages, let alone between the elderly and all of the other age groups over 20.

Spanish-origin persons have median incomes that are a little above those of elderly blacks as a whole, but both groups rank far below non-Hispanic whites. In addition, Hispanic men fare somewhat better than black men, while Hispanic women have slightly lower average incomes than black women.

Sources of Income

Most elderly people have several sources of income, though Social Security and other transfer payments are major sources for almost all. Those other transfers include railroad retirement, public assistance or welfare, Supplemental Security Income (SSI), pensions and annuities, veteran's payments, and unemployment and worker's compensation. Thus, Table 8-5 shows that well over 90 per cent of the elderly men and women receive various combinations of these transfers, though only a quarter of all older people depend on them exclusively. Therefore, the large majority also have other sources of income, including earnings from wages, salaries, and self-employment, and returns from property of various kinds. Moreover, elderly women rely more heavily than men on government transfer payments and welfare, but are only half as likely to have earnings and income from property. This places them even more at the mercy of "public" funds. Among all sources, Social Security is the single most important one for both men and women.[25]

Only about 5 per cent of all elderly families rely exclusively on Social Security, and in that sense the program meets the intent of its creators that it be only a supplement to other income. But many older people derive a much larger share of their income from it than was intended, and to that degree Social Security is more than just a protective supplement to savings and other sources. The system's creators did not envision its significant cost-of-living increases or its proliferation into other areas, such as SSI. Nor did President Franklin Roosevelt and the other founders foresee the present conflict between the insurance and welfare functions

Table 8-5. Percentages of Persons Aged 25-64 and 65 and Over Receiving Various Types of Income, by Sex, 1980

Type of Income	25-64		65+	
	Male	Female	Male	Female
Earnings	92.4	72.2	25.1	11.1
Earnings & Property Income	61.0	46.1	19.6	8.1
Government Transfer Payments	21.9	20.2	94.4	96.1
Government Transfer Payments Only	3.3	6.2	19.6	28.8
Public Assistance, SSI, or Both[a]	2.2	6.4	5.7	10.7
Social Security, Pensions, or Both	9.2	9.7	93.7	93.7
Social Security, SSI, or Both[a]	5.8	9.3	92.0	94.7

Source: U.S. Bureau of the Census, "Money Income of Households, Families, and Persons in the United States: 1980," Current Population Reports, P-60, no. 132 (1982), table 54.

[a]SSI refers to Supplemental Security Income, i.e., payments made by federal, state, and local welfare agencies to low-income persons who are 65 or over, blind, or disabled.

of the system,[26] though they did hope it would eventually provide many kinds of protection for all segments of society. In fact, the expanded role of the system is reflected in its actual name: The Old-Age, Survivors', Disability and Health Insurance Program. These and other expansions helped generate the financial difficulties of the 1980s and the reforms of 1983 to guarantee the system's long-range solvency and protections for the elderly. Those changes, which represent a compromise among proponents of various solutions to the problems, temporarily postponed one cost-of-living increase; raised Social Security taxes; increased the age for full benefits from 65 to 67 over a 27-year period beginning in 2000; brought new federal employees into the system; subjected high-income recipients to partial taxation of benefits; and changed the taxation system for self-employed persons. Even those measures may prove inadequate, however, as the numbers and proportions of elderly people grow and the burden on workers increases. Nor did these steps address the costly problems in Medicare and other programs for the aged.

About 17 per cent of all older people still do have some earnings from work, much of it part-time. Men are more than twice as likely as women to have this source, though the figures for both contrast sharply with the 81 per cent of persons aged 25-64 who receive earnings. Conversely, only 21 per cent of the younger group receive income from public sources, compared with 95 per cent of those aged 65 and older. Therefore, one of the basic difficulties is that the incomes of more and more elderly depend less on earnings than they do on non-work income, and deserved though the unearned income may be, the huge costs threaten the survival of various retirement systems and still leave a significant share of the elderly in poverty or near-poverty. Even with its escalating benefits, Social Security alone does not provide an adequate retirement for most elderly, and nearly a third of the people who rely on that source fall below the poverty threshold,[27] though the number of elderly poor would probably triple if the system did not exist.

All of the emotional and humanitarian considerations aside, the older person who could work but doesn't imposes a cost that we have not yet learned to manage adequately, either for the elderly recipients of non-work income or for those who must provide it,[28 though it is often difficult for those older people who want jobs to find them. Moreover, pension coverage from all sources combined is quite uneven and many elderly receive too little to live comfortably. Despite its large costs, even the Social Security system has gaps and flaws, while at least half of all elderly Americans are not covered by private pension plans, some of which pay only small benefits anyway.[29] Therefore, income sources vary widely within the older group, as does the relative adequacy of the total amount provide by those sources. Consequently, while some elderly are wealthy and others are desperately poor, as a whole the older group does not fare as well financially as the rest of us, and while their relative incomes are better than their absolute incomes would suggest, many still need help, especially those in their late 70s and beyond.

In view of these circumstances, it isn't surprising that the financial *satisfaction* of elderly people hasn't changed much since the 1960s, basically because most feel their income situations haven't improved enough relative to their costs. Some of this attitude reflects their expectations, which can never be fully satisfied as long as they continue to rise. Significant, too, are misperceptions among older people about their real situations relative to other members of the population.[30] But part of the financial dissatisfaction expressed by many elderly also reflects real deprivation, especially for the group living in poverty.

Income Trends

The incomes of the elderly have risen substantially for many decades, as have those of younger people. Moreover, because of improvements in the Social Security system and other sources of retirement income, the proportion of desperately poor elderly has fallen significantly, especially since 1970, though it began to rise again in the 1980s. Much of this means that the money incomes of elderly households have risen a little faster than those of all ages combined, and considerably faster than several other specific age groups.[31] (See Table 8-6.) The same is true when personal income is used as the index. Although the average elderly household does sustain a considerable drop in income when the householder and his/her spouse retire, the decline is not quite as great as it was. In 1970, for example, elderly households had 69 per cent of the incomes of those headed by people aged 55-64, while in 1980 they had 72 per cent. Some of that change is due to the early retirements of more people in the 55-64 age group, but part of it is also due to improvements in the absolute and relative income situations of those aged 65 and older. Furthermore, the rise in elderly household per capita income from $2,960 in 1970 to $7,243 in 1980 represents an increase in real income (1980 constant dollars) of about 43 per cent, compared with an increase of roughly 39 per cent for all ages. In addition, the ratio of per capita income in households with elderly heads to that in all households moved up from 72 per cent in 1970 to 94 per cent in 1980. Thus, the elderly are pushing slowly toward greater equality of income with younger people, at least by this measure.

These changes in the relative per capita income situation in the older family continue a longer trend, because for several decades the incomes of elderly families have risen faster than those of all other age groups combined, although the older ones did start with a significant disadvantage, especially during the Great Depression, when large proportions of the elderly were utterly destitute. In addition, not only are the incomes of the elderly increasing faster than those of the total population, but the proportion now protected from destitution by one or more income sources also has increased. So both income and coverage have expanded significantly.[32] The elderly have also probably been helped more than other age groups by non-cash benefits not reflected in the income data. As a result of these factors, the elderly also tend to grow somewhat more homogeneous in income and assets, despite major differences between elderly men and women and blacks and whites.

The old racial discrepancy remains a particular problem, for in 1970 older black men had 59 per cent of the median personal income of elderly white men, while in 1980 they had 58 per cent. Among elderly women the ratio of black to white personal income fell from 75 per cent in 1970 to 72 per cent in 1980. Those figures do not account for non-cash income or for

Table 8-6. Per Capita Family Income, by Age of Householder, and Percentage Change, 1970-1980

Age	Per Capita Income (Dollars)		Per Cent Change, (1970-80)
	1970	1980	
15+[a]	3,200	7,713	141.0
15-19[b]	2,743	6,327	130.7
25-35	2,798	7,082	153.1
35-44	2,736	7,131	160.6
45-54	3,660	8,527	133.0
55-64	4,305	9,969	131.6
65+	2,960	7,243	144.7

Sources: U.S. Bureau of the Census, Statistical Abstract of the United States: 1979, table 752; "Money Income of Households, Families, and Persons in the United States: 1980," Current Population Reports, P-60, no. 132 (1982), table 4.

[a]Unweighted average of the means of the age groups.

[b]Aged 14-19 in 1970.

differences in family support, of course, and it is true that the cash incomes of people of both races have grown very substantially. Regardless, the degree of inequality between older white and black people has increased somewhat, whereas the discrepancy between the elderly and other age groups has decreased, as has that between older men and women.

The Elderly Poor

It hasn't been too many decades since nearly all older people were poor or close to it, so their present overall income situation is far better than in the past. Despite these improvements, however, a significant share of the elderly still must endure extreme poverty, either for the first time in their lives or as the continuation of lifetime poverty; they lack sufficient income for even the basic necessities, and they inhabit rural slums and the deteriorating areas of large cities, somehow managing to endure. They are the "hard-core" elderly poor whose situations have improved the least. Moreover, while SSI, cost-of-living increases in Social Security, and other measures significantly reduced the percentage living in poverty, after 1978 their proportion rose somewhat and there are still about 4 million persons aged 65 and older below the official poverty line.

Indexes of Poverty

The *poverty index* now used by the U.S. Bureau of the Census was first developed by the Social Security Administration in 1964 and revised in 1969 and 1980, though the first data on the matter were published for 1959. The index now provides several *poverty income thresholds* that vary according to family size, the age of the householder, and the number of children under age 18. The poverty index is also oriented to the Consumer Price Index and is, therefore, adjusted annually so that its dollar figure changes each year for the various groups mentioned above.[33] Because of these detailed refinements, the index is a sensitive measure of how the economic well-being of the elderly compares with that of other age groups, though the index does include only money income. Moreover, the data are provided separately for persons, unrelated individuals, and families, with the last identified according to the number of members.

Older and Younger People

In 1980 about 16 per cent of the nation's elderly people fell below the poverty threshold, compared with 13 per cent of those of all ages. But the proportion for the elderly was higher than that of all other categories except persons in the very youngest years. (See Table 8-7.) In fact, the proportion in poverty falls steadily until about age 55 and then rises until the percentage for the elderly is far higher than that for people in their late 40s and early 50s. There is even a considerable increase between the ages 55-59 and 60-64, because many who retire in their early 60s are forced to do so by disability, and their pension incomes, if any, are generally well below those of people who work until age 65. The percentage of those aged 60-64 who are in poverty would be even higher if it were not for the relatively affluent group that can easily afford to retire before age 65.

This pattern by age is virtually the same for whites, blacks, and Hispanics, except that for the last group the lowest percentage of poverty is in the ages 55-59, largely because the Cuban contingent is older and wealthier on the average than are people with other Spanish backgrounds. Moreover, males and females experience similar changes with age. Therefore, no matter how the data are cross-classified, the levels of poverty tend to be very high for children, to decline steadily until late middle age, to rise somewhat after age 60, and to increase sharply after age 65. The problem is the most severe for the nation's oldest people. Moreover, since more than half the elderly population is aged 72 and older and women exceed 60 per cent of that age group, the poverty population is fairly heavily concentrated among the nation's oldest women.

The near-poor elderly. The proportion of elderly people in poverty is about 21 per cent greater than that of people in all age groups, but when the near-poor are taken into account, the difference increases. Those people have incomes that are no more than 25 per cent above the poverty threshold, and while they are not quite poor by official standards, their incomes are still inadequate. Thus, in 1980 the upper limit of income for a near-poor family of two with a householder aged 65 or over was $6,222, while that for an elderly unrelated individual was $4,937. In that year about 2.5 million older people not below the poverty line were no more than 25 per cent above it, and they accounted for about 10 per cent of all elderly. In contrast, about 5 per cent of all age groups collectively fell into the near-poor category.

When the poor and near-poor are combined, about 26 per cent of the elderly are in poverty or just above it, compared with 18 per cent of all age groups. Furthermore, people in families with an elderly female householder and no husband present fare especially badly, for 43 per cent are in poverty or near it, although in most other age groups female-headed households without husbands do not do a great deal better. All of this means that in 1980 about 6.5 million elderly people did not have sufficient income to maintain an adequate level of living, or were having to scrape by with few luxuries.

Table 8-7. Percentages of Persons Below the Poverty
Level, by Age, Sex, Race, and Spanish
Origin, 1980

Age and Sex	All Races	White	Black	Spanish Origin[a]
Male	11.2	8.7	28.7	23.5
Under 15	19.0	14.5	43.6	33.6
15-17	14.1	10.3	35.8	29.1
18-21	10.9	8.5	24.4	21.9
22-24	9.8	8.4	17.6	16.4
25-34	7.5	6.2	17.2	14.9
35-44	7.6	6.2	18.4	16.0
45-54	6.5	5.4	15.2	15.2
55-59	6.4	4.8	22.3	12.7
60-64	7.8	6.2	24.6	19.1
65+	10.9	9.0	31.5	26.8
Female	14.7	11.6	35.7	27.7
Under 15	19.3	14.8	42.6	33.9
15-17	15.8	11.1	41.5	31.0
18-21	16.0	12.3	36.5	29.2
22-24	15.1	12.0	33.6	20.9
25-34	12.8	10.0	31.1	23.9
35-44	10.6	8.3	26.8	23.1
45-54	8.9	6.7	26.3	22.4
55-59	10.6	8.2	31.8	19.5
60-64	12.6	10.3	35.8	19.6
65+	19.0	16.8	42.6	34.4

Source: U.S. Bureau of the Census, "Characteristics
of the Population Below the Poverty Level: 1980,"
Current Population Reports, P-60, no. 133 (1982),
table 11.

[a]May be of any race.

Differences by Sex

Significantly higher proportions of older women than men fall below the poverty line, though their situations vary by marital status. Thus, in 1980 about 19 per cent of all women aged 65 and older were living in poverty, compared with only 11 per cent of the men, for a ratio of 174 women for each 100 men. The ratio is greater for whites (187) than for blacks (135) and Hispanics (128) (See Table 8-7.) The poverty difference between the sexes does tend to diminish in the oldest ages, for although both sexes aged 72 and over are more apt to be poor than are the young-old, the ratio of women to men in poverty falls somewhat. That reflects the tendency toward several forms of homogeneity as people move into their 70s and 80s.

Differences by Race

The incidence of poverty among elderly blacks is roughly three times that among elderly whites. (See Table 8-7.) Consequently, just under a quarter of the whites but well over half of the blacks are either living in poverty or hovering close to it. In addition, elderly Hispanics are far more likely than the white population as a whole to be poor, but somewhat less apt than blacks to be so.

The poorest people of all in American society are elderly black women, for their incidence of poverty is significantly higher than that of elderly black men and white women. Even though they may receive somewhat more protection through the efforts of family members than do older white women, who are more apt to live alone, the average incomes of older black women are so low that a large majority live in or near poverty. And for those who do live alone or with nonrelatives, the situation is truly appalling. In 1980, for instance, 82 per cent of the elderly black women classified as unrelated individuals were in poverty or close to it, compared with 62 per cent of the black men, 47 per cent of the white women, and 38 per cent of the white men. People living in families, even if there is no spouse present, are somewhat more fortunate, but even among them the incidence of poverty and near-poverty is especially high for elderly black women. Thus, unrelated individuals and female householders are the poorest of the elderly poor; among them blacks fare worse than whites and women are worse off than men.[34] Moreover, the rates of poverty still tend to be higher among blacks who live in the South than in any other region in the nation, and also among those who reside in nonmetropolitan places rather than in SMSAs.

Despite these obvious problems, however, it is well to recall that in 1980 less than 16 per cent of all people aged 65 and older were living in poverty, that the proportion has declined significantly since the first data were complied on the topic, and th⌐t the differences among several groups of elderly tend to diminish as they age. That "leveling" helps to offset some of the effects of being old, female, and black. The concept of poverty is also relative, for many of those now classified as "poor" still have goods and services that would have been available only to the wealthy a century ago. Also, the poorest people often deal better with their problems than do members of the middle class whose incomes may plunge when they retire and who feel an acute sense of deprivation.[35]

Effects of Other Characteristics

Marital status. Among elderly men, the highest incidence of poverty occurs for those who are separated or divorced, the lowest for those who are married and living with their wives. (See Table 8-8.) Single men and widowers are about equally likely to be poor, but their rates of poverty are well over twice those of married men. Among women, the incidence of poverty is highest among those who are separated, followed by those who are divorced and who are single, and lowest for the women who are

Table 8-8. Percentages of Elderly Persons Below the Poverty Level, by Sex and Marital Status, 1980

Marital Status	Both Sexes	Male	Female
All Classes	15.7	10.9	19.0
Single	21.4	19.0	22.7
Married[a]	8.2	8.3	8.1
Spouse Absent	32.9	22.2	43.5
Separated	37.8	29.5	45.7
Other	22.7	14.4	40.5
Widowed	24.1	18.8	25.1
Divorced	27.1	21.8	30.7

Source: U.S. Bureau of the Census, "Characteristics of the Population Below the Poverty Level: 1980," Current Population Reports, P-60, no. 133 (1982), table 15.

[a]Spouse present.

married. They have a slightly lower incidence of poverty than married men, but in every other marital status category the women fare much worse than the men.

Educational status. The incidence of poverty is closely related to the levels of education people have attained and what that schooling helped produce in the way of pre-retirement income and post-retirement pensions. Therefore, the high rates of poverty in some elderly groups can be explained partly by their low levels of education, though there are still significant discrepancies between the races and the sexes for other rea-

Table 8-9. Percentages of Elderly Persons Below
the Poverty Level, by Amount of
Schooling, Race, and Sex, 1980

Years of Schooling Completed	All Groups	White		Black	
		Male	Female	Male	Female
All Levels	15.7	9.0	16.8	31.5	42.6
None	36.3	33.2	34.3	a	a
Elementary					
1-5 Years	34.4	22.8	36.9	36.7	54.9
6 & 7 Years	25.5	16.8	28.1	33.1	44.5
8 Years	17.9	9.1	22.0	33.3	36.1
High School					
1-3 Years	13.8	6.4	16.3	32.4	36.7
4 Years	8.4	4.5	9.7	16.7	30.0
College					
1+ Years	6.1	4.3	6.9	a	a

Source: U.S. Bureau of the Census, "Characteristics of the Population Below the Poverty Level: 1980," Current Population Reports, P-60, no. 133 (1982), table 13.

aPopulation base too small to compute derived measure.

sons. In 1980, however, the proportion of all elderly living in poverty declined steadily as the level of education rose, and those with no schooling had a poverty rate six times that of people who had at least one year of college. (See Table 8-9.) Moreover, the same progressive decrease was apparent for men and women, blacks and whites. Nonetheless, at each of the educational levels, men had significantly lower rates of poverty than women, and whites had far lower rates than blacks, so those differentials are partly independent of education.

Table 8-10. Percentages of People 65 and Over Below
the Poverty Level, by Selected
Characteristics, 1959-1980

Characteristic	1959	1970	1978	1979	1980
All Persons 65+	35.2	24.5	14.0	15.2	15.7
White	33.1	22.5	12.1	13.3	13.6
Black	62.5	48.0	33.9	36.3	38.1
Spanish Origin[a]	....	....	23.2	26.8	30.9
Persons in Families	26.9	14.7	7.6	8.4	8.5
Householder	29.1	16.3	8.4	9.1	9.1
Male	29.1	15.6	7.7	8.4	8.2
Female	28.8	19.9	12.2	13.0	14.0
Unrelated Individuals	61.9	47.1	27.0	29.4	30.6
Male	59.0	38.9	20.7	25.3	24.4
White	56.8	36.0	17.4	22.3	21.1
Black	77.5	59.7	37.8	44.8	45.1
Female	63.3	49.7	28.8	30.5	32.3
White	61.8	47.5	25.9	27.6	29.3
Black	84.6	79.2	62.0	65.6	66.5

Source: U.S. Bureau of the Census, "Characteristics of the Population Below the Poverty Level: 1980," Current Population Reports, P-60, no. 133 (1982), table 3.

[a]May be of any race.

Trends in Poverty Status

The proportion of elderly people living below the poverty threshold dropped by more than half between 1959 and 1980 and even the number fell from 5.5 million to 4 million, despite the substantial increase in the size of the older population. (See Table 8-10.) Those decreases represent a considerably faster rate of reduction in poverty among the elderly than among all age groups collectively, largely because of such things as Medicare, SSI, food stamps, transfer payments of other kinds for older people, and significant increases in Social Security benefits after 1972.[36]

The proportion of near-poor elderly has also decreased, but not as rapidly, partly because many people who would have been classified as poor in the 1960s and early 1970s have now moved into the near-poor category, though this should not obscure the significantly larger share of older people whose improved incomes now place them above both categories.

The proportion below the poverty level fell especially rapidly for older people living in families, though the rate of reduction was far faster among families with a male than a female householder. In 1959 male householders even had a slightly higher incidence of poverty than the females, but by 1980 the proportion of men householders in poverty had fallen 72 per cent, while that of women had dropped only 51 per cent. The same patterns hold for persons and unrelated individuals; that is, the incidence of poverty declined significantly for both sexes, but more for men than for women.

The incidence of poverty among the elderly also dropped more drastically for whites than for blacks. Between 1959 and 1980 all elderly white persons witnessed a 59 per cent decrease in poverty, blacks only a 39 per cent drop. For those living in families and for unrelated individuals the proportion living below the poverty threshold also fell more slowly for blacks than for whites, who had the advantage to begin with.

When the situations of the sexes and the races are considered together, it is clear that the great financial disadvantage of elderly black women is a persistent one despite some improvements, and they are still more likely than black men and whites of both sexes to be poor. In addition, the rate of improvement has been slowest for those who were the poorest in 1959 — elderly black women living alone or with nonrelatives. Two-thirds of them are still below the poverty line, and while the poverty rate for all unrelated individuals was cut in half, their rate fell only 21 per cent.

Table 8-10 shows that there has been some tendency for the incidence of poverty to rise since about 1978. A small part of that increase is due to revisions in the definition of ''poverty,'' but inflation and other factors are also involved. It is too early, however, to tell whether the economic constraints of the early 1980s will cause the percentage of poverty-stricken elderly persons to rise significantly, or whether the increases since 1978 will prove temporary. The data for 1982 and 1983, though, show that the proportion of elderly persons in poverty dropped slightly. Even so, in our attempt not to underestimate the economic well-being of the elderly, we don't want to overestimate it, because a significant share of older people who don't fall below the official poverty line don't live very comfortably either, and major improvements are still needed in some groups, especially that of older women living alone. Many of them are not quite poor enough to be eligible for Medicaid, which can prove a costly omission, and the problem is intensified by the tendency to eliminate hospitals that treat the poor and near-poor at subsidized rates.

Women have also suffered from the practice of reducing their benefits from private pension plans because of their greater longevity, even though benefits were not increased for groups with relatively short life expectancy such as black men.[37] Under the recent Supreme Court ruling, however, the situation for women should gradually improve. Even so, each race and sex category still has significant numbers in poverty and others above that level who lack an overall income in cash and other benefits to provide what the federal government defines as a moderate standard of retirement living (now about $6,500 for single people and $9,800 for couples).[38] At present, that situation includes well over half of all elderly persons and more than a third of the couples.

The great proportional decrease in poverty during the 1970s represents a unique combination of legislation and other advantages that we are unlikely to match in the 1980s. The elderly could even lose ground because of changes in the Social Security system to overcome its financial problems, other budgetary constraints, and the shift of priorities away from "social programs" in order to deal with budgetary deficits created by higher military spending and reduced revenues because of high unemployment. At the same time, prices for most of the things that use most of the funds of elderly people — food, fuel, utilities, and medical care — are still rising, and the elderly are more affected by the increases than are many younger people. Therefore, new millions of the elderly could become officially poor or at least poorer than they had expected. It simply is not true that the bulk of elderly Americans live well enough to withstand major cuts in benefits or rapid inflation and not suffer, for while that assumption might have some credibility if the income trends of the 1970s had continued, it had little during the economic reversals of the early 1980s.[39] For some elderly any failure to provide regular increases in Social Security benefits will produce hardships and perhaps even a class of new poor among them.

Summary

Most elderly are often thought to be poor, but while some are deep in poverty, most manage to get by and a minority live well. The actual income situation of elderly persons depends in part on whether they live in families or alone, for while the average income of elderly families is substantially below that of all families, the older ones have fewer members and their per capita income is relatively close to that received by all families. But the picture is far less favorable for those who live alone or with nonrelatives and for women who head households without a husband present. The incomes of the elderly in those categories are far below the ones received by people of all ages collectively, although virtually all older people have some source of income.

Typically, elderly women have significantly smaller incomes than elderly men, no matter what the living arrangements, and older blacks receive considerably less than older whites. Therefore, the poorest elderly poor in American society are black women, especially those who live alone or with nonrelatives. At the same time, more black than white women are apt to be taken into a family and to share in its resources, no matter how meager.

Income and poverty status are also heavily influenced by marital status and education. The incidence of poverty is far less for married people with a spouse present than for those in all of the nonmarried categories, especially the ones who are separated or divorced, and the women in those groups are much more likely than the men to be poor. Income also rises as the level of education rises, and the incidence of poverty decreases accordingly. Nevertheless, the income and poverty disparities between men and women and blacks and whites persist even at the same levels of schooling, thus reflecting pervasive patterns of discrimination that have affected the wages of those groups and still influence their retirement incomes.

Income and poverty trends have been quite favorable for the elderly, especially since the early 1970s when various kinds of government benefits were increased significantly. Therefore, the incomes of older people rose faster between 1970 and 1980 than did those of all other groups collectively, and the disparity between the elderly and younger wage earners decreased. At the same time, the incidence of poverty fell dramatically, though the greatest reductions took place before 1975 and it rose a little after 1978.

NOTES

1. Charles S. Harris, *Fact Book on Aging: A Profile of America's Older Population.* Washington, DC: National Council on the Aging, 1978, pp. 37-38. See also Beth J. Soldo, "America's Elderly in the 1980s," *Population Bulletin* 35 (1980): 21.

2. Fred C. Cottrell, *Aging and the Aged.* Dubuque, IA: Wm. C. Brown, 1974, pp. 23-24.

3. Kingsley Davis and Pietronella van den Oever, "Age Relations and Public Policy in Advanced Industrial Society," *Population and Development Review* 7 (1981): 9.

4. The term *householder* has replaced the designations *head of household* and *head of family*. See U.S. Bureau of the Census, "Money Income of Households, Families, and Persons in the United States: 1980," *Current Population Reports,* P-60, no. 132 (1982): 223.

5. For the data, see U.S. Bureau of the Census, "Estimating After-Tax Money Income Distributions Using Data from the March Current Population Survey," *Current Population Reports,* P-23, no. 126 (1983): 12.

6. Use of the per capita index is adapted from Davis and van den Oever, *op. cit.,* pp. 9-10. See also U.S. Bureau of the Census, "Demographic Aspects of Aging and the Older Population in the United States," *Current Population Reports,* P-23, no. 59 (1978): 53.

7. Fred C. Pampel, *Social Change and the Aged.* Lexington, MA: Heath, 1981, p. 18.

8. George F. Patterson, "Income," in U.S. Bureau of the Census, "Population of the United States, Trends and Prospects: 1950-1990," *Current Population Reports,* P-23, no. 49 (1974): 163.

9. Bernice L. Neugarten, "The Rise of the Young-Old," in Ronald Gross, Beatrice Gross and Sylvia Seidman, eds., *The New Old: Struggling for Decent Aging.* Garden City, NY: Doubleday, 1978, p. 48.

10. U.S. Bureau of the Census, "Money Income of Households...," *op. cit.,* pp. 221-222.

11. For an analysis of the problems in using income data, see Oskar Morgenstern, *National Income Statistics: A Critique of Macroeconomic Aggregation.* Washington, DC: Cato Institute, 1979.

12. James C. Schulz, "Income Distribution and the Aging," in Robert H. Binstock and Ethel Shanas, eds., *Handbook of Aging and the Social Sciences.* New York: Van Nostrand, 1976, p. 563. Cf. Juanita M. Kreps, "The Economy and the Aged," in Binstock and Shanas, *ibid.,* pp. 273-276.

13. Pampel, *op. cit.,* pp. 107-108; 122-123.

14. Soldo, *op. cit.,* pp. 23-24.

15. William C. Greenough and Francis P. King, *Pension Plans and Public Policy.* New York: Columbia University Press, 1976, p. 235.

16. Harris, *op. cit.,* pp. 63-64.

17. Soldo, *op. cit.,* p. 24.

18. Gordon F. Streib, "Social Stratification and Aging," in Binstock and Shanas, *op. cit.,* p. 163.

212

19. U.S. Bureau of the Census, "Money Income of Households...," *op. cit.,* table 61.

20. Patterson, *op. cit.,* pp. 170-171.

21. Nancy Hicks, "Life After 65," in Kurt Finsterbusch, ed., *Social Problems 81/82.* Guilford, CT: Dushkin, 1981, p. 161.

22. Jacquelyne Johnson Jackson, *Minorities and Aging.* Belmont, CA: Wadsworth, 1980, p. 144. For another analysis of coping networks and mechanisms, see Rose C. Gibson, "Blacks at Middle and Late Life: Resources and Coping," *Annals of American Academy of Political and Social Science* 464 (1982): 79-90. Cf. Ronald Angel and Marta Tienda, "Determinants of Extended Household Structure: Cultural Patterns or Economic Need?" *American Journal of Sociology* 87 (1982): 1360-1383.

23. National Caucus on the Black Aged, "A Generation of Black People," in Gross, Gross and Seidman, *op. cit.,* pp. 281-282.

24. Pampel, *op. cit.,* pp. 150-152.

25. Soldo, *op. cit.,* p. 21.

26. For an analysis, see Peter J. Ferrara, *Social Security: The Inherent Contradiction.* Washington, DC: Cato Institute, 1982.

27. Mary Barberis, "America's Elderly: Policy Implications," *Population Bulletin* 35 (1981): 6.

28. Davis and van den Oever, *op. cit.,* pp. 8-9.

29. Barberis, *op. cit.,* p. 7.

30. Pampel, *op. cit.,* p. 182.

31. Davis and van den Oever, *op. cit.,* p. 12.

32. R. Meredith Belbin, "Retirement Strategy in an Evolving Society," in Carp, *op. cit.,* p. 177.

33. For this description of the poverty index, see U.S. Bureau of the Census, *Statistical Abstract of the United States: 1982-83.* Washington, DC: U.S. Government Printing Office, 1982, p. 417. For the specific dollar variations among different groups in 1980, see U.S. Bureau of the Census, "Characteristics of the Population Below the Poverty Level: 1980," *Current Population Reports,* P-60, no. 133 (1982): 3-4.

34. For discussions of this matter, see Soldo, *op. cit.,* pp. 21-23; Jackson, *op. cit.,* pp. 166-169; and Philip Janson and Karen Frisbie Mueller, "Age, Ethnicity, and Well-Being," *Research on Aging* 5 (1983): 353-367.

35. Cottrell, *op. cit.,* pp. 23-24.

36. Harris, *op. cit.,* p. 51. Cf. U.S. Bureau of the Census, "The Social and Economic Status of the Black Population in the United States: An Historical View, 1790-1978," *Current Population Reports,* P-23, no. 80 (1979): 29.

37. Phyllis W. Berman and Estelle R. Ramey, eds., *Women: A Developmental Perspective.* Washington, DC: National Institutes of Health, 1982, p. 408.

38. Cyril F. Brickfield, "Rags to Riches — or Reality? Economic Prospects for the Elderly in the 1980s," in Kurt Finsterbusch, ed., *Social Problems 82/83.* Guilford, CT: Dushkin, 1982, p. 132.

39. *Ibid.,* p. 133.

Chapter 9

Mortality Levels, Differentials, and Trends

The first three chapters dealt with the ways in which mortality affects the growth of the older population, the distribution of people among the various elderly age categories, and the sex composition of the older population. Now, however, the analysis turns to mortality per se, and especially the ways in which it has changed for various groups in the elderly population, including its rates, differentials, and causes.

Measures of Mortality

Mortality can be gauged by a large variety of rates, ratios, and other indexes, but this study concentrates principally on three:

1. Age-specific death rates are mortality levels computed separately for persons in various age categories, usually five-year or 10-year ranges. This index is related to the *age-adjusted death rate,* which shows what the level of mortality would be if the age composition of a population remained unchanged from year to year, and which uses the age distribution for a given year as the standard.

2. Life expectancy is usually expressed in two ways. The expectation of life at birth is the average number of years a group of newborn infants would live if their survival were governed by the age-specific death rates that prevailed when they were born. The expectation of life at 50, 65, 80, or any other age is the average lifetime remaining to persons who have reached those ages, also assuming unchanging age-specific death rates.

3. Age-specific death rates by cause result from heart disease, cancer, stroke, accidents, and other causes, and are a way to report the relative importance of the events from which people actually die and the changes in their importance over time.

213

All of these indexes are also reported separately for men and women, blacks and whites, and other groups in the population.[1] The vital statistics registrations on which they and the long-term trends are based are available for as early as 1900-1902, but it was not until 1933, when the last state (Texas) was added to the registration area, that the data applied to the nation's total population. For that reason and because the quality of the data has improved greatly since the early decades, this chapter will trace most trends from 1940 to the early 1980s. It is worth noting, however, that since 1900 the death rates of all age, race, and sex groups dropped dramatically, though there were fluctuations, including increases, at various times.

Indexes of *morbidity* (illness, injury, and disability) are also available, though more difficult to create and use; the line between wellness and illness is often unclear, while specific older persons are often afflicted by several maladies at the same time. In addition, the information on this topic is generally less adequate than mortality data for earlier decades, partly because the morbidity materials depend on the person's own assessment of his/her state of physical well-being. Nonetheless, health surveys have improved greatly in recent years and do enable the use of *morbidity factors,* such as the number of days one is hospitalized or bedridden, the time during which one's activity is restricted by certain degrees, the number of sick days one suffers during a year, and the person's own report on illnesses and their severity. But morbidity is a large study in itself and beyond the scope of this book, though we will allude to it at points where it is inseparable from a consideration of mortality.

Differences in Age-Specific Death Rates

Death rates are relatively high for infants, but they drop to a low point for children aged 5-14 and then begin their virtually uninterrupted rise toward the oldest ages, though the change in the ages 20-34 is slight. (See Table 9-1.) It isn't until about age 60 or so, however, that the death rate again reaches the one for infants, so while the first year of life is still rather hazardous, the several decades that follow have very low death rates. In fact, disease control is so effective that until people reach their mid-30s, accidents are the chief cause of death, and the chances that a person in late middle-age will die from most of the major causes of death are not drastically greater than those of an infant.[2]

Despite that situation, however, after about age 40 the death rate rises by at least 50 per cent for each of the succeeding five-year age groups, and the climb is especially rapid in the 80s. As a result, the death rate of people aged 85 and older is more than six times that of people aged 65-69.

Table 9-1. Age-Specific Death Rates, by Race and
Sex, 1980

Age	Deaths per 1,000			
	White		Black	
	Male	Female	Male	Female
All Ages	9.8	8.1	10.3	7.3
Age-Adjusted	7.5	4.1	11.1	6.3
Under 1	12.3	9.6	25.9	21.2
1-4	0.7	0.5	1.1	0.8
5-9	0.3	0.2	0.5	0.3
10-14	0.4	0.2	0.5	0.3
15-19	1.4	0.5	1.4	0.5
20-24	1.9	0.6	2.9	0.9
25-29	1.7	0.6	3.7	1.3
30-34	1.7	0.7	4.6	1.7
35-39	2.1	1.1	5.9	2.5
40-44	3.2	1.7	8.1	4.1
45-49	5.2	2.8	12.0	6.3
50-54	8.7	4.5	17.6	9.1
55-59	13.8	7.0	24.6	13.1
60-64	21.4	10.8	33.8	18.6
65-69	33.1	16.4	44.8	25.4
70-74	50.2	25.9	60.5	37.6
75-79	74.7	41.9	80.9	52.4
80-84	112.7	72.4	115.5	80.3
85+	191.0	149.8	161.0	123.7

Source: National Center for Health Statistics,
"Advance Report of Final Mortality Statistics,
1980," Monthly Vital Statistics Report, vol. 32,
no. 4 (1983), tables 1 and 9.

These patterns together mean that the median age of death is quite high and that the average young-old person enjoys reasonably good health and can anticipate several more years of life.

Even though the current death rates in the ages 60-64, 65-69, and 70-74 are much lower than those of earlier decades and large proportions of people reach the late 70s and the 80s, people eventually die of something. Therefore, the oldest population is faced with the paradox of declining death *rates* and a large *number* of deaths concentrated in their ages. For example, in 1980 people aged 80 and over accounted for 46 per cent of all deaths in the population aged 65 and older, even though they made up only 20 per cent of the elderly group. Consequently, the probability of dying has continued to shift upward in the age scale and has helped enlarge the population of the old-old faster than that of any other group, because far more of the young-old now survive to those oldest ages than was true in earlier generations.

Some International Comparisons

The death rates of America's elderly compare favorably with those in most other highly technological societies, including Japan and most European countries. Table 9-2 shows that the rates for American men and women both fall below the means and medians for the other nine representative countries collectively in all of the elderly age groups, except the 65-69 category. The rates in the United States are especially low for persons aged 75 and older, though those low figures are partly due to differences in the age structures of the 85-and-over group. Japan, Norway, and Sweden also have excellent overall records of low mortality among the elderly, and in the young-old categories those countries are superior to the United States. Moreover, those three countries, along with a few others, have higher life expectancy at birth than does the United States, both for males and females.

Other developed countries, for which the data are not quite as recent as those in Table 9-2, also have relatively low death rates among their various groups of elderly; they include Canada, Hong Kong, Israel, New Zealand, and several European nations. In each of them life expectancy at birth for males approaches or even exceeds 70 years, while for females it is in the upper 70s, just as is true of most countries in Table 9-2. In the developing nations, on the other hand, the often incomplete data that are available show substantially higher death rates among the elderly and life expectancy at birth that is many years below that in the industrialized countries. At the same time, the average expected years of life remaining to people who do reach age 65 is often only a few years less in the developing countries than in the developed ones.[3]

217

Table 9-2. Age-Specific Death Rates for the
Elderly Populations of Selected
Developed Countries, by Sex, 1980

Country and Sex	Deaths per 1,000				
	65-69	70-74	75-79	80-84	85+
Male					
Austria	36.1	58.3	94.7	146.8	225.1
Denmark	33.6	54.2	84.0	121.9	216.7
Finland	41.0	61.7	92.2	142.7	230.7
France	28.7	49.3	79.5	133.8	232.2
Germany, East	40.5	67.5	107.8	167.2	288.8
Germany, West	35.8	58.9	93.2	140.9	222.5
Japan	25.4	43.8	75.6	123.5	209.4
Norway	31.0	46.7	76.7	117.7	200.8
Sweden	28.4	47.0	75.9	123.7	222.0
UNITED STATES	33.9	50.8	74.8	112.4	188.0
Female					
Austria	17.6	32.1	60.0	109.1	207.0
Denmark	17.0	27.9	46.8	83.7	172.1
Finland	16.4	30.4	53.1	97.3	187.8
France	11.7	22.7	42.9	83.3	187.4
Germany, East	22.2	39.8	73.1	128.8	244.7
Germany, West	16.9	30.5	56.3	100.3	191.4
Japan	13.5	25.0	47.7	87.8	176.3
Norway	13.7	25.0	45.8	83.2	167.2
Sweden	14.0	24.7	46.0	84.2	173.9
UNITED STATES	17.2	26.7	42.6	72.6	147.5

Sources: United Nations, Demographic Yearbook, 1981, table 14; National Center for Health Statistics, "Advance Report of Final Mortality Statistics: 1980," Monthly Vital Statistics Report, vol. 32, no. 4 (1983), table 1.

Sex Differences in the United States

At every age from birth to age 85 and older the death rates of males are significantly higher than those of females, just as they are in all other technologically advanced countries and most developing ones as well. These differences are apparent in Tables 9-1 and 9-2. Therefore, second only to age, sex is the most significant variable in mortality analyses, and age-specific death rates must also be made sex specific for even reasonable accuracy. Moreover, the lower the general death rate, the greater the difference between the sexes, so the gap is narrower in the developing countries than in the industrialized ones.[4] In turn, differences in the mortality sex ratio produce significant variations in the overall sex ratio, as we saw earlier.

But the death rates of the sexes still vary widely by age, for among infants and young children males are only about 25 per cent more likely than females to die, while in the ages 20-24 the difference is over 300 per cent. The gap then narrows somewhat, but from the middle 30s until the middle 70s the death rates of men remain nearly twice as high as those of women. Finally, in the oldest ages the difference declines, until at 85 the death rates of men are only about 27 per cent higher than those of women. The mortality sex ratio also declines into the oldest ages among the various racial and ethnic groups in the United States.[5]

Men also have higher mortality rates from the leading causes of death, though larger percentages of women are likely to be disabled when ill, perhaps because more are willing to seek treatment and take time to recuperate when illness strikes. Moreover, men appear more often in the morbidity categories that result in high death rates, whereas women show up more frequently in those that produce chronic illness.[6] Nor have the sexes shared equally in the mortality-reduction advances of the twentieth century, for in 1900 females had only a slight advantage over men in mortality rates, whereas now their advantage is considerable.[7]

The reasons for the male-female difference are not fully known, though both the environmental and biological explanations considered in Chapter 3 have credibility. Perhaps most convincing is the hypothesis that women have greater potential durability because of various biological advantages, and with the great reductions in death rates from infectious and parasitic diseases and childbirth, that biological superiority has become more fully manifest, though a range of environmental factors also operates.[8] No matter what the reasons, however, black and white females of all ages have far lower death rates than males, though the sex differential does diminish some in the oldest years and is not as great for blacks at most ages as it is for whites.[9] Furthermore, while the mortality sex ratio may decrease in the future as environmental factors grow more alike for males and females, it is likely that women's biological advantage will still keep the death rates of the sexes from becoming identical.[10]

Racial Differences in the United States

The death rates of blacks in all but the ages 15-19 and those 85 and over are significantly higher than the rates of whites, though the racial gap has been narrowing while that between the sexes in both racial groups has been widening.[11] Thus, Table 9-1 shows that the death rate of black infants is about twice as high as that of white infants, but that the black-white mortality ratio then declines steadily to 100 in the ages 15-19. That happens largely because the death rate from motor vehicle accidents is more than twice as high for whites in those ages as it is for blacks, and the higher black death rates from other causes are not sufficient to offset the large discrepancy in motor vehicle deaths. By age 20, however, the mortality disadvantage of blacks is again substantial, and from age 25 to 54 their death rates are at least twice those of whites. At the same time, of course, the death rates of members of both races rise significantly with age, especially after 50.

In the older years the racial differential does decline substantially, and among people in their 80s the "crossover" occurs, in which the reported death rates of blacks of both sexes fall below those of whites. The data for those oldest years are less than perfect, however, especially for blacks, and the census bases and the reported numbers of deaths contain enough errors to account for at least part of the crossover.[12] Medicare data, which substantiate the crossover, do seem more reliable and allow some revisions in the materials compiled by the National Center for Health Statistics, but they are not specific for causes of death and go back only to 1966. To complicate matters further, there are differences btween the races as a whole in education, income, and other aspects of socioeconomic status that affect mortality rates, though they generally work to the disadvantage of blacks; those factors would reduce their chances of reaching age 65 and diminish the crossover phenomenon.

Therefore, despite some data inaccuracies, perhaps the blacks who have made it to the older years in spite of more severe environmental stress "may be destinted by natural selection to live an especially long life,"[13] though it is easy to carry this Darwinian notion too far and thereby miss other possible explanations. Nonetheless, the racial mortality similarities in the older years probably do reflect greater similarities of other kinds among people who survive to those ages than exist among the cohorts at birth and in middle age, when the racial mortality discrepancies are the greatest.[14] In addition, larger proportions of elderly blacks than whites live with relatives instead of alone, and that probably contributes to longevity, though there is still much to be learned about the precise causes and actual magnitude of the crossover phenomenon.[15]

The longevity advantage that women have over men shows up in the racial comparisons long before the crossover in the 80s. Thus, the death rate of black females, which is substantially below that of black males at every age, also falls below that of white males in the ages 10-14 and remains lower until the early 30s. It then rises somewhat above the rate for white men until the late 50s, and thereafter it falls below and remains there through the ages 85 and older. That comparison further demonstrates that while the age-specific death rates of blacks and whites have tended to converge because the black rates have fallen faster than the whites, the differences between males and females of both races have increased substantially. As a result, the life expectancy at birth of black females now exceeds that of white males and is approaching that of white females, while the life expectancies of the sexes remain several years apart, even though black males are slowly nearing white males.[16] Some discrepancy between the races will persist as long as average socioeconomic levels differ, but the long-term racial convergence in death rates does imply significant improvements during the twentieth century. They are also reflected in the increasingly good data on morbidity, health care usage, levels and periods of disability, and similar indexes.

Differences by Socioeconomic Characteristics

The racial differentials in mortality reflect variations in average levels of education, especially of older people, and other aspects of socioeconomic status that were shaped by historical circumstances. Therefore, mortality variations by education, income, and occupation are also important, though space and the available data enable only a cursory look at these influences. Moreover, the situation of the elderly cannot easily be separated from that of the population as a whole according to these characteristics.

Education. The level of schooling attained is probably the single best socioeconomic variable to analyze mortality differentials between men and women, because it is applicable to all people and changes little in the older years. In general, there is a strong inverse relationship between the amount of schooling people receive and their age-specific death rates, though it is less consistent for elderly persons than for those aged 25-64. The relationship also pertains to both major races and to men and women. It is particularly strong for the sexes, though they are more alike in this respect after age 65 than they are in the younger ages.[17] Given these mortality differentials by education, as better-educated cohorts enter the older years, their death rates will probably decrease even more because of the various advantages that accompany higher levels of schooling. In fact, the significant drop in the age-specific death rates of the elderly after 1968 was related in part to the rapidly rising average level of education among that age group. As a result, they are better informed about health, nutrition, and other conditions that prolong life, though the impact of education is not that simple, for it also relates to the ability to afford medical care and to other variables.

Income. Age-specific death rates also fall as income rises, though this inverse relationship is closely tied to the one between mortality and education. The latter helps determine the level of income, and people in the higher income brackets are better able to afford good nutrition, housing, privately financed health care, rising Medicare premiums and deductibles, and other things that help prolong life. Therefore, significant improvements in Social Security coverage and the advent of cost-of-living increases also help account for the renewed downward trend in the elderly death rate after 1968, though the enactment of Medicare on July 1, 1965, was also a major part of that process. Its significance is reflected in the fact that between 1965 and 1970 health expenditures by people aged 65 and older almost doubled, while public payment of those costs rose from 30 per cent in 1965 to 61 per cent in 1970.[18] Furthermore, over nine-tenths of all elderly men and women discharged from short-stay hospitals expect Medicare to be the principal source of payment;[19] that also signifies the extent to which public funds have helped provide the better health care that lowers the death rate of the elderly.

Occupation. The death rates of elderly people are at least indirectly related to the occupations at which they worked, though levels of education and income are also part of that relationship. Some occupations produce relatively high rates of death from specific causes, such as "black lung" in coal mining, "brown lung" in textile manufacturing, and "asbestosis" in certain insulation jobs; many who do survive to 65 are apt to have serious chronic illnesses and abnormally short life expectancies. Other occupations, such as logging and mining, are unusually subject to accidents, and some elderly survivors may also succumb rather soon to disabilities incurred earlier. In general, however, the lowest mortality rates occur among elderly persons who had been professional and technical workers, the highest among laborers of various kinds, while other categories are intermediate.[20] As a result, though the occupations themselves probably play some part, they seem less directly related to mortality rates than are the levels of living they provide. Moreover, in some occupations the direct danger is partly offset by high levels of physical activity that may lower mortality rates, whereas the safer conditions of others may be partially countered by their sedentary nature, which tends to increase mortality indirectly. In fact, many apparent occupational differentials in mortality can be explained by other socioeconomic factors that affect the type of job one gets and the amount of income it pays.

Trends in Age-Specific Death Rates

The long-term decline in death rates throughout the world really began after the *age of pestilence and famine* brought high death rates and life expectancy of only 20 or 25 years. That era extended from prehistory to the eighteenth century in the developed countries and to the twentieth century in many developing ones. The next *age of receding pandemics* saw less massive decimation of populations and increases in life expectancy at birth to about 50 years. It was followed by the *age of degenerative and human-made diseases,* in which the death rate fell to a low and relatively stable level and life expectancy at birth reached 70 or more years. That stage prevails now in the developed countries.[21]

Over a much shorter time than this entire three-stage *epidemiologic transition,* mortality trends in the United States also followed three fairly distinct periods according to the pace at which the death rate fluctuated. From about the middle of the last century until 1954 the rate fell steadily, interrupted significantly only by the disastrous influenza epidemic of 1917-1918. Between 1954 and 1968, however, the death rate became so static that no further decline was expected; but from 1968 to the late 1970s it fell steadily once again.[22] Table 9-3 shows how various groups in the 65-and-over category were affected by these changes.

Between 1979 and 1980 the death rates for all age groups in the elderly category rose significantly because of new outbreaks of influenza, but in 1981 they began to move downward once again, especially among people aged 75-84. Despite the fluctuations, however, the substantial fall in the elderly age-specific death rates between 1940 and 1980 helps account for the rapid growth in the numbers of older people, particularly women, and for increases in their life expectancy. These changes, especially the renewed mortality drop after 1968, represent improvements not only in the "quantity" of life, reflected in such things as greater longevity, but also in the "quality" of life, mirrored in decreased rates of illness, disability, and hospitalization.[23] Therefore, the changes are related to improvements in the delivery of health care services, such as Medicare and the programs developed to screen for high blood pressure, and to alterations in people's life styles. The significant reductions in deaths from heart disease are closely associated with these developments, although the precise causes of the swings in death rates from 1940 to the present are still not fully understood.[24] What is clear is that the death rates of the elderly in the United States are now declining faster than those in the other industrialized countries, except Japan.[25]

Despite the significant long-term decreases in the death rates among the elderly, the reductions among several other age groups have generally been greater, because young children have benefited most as deaths from infectious diseases have diminished, while the elderly, especially men, are the chief victims of the chronic and degenerative illnesses that have taken on greater proportional significance.[26] Thus, the death rates of people in the five age-groups that make up the 65-and-over age category have fallen more slowly than those of children and young adult women, and often they have not decreased as rapidly as the rates among middle-aged persons. The rates for elderly black men have even gone up, as have those of young adult males, whose mortality levels from motor vehicle accidents have grown significantly.

Table 9-3. Average Annual Percentage Change in the Death Rates of Elderly People, by Age and Sex, Selected Years

Sex and Age	1940-54	1955-67	1968-78	1979-80
Male 65+[a]	-1.1	+0.2	-1.5	+2.9
65-69	-0.7	+0.1	-2.2	+2.1
70-74	-1.0	+0.2	-1.5	+0.3
75-79	-1.1	+0.2	-0.9	+3.2
80-84	-1.3	-0.4	-1.2	+2.2
85+	-1.5	+0.9	-2.2	+6.8
Female 65+[a]	-2.0	-1.0	-2.3	+4.0
65-69	-2.3	-1.1	-2.6	+4.5
70-74	-2.2	-1.3	-2.0	+2.1
75-79	-1.9	-1.2	-1.7	+3.1
80-85	-1.9	-1.1	-2.3	+3.1
85+	-1.3	0.0	-3.0	+7.0

Sources: Lois A. Fingerhut and Harry M. Rosenberg, "Mortality Among the Elderly," in National Center for Health Statistics, Health, United States, 1981, PHS Pub. no. 82-1232 (1981), p. 17; National Center for Health Statistics, "Advance Report of Final Mortality Statistics, 1979," Monthly Vital Statistics Report, vol. 31, no. 6 (1982), table 1; "Advance Report of Final Mortality Statistics, 1980," Monthly Vital Statistics Report, vol. 32, no. 4 (1983), table 1.

[a]Age-adjusted rates.

On the other hand, data collected since 1980 show that the death rates of the elderly are falling a little faster than those of some middle-aged groups, but still not as rapidly as those of infants, children, or people in several other age groups. Therefore, while declining death rates of older people over several decades have added greatly to their numbers, the slower pace of reduction has actually retarded rather than accelerated the aging of the total population. That process, as we have seen, is due primarily to major reductions in the birth rate since 1960. Moreover, the average life expectancy of the whole population has increased significantly because larger percentages of infants can expect to reach the older ages, while life expectancy of the elderly themselves has increased more modestly, given the smaller reductions in their death rates.

Trends by sex. Reductions in the death rates of infants and very young children have not varied greatly by sex, but at most ages the death rates of females have fallen more than those of males. That is particularly true of the elderly, and the mortality sex ratio of people in all of the age groups over 65 has increased substantially. (See Table 9-4.) That ratio has risen most rapidly for people 70-74, followed by those 65-69 and people in the three oldest age ranges. The ratio among people age 85 and older has also increased, but the death rate of men in that group is still only 27 per cent higher than that of women, whereas among people 65-69 the male death rate is more than twice that of females.

But the rates at which the mortality sex ratio is rising in most age groups under 80 is less now than it was in earlier decades, and the white figure in the ages 65-69 has even fallen slightly. This deceleration suggests that the death rate differential between older men and women won't increase in the future as it has in the past. It will probably decrease, perhaps significantly, though there is little likelihood that the death rates of the sexes will again converge to the ratios of 1900 or 1940.[27] Moreover, even if the environmental differences between the sexes were eliminated, biological factors would still preserve a significant mortality difference between males and females, though a smaller one than exists now. But the largest increases in the mortality differential by sex seem about over for young-old whites, though not yet for the old-old. In the black group, however, the mortality sex ratio is still rising for all age groups 65 and over, and the rate of increase is also the greatest among the oldest people. It is likely, however, that for both races the pace of divergence in death rates by sex will slow and even give way to some convergence as elements in the socioeconomic environment become more similar for men and women.

Trends by race. Tracing the long-term mortality trends for blacks is discouraging methodologically, because even now many vital statistics are

Table 9-4. Male to Female Death Rate Ratios Among
the Elderly, by Age and Race, 1940-1980

Race and Year	Death Rate Ratio, by Age				
	65-69	70-74	75-79	80-84	85+
All Races					
1940	1.34	1.25	1.20	1.15	1.08
1950	1.58	1.40	1.29	1.21	1.13
1960	1.83	1.62	1.42	1.26	1.11
1970	2.02	1.82	1.61	1.41	1.15
1980	1.98	1.90	1.76	1.55	1.27
White					
1940	1.36	1.26	1.19	1.14	1.07
1950	1.62	1.42	1.29	1.20	1.12
1960	1.88	1.65	1.43	1.27	1.12
1970	2.10	1.86	1.62	1.42	1.16
1980	2.02	1.94	1.78	1.56	1.27
Other Races					
1940	1.20	1.20	1.28	1.33	1.25
1950	1.28	1.23	1.28	1.30	1.20
1960	1.47	1.37	1.30	1.30	1.18
1970	1.52	1.46	1.47	1.33	1.12
1980	1.74	1.58	1.53	1.45	1.32

Sources: Robert D. Grove and Alice M. Hetzel,
Vital Statistics Rates in the United States, 1940-1960 (Washington, D.C.: National Center for Health Statistics, 1968), table 55; National Center for Health Statistics, Vital Statistics of the United States, 1970, vol. 2, Mortality, part A (1974), table 1-8; "Advance Report of Final Mortality Statistics, 1980," Monthly Vital Statistics Report, vol. 32, no. 4 (1983), table 1.

compiled only for the categories *white* and *all other* or *other races*. That tends to obscure the actual situation of blacks, even though they are well over 90 per cent of the ''other-races'' group. In many earlier years, the designations were *white* and *nonwhite,* which were no more helpful and even implicitly racist.[28] Therefore, in order to trace trends only for the two major races, we have used data for 1960 and 1980, which do separate blacks from other races.

The age-adjusted death rates for the black population as a whole fell faster between 1960 and 1980 than did those of whites, but that was true only because of reductions in early childhood and several other ages up to 70, whereas the death rates of black infants and elderly people did not drop as fast as those of whites.[29] Nevertheless, the more rapid decreases in the death rates of blacks under age 70, especially women, significantly accelerated the proportions who entered the older years, and blacks rose from 7.2 per cent of the nation's elderly in 1960 to 8.2 per cent in 1980. At the same time, however, there is also a tendency for the mortality levels of the oldest whites to fall faster than those of the oldest blacks, so while the death rate crossover persists, the difference in favor of blacks is growing smaller. In fact, the death rate of black men aged 85 and older was 32 per cent lower than that of white men in 1960, but only 16 per cent lower in 1980; for women the difference declined from 33 per cent to 17 per cent. Some of the change, however, was due to improvements in the quality of the data.

Life Expectancy

At the turn of the century, when life expectancy at birth was only 49 years, relatively few Americans could expect to live to age 65. But the situation has changed so much that death is now primarily a phenomenon of those past age 65, rather than an event that occurs more evenly over the age span.[30] Moreover, deaths of the elderly are disproportionately concentrated in the oldest ages. These changes have occurred largely because greater proportions of the newborn survive to the older ages, but also because the life expectancy of older persons has increased, even if rather modestly. Thus, in 1981 the expectation of life at birth for the total population was 74.1 years, which was an all-time high and an increase of almost 25 years over 1900-1902, although there were periodic decreases for some groups during the 80-year period, especially in 1917-1918. (See Table 9-5.) In the 1980s the expectation of life at birth was still moving upward and represented a 57 per cent increase over 1900-1902. This spectacular progress has close parallels in the other industrialized countries. The increase in the United States indicates very significant progress in health status during the twentieth century, and while in 1900-1902 only

41 per cent of the newborn could expect to reach age 65, by 1981 about 77 per cent could anticipate surviving that long — a gain of 36 elderly people for each 100 infants.

Variations by Race and Sex

In the first 80 years of the century, life expectancy at birth increased by the largest percentage for white females, followed closely by black females. However, the latter actually added more years to their life expectancy because their situation was so much poorer in 1900-1902. Black males also added more years than white males to their life expectancy, and their proportional improvement was greater. Even so, the life expectancy at birth of black males is still well below that of the other three race and sex categories.[31]

Table 9-5. Years of Life Expectancy at Birth, by Race and Sex, 1900-02 to 1980-81

Years	All Groups	White		Other Races	
		Male	Female	Male	Female
1900-02[a]	49.2	48.2	51.1	32.5	35.0
1909-11[a]	51.6	50.3	53.7	34.2	37.7
1919-21[a]	56.5	56.6	58.6	47.2	47.0
1929-31	59.3	59.2	62.8	47.5	49.5
1939-41	63.8	63.3	67.2	52.4	55.4
1949-51	68.2	66.4	72.2	59.1	63.0
1959-61	68.9	67.6	74.2	61.5	66.5
1969-71	70.7	67.9	75.5	61.0	69.1
1980-81	73.9	70.8	78.4	65.7	74.8

Sources: National Center for Health Statistics, Vital Statistics of the United States, 1978, vol. 2, sec. 5, Life Tables (1980), tables 5-A and 5-5; "Annual Summary of Births, Deaths, Marriages, and Divorces: United States, 1981," Monthly Vital Statistics Report, vol. 30, no. 13 (1982), pp. 3-4 and 15.

[a]Death-registration states only.

The most spectacular change of all has been the divergence between males and females in life expectancy. In 1900-1902, white females already had an edge of 2.9 years over white males, but in 1980-1981 the difference was 7.6 years. This reflects the superior progress in mortality control that has accrued to white females as compared with any other group in the population, for their life expectancy still exceeds by 3.6 years that of their nearest competitor — black females — though the latter are moving up fast. But blacks also experienced an even more significant divergence between the sexes, and in 1900-1902 life expectancy for black females was 2.5 years higher than that for black males, while by 1980-1981 the gap had increased to 9.1 years. In fact, about 1965 the life expectancy of black females even surpassed that of white males, and by 1980-1981 the difference had grown to 4.0 years.

At the extremes, white females can now expect to live an average of 12.7 years longer than black males, though the discrepancy is not as great as it was in 1900-1902, when 18.6 years separated those groups. So despite the great divergence by sex, there are also certain convergences underway, and it is likely they will continue until the life expectancy of males and females and blacks and whites grow at least somewhat more alike.

Changes in Life Expectancy of the Elderly

The expectation of life at age 65 has changed much less than that at birth, because the most spectacular mortality reductions have occurred at the younger end of the age scale. Therefore, expectation of life at birth doesn't provide a true picture of what really happened to the average remaining lifetimes of older people, but shows, instead, that much larger percentages of infants survive to the older ages. Consequently, it is necessary to examine life expectancy for each of the age-groups in the elderly population.[32]

For all race and sex groups together, life expectancy at age 65 rose from 11.9 years in 1900-1902 to 16.7 years in 1980, for a difference of 4.8 years, which is a far smaller increase than the 24.7 years at birth in the same period. Furthermore, the life expectancy of elderly women of both races has increased significantly more than that of men in each of the five-year age groups that make up the 65-and-over age category, as shown in Table 9-6. White women registered the largest gains, followed by black women, black men, and white men, in that order. The only exception was the nearly equal increase among black and white women at age 65. There were even occasions during the 80-year period when the life expectancy of elderly white men dropped slightly, whereas in most instances that of the other three groups continued to rise, except in 1917-1918, when the influenza epidemic caused life expectancy to fall for all of the groups.

Early in the 80-year period, life expectancy tended to rise most rapidly for the young-old, but because of the dynamics of the last few decades, the rate of increase has become substantial for the old-old. As a result, the pace of increase during the twentieth century has been greater for men of both races at age 85 than for those aged 65. Life expectancy for the oldest white women has also increased slightly faster than that for the young-old, while the reverse is true for black women. In total, however, the elderly population is becoming increasingly concentrated in the oldest ages, which profoundly affects the kinds and costs of services that are necessary.

In summary, the life expectancy of Americans of all ages has increased dramatically since 1900, but while much of the change is due to rapid

Table 9-6. Years of Life Expectancy at Various Elderly Ages, 1900-02 and 1980

Year and Age	White		Black	
	Male	Female	Male	Female
1900-02[a]				
65	11.5	12.2	10.4	11.4
70	9.0	9.6	8.3	9.6
75	6.8	7.3	6.6	7.9
80	5.1	5.5	5.1	6.5
85	3.8	4.1	4.0	5.1
1980				
65	14.2	18.5	13.5	17.3
70	11.3	14.8	11.1	14.2
75	8.8	11.5	8.9	11.4
80	6.7	8.6	6.9	9.0
85	5.0	6.3	5.3	7.0

Sources: National Center for Health Statistics, Vital Statistics of the United States, 1978, vol. 2, sec. 5, Life Tables (1980), table 5-4; "Advance Report of Final Mortality Statistics, 1980," Monthly Vital Statistics Report, vol. 32, no. 4 (1983), table 2.

[a]Death-registration states only.

improvements in the survival potential of infants, the elderly have also experienced important if more modest increases in the expectation of life. The improvements have been particularly significant for women and for persons aged 75 and older. In Chapter 11 we will consider the impact on longevity of new technologies, especially those that may lengthen the life span, which has long been thought to be a fixed attribute of the human species, and will look at the prospective changes in life expectancy and the impact they will have on the future of American society.

Cause of Death

The three major causes of death of elderly people are heart disease, cancer, and stroke, though individual deaths often result from multiple causes and the average person suffers from more than one chronic illness. For example, pneumonia finally kills some patients disabled by strokes or bedridden with osteoporosis, because these and other chronic deteriorative diseases often reduce resistance to the point where people are susceptible to fatal infections, often of the lungs and blood.[33] Numerous victims of fatal heart attacks have also endured years of hypertension, emphysema, arthritis, or other maladies, and many suicides among the elderly are motivated at least partially by serious health problems. Thus, while the data on the eventual cause of death are useful, especially in tracing long-term changes in the importance of various causes, they do not reveal the several chronic maladies that may combine to bring about the deaths of specific individuals or cause suffering before death.

Age Differences

The causes of death vary greatly in importance by age, and those that claim most elderly lives are not the same ones that account for most deaths of infants, children, and young adults. For example, infants are most likely to die from birth defects, accidents, and pneumonia and influenza, but for children aged 1-14, accidents are the chief cause of death, followed by cancer, especially leukemia, and the lingering effects of birth defects. People aged 15-34 also succumb most often to accidents, especially those involving motor vehicles, but homicide and suicide are the second and third most important causes. Those aged 35-54 die most often from cancer, followed by heart disease and accidents. From there on, however, heart disease assumes first place, cancer second position, and cerebrovascular disease (stroke) third place. There is no change in that ranking with increasing age, except that stroke is in second place for people aged 85 and over, while cancer is third. Moreover, until the ages

55-64 heart disease and cancer are about equally important, but heart disease then pulls far ahead despite its declining rate in recent years, and by the ages 75-84 it kills well over twice as many people as cancer; at age 85 it takes more than three times as many lives as stroke, its nearest competitor.

It is also worth noting, however, that while accidents account for a larger *percentage* of deaths among young people than among any other age group, the *death rate* from that cause is highest for those aged 65 and older. The majority do not involve motor vehicles, whereas for young adults the reverse is true, and for people aged 85 and older the death rate from other accidents is 10 times that from vehicular accidents. Both men and women are especially likely to die from falls, though motor vehicle accidents are in second place, fires in third, and the inhalation or ingestion of food in fourth.[34]   Since 1968-1969, however, the death rate from accidents among the elderly has declined by about a third, though older people still account for twice their fair share of all fatal accidents.

These and other major killers of elderly people appear in Table 9-7, which shows the 10 leading causes of death and the rates from each in 1980.[35] Those data emphasize the significant gap between the three top killers of the elderly and all of the other causes, for heart disease, cancer, and stroke account for 75 per cent of all deaths among persons aged 65 and older. The proportion is the same for those aged 65-84, but it drops to 73 per cent in the oldest ages, when people are somewhat more likely to succumb to a wider range of causes, especially pneumonia and influenza, atherosclerosis, accidents, and chronic pulmonary diseases, particularly emphysema.

The list of major causes of death among the elderly is also significant for what it does not include. Especially scarce are most of the infectious and parasitic diseases and the effects of nutritional deficiency, all of which were far more significant earlier in the century. For example, the death rates from tuberculosis, syphilis, intestinal infections, and hepatitis are a small fraction of what they were in 1940, and despite the 1980 influenza epidemic the death rates from that disease and pneumonia were less than half what they were in 1940. The death rates from other controllable maladies, such as appendicitis, also have fallen faster than the overall death rate of the elderly. Therefore, the major causes have become more heavily concentrated among the degenerative illnesses that are much more difficult to control than are infectious and parasitic diseases, and which are typical of any population with low overall mortality rates and a high percentage of elderly people.

232

Table 9-7.   Death Rates of People 65 and Over for
the Ten Leading Causes, by Age, 1980

Cause of Death[a]	Deaths per 100,000			
	65+	65-74	75-84	85+
All Causes	5,253	2,995	6,693	15,980
Diseases of Heart	2,331	1,219	2,993	7,777
Malignant Neoplasms	1,012	818	1,232	1,595
Cerebrovascular Diseases	573	220	789	2,289
Pneumonia & Influenza	178	56	220	886
Chronic Obstructive Pulmonary Diseases	171	129	224	274
Atherosclerosis	110	24	126	657
Diabetes Mellitus	99	65	131	222
Accidents	97	58	120	293
Motor Vehicle	22	19	28	28
Other	75	39	92	265
Nephritis & Other Kidney Diseases	60	25	68	174
Chronic Liver Disease & Cirrhosis	37	43	31	20
All Other Causes	585	280	639	1,500

Sources: National Center for Health Statistics,
"Advance Report of Final Mortality Statistics:
1980," Monthly Vital Statistics Report, vol. 32,
no. 4 (1983), tables 4 and 5;   U.S. Bureau of the
Census, 1980 Census of Population, Supplementary
Reports, PC80-S1-1, Age, Sex, Race, and Spanish
Origin of the Population by Regions, Divisions,
and States: 1980 (1981), table 1.

[a]Ninth International Classification, 1975.

Cause-of-Death Differences by Sex

The death rates for elderly men attributable to heart disease and cancer are far higher than those for elderly women, though the toll from hypertensive heart disease (associated with high blood pressure) is somewhat greater among women. Men are much more likely to die of ischemic (coronary) heart disease, though it also accounts for the great majority of heart disease deaths among women. Cancer, which is the only major cause of death for which the mortality rates among the elderly have continued to rise since 1900,[36] also takes a much higher toll of elderly men than women, particularly cancer of the digestive and urinary organs, the respiratory system, and the mouth, throat, and larynx, largely because of a higher incidence of long-term smoking among the men. Conversely, cancer of the breast is almost exclusive to women, and their death rates are also higher for cancer of the genital organs.

Men are also considerably more likely to die from influenza and pneumonia, accidents, and the chronic obstructive pulmonary diseases, principally bronchitis, emphysema, and asthma. The death rates from kidney diseases are also about twice as high among elderly men as among women, and so are those from liver diseases, partly because of long-established cultural differences between the sexes in the use of alcohol. Cerebrovascular disease also tends to produce higher rates among men close to age 65, but as people approach their 80s the gender differential diminishes substantially, and for the whole group 65 and over the death rate from this cause is somewhat higher for women than for men. The same is true for atherosclerosis. Women are also somewhat more likely to die of diabetes mellitus, but even that crossover doesn't occur until about age 70.

In short, most of the causes of death reflect the greater survival potential of women, as does the fact that their death rates from most of the major causes have declined faster than those of men. Even in the case of cancer, the death rates of men have gone up sharply and steadily, whereas the rates among women have escalated far less and only since the mid-1960s, particularly because of the change in their smoking habits.

Cause-of-Death Differences by Race

In the elderly population as a whole, the differences between the races in rates of death from the leading causes are generally smaller than those between the sexes, though certain causes are particularly hard on one race or the other. For example, elderly blacks have lower rates from bronchitis, emphysema, and asthma and from cirrhosis of the liver, and their suicide rate is far below that of whites. Conversely, the rates for blacks are considerably higher for diabetes and infections of the kidney, and especially homicide. But the races are fairly similar in their susceptibility to most of the major causes of death.

The relationship is strongly influenced by the age distributions within the 65-and-over group, however, and by differences in the sex ratio by race, and it is necessary to account for both of those variables. Thus, among men aged 65-74 the death rates are significantly higher for blacks than for whites from most of the major causes, except bronchitis, emphysema, and asthma, and cirrhosis and suicide, while the rate from cancer is somewhat higher for blacks and that from heart disease is a little lower. The black men are nearly six times as likely as whites to die from homicide, but less than a third as likely to take their own lives. Among women aged 65-74 most of the same relationships between the races apply, except that death rates of black women are much higher than those of white women from heart disease, cerebrovascular disease, and diabetes. But the black women are less often the victims of motor vehicle accidents and their suicide rate is especially low.

In the ages 75-84 the mortality levels for blacks from about half the causes drop below those of whites, though the differences are relatively small. These are the ages in which the death rate crossover appears. Thus, black men aged 75-84 are considerably less likely than whites to die of heart disease, bronchitis and related diseases, atherosclerosis, cirrhosis, and suicide, while their rates from kidney disease and homicide remain relatively high. At about age 80 the death rate from cancer among black men drops slightly below that among white men. Black women aged 75-84 follow many of the same patterns, except that their heart disease death rate is about the same as that of white women, while their rates from cerebrovascular disease, diabetes, and kidney problems remain relatively high. As with black men, the homicide rate of the women is far above that of whites.

In the ages 85 and older the reported data suggest that the death rates of blacks from virtually all causes have fallen well below those of whites, both for men and women. The only exception is the homicide rate of black men, which is still nearly four times that of white men. Moreover, the rates are about the same for blacks and whites of both sexes from kidney infections, while the women of both races have nearly similar rates from diabetes and homicide. Because of distortions in reporting, however, the comparisons in the oldest ages should be treated with caution.

In general, then, heart disease is the major cause of death for the elderly of both races and sexes, followed by cancer and cerebrovascular disease. Moreover, blacks and whites are gradually tending to succumb to more of the same causes at more similar rates, because the diseases associated with low levels of living and poor medical care have declined greatly during the twentieth century and no longer take the disproportionate toll of blacks they once did. But while blacks are increasingly like whites in the tendency to die from the major degenerative illnesses of old age, the changes have not totally obliterated the mortality differences between the races, and a few causes are still much more lethal for elderly people in one race or the other.

Cause-of-Death Trends

Since 1900 the infectious diseases have diminished greatly in importance as causes of death of Americans of all ages. In that year, influenza and pneumonia and tuberculosis led the list of killers and accounted for 23 per cent of all deaths, compared with less than 3 per cent in 1980. They were followed in order by diarrhea and enteritis, heart disease, stroke, nephritis, accidents, diseases of early infancy, cancer, and senility.[37] Other significant causes were syphilis, the death rate from which fell 98 per cent, and typhoid and paratyphoid, which have almost disappeared, as has diphtheria.

Changes in the causes of death among the elderly have paralleled those in the whole population, and in fact the changes are closely associated with the aging of the population and significant increases in life expectancy at birth. But the classification of causes of death has changed over time and record keeping has improved, so it seems best to look at changes in the causes of death that occurred among the elderly between 1950 and 1980. Even during that time the International Classification of Diseases has been revised, but the data are reasonably comparable or can be made so statistically. They show that by 1950 heart disease, cancer, and stroke already accounted for three of every four deaths of elderly people, just as they did in the 1980s, though the relative importance of these three major causes has changed during the period. Table 9-8 shows that while the death rates from heart disease and stroke have fallen significantly, that from cancer has risen, especially since 1970.

Heart disease. This cause is so significant that its trends greatly affect mortality trends in general. It was, of course, by far the leading cause of elderly deaths in 1950 as it is now, but it has been decreasing in importance since the mid-1960s, largely because of reductions in the death rate from coronary heart disease. Furthermore, while the rates have fallen for both sexes and races, they have generally done so fastest for white women, followed by black men and women, and trailed by white men. Between 1950 and 1980, however, the mortality sex ratio for heart disease deaths among the elderly rose significantly, so the advantage that women enjoy relative to men in deaths from this major cause is growing.

Malignant neoplasms. The death rate of the elderly for cancer has risen since 1900 and the increase continued at a substantial pace after 1950. But the situations of men and women are quite different: The former experienced virtually uninterrupted increases, while the rates for women fell until 1965 and then began to move upward. The cancer category includes many types of malignancies, however, and only a few are responsible for the overall increase in death rates from this cause. The dramatic increase in lung cancer is most at fault for both sexes in all of the older age categories, and cigarette smoking is now responsible for more than 80 per cent of the lung cancer deaths among the men and more than 40 per cent of those among the women.[*38*] In addition, death rates from cancer of the colon have risen among men but decreased among women. The relative significance of breast cancer also increased somewhat among women aged 65-74, but decreased in the older ages. As a result of these dynamics, the mortality sex ratio for cancer among the elderly rose significantly between 1950 and 1980, though the rate of increase slowed after the mid-1960s because of the rapidly increasing incidence of lung cancer among women. Those changes coincided with an increase in the percentage of women smokers and a decrease in the proportion of men who smoke, though the latter who continue tend to consume more cigarettes daily than they did.

Much progress has also been made in curing or arresting some malignant neoplasms, such as cervical cancer, and in increasing the average survival time of treated victims. But these advances have not yet been sufficient to offset the increases from other types of the disease, especially lung cancer, but also genital and colon cancer among men.

Cerebrovascular disease. Death rates for stroke among the elderly have decreased even faster than those for heart disease, especially since 1970 and among women aged 65-74, largely because of substantial improvements in the control of hypertension. In the two older age groups the 1970-1980 decrease has been nearly the same for men and women. As a result, strokes still take a somewhat higher toll of men than women in the ages 65-74, but the reverse is true above age 85.

Not only have the infectious, parasitic, and deficiency diseases become less significant as causes of death among the elderly while the degenerative illnesses have become more important proportionately, but the large majority of elderly people suffer from one or more chronic illnesses, especially arthritis, heart ailments, high blood pressure, and diabetes.[*39*] They are the price paid for long life expectancy, and while certain chronic diseases may be even better controlled in the future and death rates for them lowered further, they will remain the principal maladies of the older years, and the present major killers of elderly people are apt to be the same in the foreseeable future. Consequently, health-care efforts for the elderly require better daily care for people whose chronic illnesses, unlike the acute ones, are not very responsive to dramatic measures and sophisticated medical technology.[40]

Various chronic diseases will persist in the older population even if the three major killers are much better controlled. For example, Alzheimer's Disease, which produces progressive mental disability, is poorly understood and its cause still unknown. As the population ages, the incidence of that disease is likely to rise dramatically from the 1.5 million people who now suffer from it. It is also costly of a family's financial and emotional resources, because care for its increasingly disoriented victims can extend

Table 9-8. Changes in the Death Rates of Elderly People for the Three Leading Causes of Death, by Age and Sex, 1950-1980

Cause and Age	Per Cent Change		
	1950-60	1960-70	1970-80
Heart Disease			
65-74	-5.4	-10.5	-21.8
75-84	-5.1	-9.9	-18.8
85+	+1.8	-9.1	-8.2
Malignant Neoplasms			
65-74	+3.1	+5.6	+8.5
75-84	-2.2	+3.7	+5.4
85+	-0.1	-2.3	+12.6
Respiratory Cancer			
65-74	+69.1	+49.0	+39.9
75-84	+48.5	+70.2	+54.5
85+	+23.6	+54.0	+31.0
Cerebrovascular Diseases			
65-74	-14.6	-18.1	-42.7
75-84	-0.6	-15.9	-37.1
85+	+23.1	-12.1	-29.2

Sources: National Center for Health Statistics, Health, United States, 1982, PHS Pub. no. 82-1232 (1982), tables 16-19; "Advance Report of Final Mortality Statistics, 1980," Monthly Vital Statistics Report, vol. 32, no. 4 (1983), table 6.

over several years before death follows. Alzheimer's Disease will increase the need for nursing home facilities, although the large majority of victims are cared for at home and the total cost of that care will rise. Therefore, this one example illustrates the fact that even with better control of heart disease, cancer, and stroke, it will be a long while before the aging clock can be turned back and more years of *healthy and vigorous* existence added to the life span. In the meantime, the quality of life for the nation's elderly may even deteriorate in the sense that we will have larger numbers and percentages of people in the oldest ages suffering from the chronic illnesses, many of which develop over a long period, not just because of environmental conditions that could be controlled, but also because of less manipulable genetic factors. Therefore, the health and longevity of a rapidly growing population of old-old still pose perplexing questions.

Summary

In the 100 years from 1900 to 2000 America's elderly population will have grown from 3 million to 35 million, and while fertility changes are a principal reason, reductions in mortality have also played an equally significant part. Because of sophisticated mortality controls, the death rate among infants is not reached again until about age 60, and while the mortality levels of children and young adults haven't fallen to their absolute limits, they have come close to it. Furthermore, the mortality rates of elderly persons are quite low compared with those of earlier decades, and death is more a phenomenon of the very old. In that sense, the United States compares favorably with other urban-industrial societies, though the death rates of elderly women are significantly lower than those of elderly men, while the older black population still has higher rates than the older white group. Even so, the death rates of elderly black and white people have been converging, while those of men and women have been diverging. The racial convergence even results in the well-known cross-over effect, in which the reported death rates of blacks over age 80 are lower than those of whites, partly because of inaccuracies in the data, but also because blacks who do manage to reach the oldest ages seem to have a somewhat higher survival potential than whites in the advanced years. The mortality variations also reflect higher death rates among the most poorly educated Americans and those with the lowest incomes.

Given these differences in death rates, it is logical that vastly more people reach the older ages now than ever before, and that life expectancy is longer for women than for men and greater for whites than for blacks. Despite these variations, however, in 1981 Americans could expect an average lifetime at birth of 74.1 years, while people aged 65 could anticipate an average of 16.7 more years of life (by 1984, the figures were 74.7

and 16.8, respectively). Both figures are record highs in longevity and both reflect the progress in saving lives at all ages, though the incremental increases in life expectancy are smaller among the elderly than the young, because life-saving technology has had more effect at the lower than the upper end of the age scale. Moreover, the increases in life expectancy are due more to the large proportions of the newborn who reach the older years than to prolongation of life among elderly persons, though the latter improvement has also occurred at a modest rate.

The question as to whether or not life expectancy of the elderly will increase at the rate it has in the past is still open, though medical advances now underway could increase it considerably. They could even expand the historically inexpansible life span — the biological potential for people to survive only a certain number of years, generally 100 or so.

The major causes of death have become fewer in the sense that infectious, parasitic, and nutritional diseases have diminished greatly as causes, leaving heart disease, cancer, and stroke as the major causes of death of the elderly. This is typical of an aging population, in which most people are cut down by the degenerative diseases. There are race and sex variations, but the basic causes of death of elderly Americans reflect a high degree of control over the contagious illnesses of earlier times. They also mirror the effects of excessive smoking, inadequate physical activity, and other contributing factors that could potentially be controlled.

NOTES

1. For detailed accounts of mortality measurement procedures, see Henry S. Shryock and Jacob S. Siegel, *The Methods and Materials of Demography.* v. 2. Washington, DC: U.S. Government Printing Office, 1973, chapters 14 and 15.

2. U.S. Bureau of the Census, "Some Demographic Aspects of Aging in the United States," *Current Population Reports,* P-23, no. 43 (1973): 20.

3. See the international comparisons in Lois A. Fingerhut and Harry M. Rosenberg, "Mortality Among the Elderly," in National Center for Health Statistics, *Health, United States, 1981.* PHS Pub. no. 82-1232 (1981), pp. 20-22.

4. Shryock and Siegel, *op. cit.,* p. 401.

5. Fingerhut and Rosenberg, *op. cit.,* pp. 21-22.

6. U.S. Bureau of the Census, "A Statistical Portrait of Women in the U.S.," *Current Population Reports,* P-23, no. 58 (1976): 8.

7. For a discussion of these points, see U.S. Bureau of the Census, "Demographic Aspects of Aging and the Older Population in the United States," *Current Population Reports,* P-23, no. 59 (1976): 28-29.

8. *Ibid.,* p. 30.

240

9. See the discussion by Estelle R. Ramey, "The Natural Capacity for Health in Women," in Phyllis W. Berman and Estelle R. Ramey, eds., *Women: A Developmental Perspective.* Washington, DC: National Institutes of Health, 1982, pp. 3-12, especially pp. 4-6.

10. Jacob S. Siegel, "On the Demography of Aging," *Demography* 17 (1980): 350.

11. Beth J. Soldo, "America's Elderly in the 1980s," *Population Bulletin* 35 (1980): 15.

12. Lois A. Fingerhut, "Changes in Mortality Among the Elderly: United States, 1940-78," *Vital and Health Statistics,* Analytical Studies, series 3, no. 22 (1982): 15-18.

13. U.S. Bureau of the Census, "Demographic Aspects of Aging...," *op. cit.,* p. 32.

14. Jacquelyne Johnson Jackson, *Minorities and Aging.* Belmont, CA: Wadsworth, 1980, p. 64.

15. For a discussion of the crossover phenomenon, see Charles B. Nam, Norman L. Weatherby and Kathleen A. Ockay, "Causes of Death Which Contribute to the Mortality Crossover Effect," *Social Biology* 25 (1978): 306-314.

16. John Reid, "Black America in the 1980s," *Population Bulletin* 37 (1982): 14-15.

17. Paul C. Glick, "Differential Mortality," in U.S. Bureau of the Census, "Population of the United States, Trends and Prospects: 1950-1990," *Current Population Reports,* P-23, no. 49 (1974): 45; 46-47.

18. National Center for Health Statistics, *Health..,* p. 210.

19. Edmund Graves and Robert Pokras, "Expected Principal Source of Payment for Hospital Discharges: United States, 1979," in National Center for Health Statistics, *Advance Data from Vital and Health Statistics,* no. 75 (1982): 3.

20. Shryock and Siegel, *op. cit.,* pp. 409-410.

21. Regina McNamara, "Mortality Trends," in John A. Ross, ed., *International Encyclopedia of Population.* v. 2. New York: Free Press, 1982, p. 461; adapted from Abdel R. Omran, "The Epidemiologic Transition: A Theory of the Epidemiology of Population Change," *Milbank Memorial Fund Quarterly* 49 (1971): 509-538.

22. Jean van der Tak, "U.S. Population: Where We Are; Where We're Going," *Population Bulletin* 37 (1982): 15.

23. U.S. Bureau of the Census, "Demographic Aspects...," *op. cit.,* p. 25.

24. Siegel, *op. cit.,* p. 348.

25. Lois A. Fingerhut, "Chartbook," in National Center for Health Statistics, *Health, United States, 1982,* PHS Pub. no. 83-1232 (1982): 34.

26. Soldo, *op. cit.,* p. 16.

27. For projections to 2000 that anticipate reductions in the mortality sex ratio, see Shryock and Siegel, *op. cit.,* p. 780, table 24-4. Cf. Siegel, *op. cit.,* p. 350.

28. For an effort to overcome some of this problem, see Jacquelyne Johnson Jackson, "Death Rate Trends of Black Females, United States, 1964-1978," in Berman and Ramey, *op. cit.,* pp. 23-35.

29. For the data, see National Center for Health Statistics, *Health, 1981, op. cit.,* table 8; and National Center for Health Statistics, "Advance Report of Final Mortality Statistics, 1980," *Monthly Vital Statistics Report* 32 (1983), table 1.

30. Richard A. Kalish, "Death and Dying in Social Context," in Robert H. Binstock and Ethel Shanas, eds., *Handbook of Aging and the Social Sciences.* New York: Van Nostrand, 1976, p. 484.

31. For a discussion, see Reid, *op. cit.,* pp. 14-15.

32. U.S. Bureau of the Census, "Demographic Aspects...," *op. cit.,* p. 27.

33. Kenneth G. Manton and Eric Stallard, "Temporal Trends in U.S. Multiple Cause of Death Mortality Data: 1968 to 1977," *Demography* 19 (1982): 539.

34. Metropolitan Life Foundation, *Statistical Bulletin* 63 (1982): 12.

35. Causes are from World Health Organization, *Manual of the International Statistical Classification of Diseases, Injuries, and Causes of Death, Ninth Revision.* Geneva: WHO, 1977.

36. National Center for Health Statistics, *Health, 1981, op. cit.,* p. 18.

37. van der Tak, *op. cit.,* p. 16.

38. American Cancer Society, *Cancer Facts and Figures.* New York: American Cancer Society, 1983.

39. Mary Barberis, "America's Elderly: Policy Implications," *Population Bulletin* 35 (1981): 8.

40. *Ibid.,* p. 12.

Chapter 10

Internal Migration of the Elderly

Migration within the United States is the third major population process that determines the size, proportional significance, and distribution of the elderly population in particular places, although movement from abroad also has some impact. Despite recent attention to the movement of older retired persons to Florida, California, and other Sunbelt areas, however, movements of the elderly are not new in industrial societies, for they have long altered the lives of millions, while they have helped re-distribute the older population in general.[1] Nevertheless, migration is mostly an activity of young adults, and older people are far more likely to stay where they are because of social ties, familiar settings, or prohibitive costs. Therefore, the focus on the minority who do migrate tends to divert attention from problems in the areas where most older people remain after they retire, especially the rural communities, the deteriorating urban areas, and some aging suburbs.[2] Some of these places have become elderly enclaves, not because of migratory influxes of old people, but because the exodus of younger ones has left behind a high concentration of the elderly.

There is a growing body of literature on the minority who do migrate, however, and it deals with their characteristics, the places they leave and those they enter, and the reasons they move. These studies, most done since 1960, show that elderly migrants are not representative of the entire older population, but rather that the process selects for certain kinds of people. Even most of those who do move don't go very far, because well over half remain in the same county, while only a fifth depart for another state. The young-old also tend to migrate for different reasons than the old-old; the former often seek better recreational opportunities and climate, whereas the latter frequently relocate for health reasons or to be with adult offspring, sometimes returning to an original home area.[3] In any case, elderly migration is now studied intensively, and while the phenomenon lacks an adequate explanatory theoretical framework, there are many specific contributions toward that end.[4]

Measuring Migration

Migration is assessed by counting either the number of people who move from place to place on a relatively permanent basis within a given period, or the number of moves specific persons make. Data for the United States better enable the first measurement than the second.[5]

Sources of Data

There are two basic sources of data on migration in the United States: the decennial census of population and the Current Population Survey, which has collected statistics on the spatial mobility of the population each year since 1948. Both sources provide information on the numbers of people who enter and leave various places, usually during periods of one year or five years. But these sources account for only one move per person during the specific period, and thus neglect multiple moves and seasonal shifts — a methodological problem created by the assumption that the person has a "usual place of residence."[6] Nevertheless, the materials do include considerable detail on movement by age, sex, marital status, and other characteristics. They also describe the migration of people between counties, states, and major regions, as well as more localized moves within counties and Standard Metropolitan Statistical Areas (SMSAs) and their components.

These data fail to reveal much about the social environments that people leave and enter, however, and while one can infer some things about the elderly who move from the Northeast to South Florida, what do shifts from North Carolina to South Carolina mean, or from one Iowa county to another? Therefore, while the data describe several types of physical movement, other kinds of studies must provide the information about changes in social settings and status, the reasons people move, the kinds of adjustments they and the receiving areas make, and other crucial matters. This is one reason why the last two decades have seen numerous investigations of elderly migration.[7]

Other more limited sources of migration data include sample surveys of changes in people's places of employment, taken by the Social Security Administration; the Health Interview Survey of the National Center for Health Statistics, which began to ascertain residential mobility in 1979; the Study of Housing Adjustments of Older People, conducted in a few areas as part of the Annual Housing Survey; and several surveys that determine the home areas of the institutionalized population.[8] These materials have specific usefulness as well as limitations in coverage, but used with censuses and Current Population Survey data, they help enlarge our view of elderly migration. In its diversity, that phenomenon includes the migration of older workers because of job relocation; retirement migration; residential changes necessitated by deteriorating health or other aspects of the aging process; shifts of the elderly poor who are evicted from rental housing; migration in pursuit of a better environment or to be near children; and temporary moves, usually on a seasonal basis because of climate.[9] Thus, while most elderly long-distance movers go to retirement areas, the whole phenomenon of migration is far more complex than that and has a qualitative dimension that is not easily detected in the quantitative data on who went where.[10]

Concepts and Indexes

The vocabulary of migration in the United States is quite specific, and because certain terms used in this chapter will have those specific meanings, it is well to clarify them briefly:

Mobility status is ascertained by comparing where people lived when they were surveyed with where they resided a given number of years earlier, usually one or five. *Nonmovers* are people who were living in the same residence at the beginning and the end of the period, though any who left and returned to the same house in the interim are classified as nonmovers. *Movers* are all persons who lived in a different house at the end of the period than at the beginning. They are classified further according to whether or not they were living in the same county, state, or region; had moved from abroad; lived in the same or a different central city or SMSA; or had made any other type of move.[11] Thus, people can be identified as intracounty movers, movers between counties in the same state, interstate migrants to contiguous or noncontiguous states, and interregional migrants.

In addition, *in-migrants* are people who enter an area, while *out-migrants* are those who leave, and the balance between them is *net migration*. *Migration streams* flow from one area to another, and each has a *counterstream,* either larger or smaller; the two produce the *net interchange* between the two areas, represented as a net gain for one and a net loss for the other. Finally, *return migration* refers to people who move back to their origins, though they are usually classified simply as movers.[12]

Differentials in Internal Migration

The elderly people who do move differ from those who do not according to several personal, social, and economic characteristics, which also vary by the distance covered, the reasons people move, and their destinations. Therefore, interstate migration and local movement are selective of different types of older persons. Specifically, migrants who cover relatively long distances tend to be the young-old, and to be married, affluent, and relatively well educated, whereas those who move locally are more apt to be poor and dependent.

The following sections consider the various characteristics of the elderly people who do move. The discussion of age compares their migration patterns with those of younger people, while the sections on selectivity by sex, race, and other characteristics focus only on the older population.

Differentials by Age

The demographic characteristic that most influences the rate of migration is age, and the elderly are far less likely than younger people to move from region to region, state to state, county to county, or even house to house within the same county.[13] Figure 10-1 shows that the migration rate of children aged 6 or 7 is relatively high, because they share the high rates of their parents, who are generally in their late 20s or early 30s. The rate falls off steadily from early childhood until age 18, when most people have finished high school and many leave home for college, new jobs, or their own marriages and households.[14] Thus, the proportion who moved between 1975 and 1980, added to those who came from abroad, reached a peak of 83 per cent at age 27. By age 35 the rate falls sharply, because adults become increasingly committed to particular jobs, homes, and social contacts, and because their older children are more likely to resist moving than are younger ones.[15]

The migration rate reaches a low point about age 61, but rises somewhat between 62 and 64, when some of the people who can afford early retirement move to better climates and recreational opportunities. There are additional increases among people in their late 60s, reflecting the movement of those who retire at age 65, some of whom migrate long distances in search of amenities or to be near children, while others move only within their home counties. Finally, people aged 75 and older also have higher rates of interstate migration than do those slightly younger, and people aged 85 and over have even higher rates, because many can no longer live alone and must migrate to be with adult children or to enter nursing homes near those children.[16] Much of the migration among people of any elderly age, however, represents an effort to find better living conditions, especially housing, and is far less affected by employment factors than is the movement of younger people.[17] In fact, involvement in the labor force is a minor influence in elderly migration, though some retired people might seek part-time jobs in their new locales.

Figure 10-2 shows the details of the various movements of people from age 55 to 75 and older, though these migration rates by single years of age refer to moves that people made at any time in the 1975-1980 period. Consequently, someone aged 65 who is classified as a mover could have made the shift at any age from 60 to 65 and could have moved more than once.

Almost four-fifths of the people aged 65 and older did not move at all between 1975 and 1980, though the ones who did represent 5 million individuals and the interstate migrants among them numbered 1 million. Furthermore, in every age category from 5 to 75 and over, smaller per-

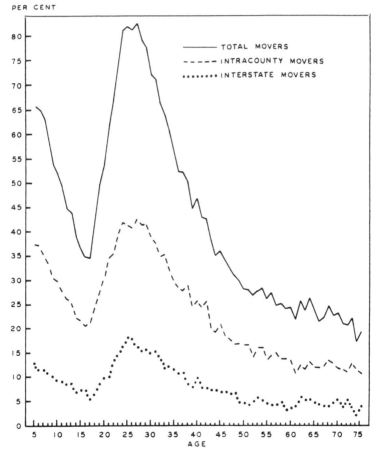

Figure 10-1. Percentages of American People Who Made Specified Moves Between 1975 and 1980, by Single Years of Age in 1980
Source: U.S.Bureau of the Census, ''Geographical Mobility: March 1975 to March 1980,'' *Current Population Reports,* P-20, no. 368 (1981), table 5.

centages of people were intercounty and interstate movers combined than were intracounty movers. In the age group 65 and over, 57 per cent of those who moved stayed in the same county, while 20 per cent went to another state; but three-quarters of them went to noncontiguous states, often in the Sunbelt. In fact, the elderly began moving to the Sunbelt long before the large flow of younger people to those states got underway. They were also the harbingers of the reversal in metropolitan-

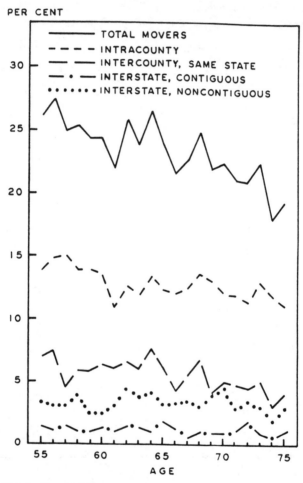

Figure 10-2. Percentages of Older American People Who Made Specified Moves Between 1975 and 1980, by Single Years of Age in 1980
Source: U.S. Bureau of the Census, "Geographical Mobility: March 1975 to March 1980," *Current Population Reports*, P-20, no. 368 (1981), table 5.

nonmetropolitan migration, for while large numbers in other age groups started moving to small towns and other nonmetropolitan areas after 1970, the elderly had begun that movement in the 1960s. Furthermore, although elderly interstate migrants tend to cover shorter distances than other age groups, those who move to Florida, Arizona, and California often come from quite far away.[18]

Actual rates of migration tell little about the elderly people who would like to move but cannot for various reasons, often financial. Therefore, low mobility rates are not evidence that all of the nonmovers are satisfied with their settings. On the contrary, many are not content and even hope to move, and when opportunities present themselves many older people actually do migrate. Fairly small percentages get those opportunities, however, and when people feel they have no alternatives, they may even say they are satisfied in unpleasant or even dangerous surroundings. Thus, actual movement is a poor indicator of people's satisfaction with their situations, just as expressed intentions about migration are a faulty way to predict actual movement, because the interplay of aspirations and circumstances, opportunities and constraints is very complex.[19]

Differentials by Sex

There is relatively little difference between the internal migration rates of men and women, including the elderly, though women have somewhat higher rates in their late teens and early twenties, and somewhat lower rates from then through their early 50s. (See Figure 10-3.) The peak age of probability for women to migrate is 24, while that for men is 26 or 27, though even that difference may reflect the persistent tendency for women to marry men who average a couple of years older and with whom they then migrate.[20]

In the ages 65 and over, there is also not much difference in mobility rates by sex, because 20 per cent of the men and 21 per cent of the women moved between 1975 and 1980. There are significant variations in the ages 70 and over, however, as the proportion of widows increases and many give up their homes and move to be with children, to enter retirement facilities or nursing homes, or to return to areas where they grew up. (See Table 10-1.) Those changes account for the higher rate of intracounty movement among women than men in the ages 70 and over, while the rates of interstate migration don't vary a great deal.

The *number* of elderly women who move, of course, is much greater than that of elderly men because of the low sex ratios in the older ages. Thus, between 1975 and 1980, about 2 million men aged 65 and older but 3 million of the women made a move of some kind. Therefore, the currents of movement within and between counties contain larger numbers of older

250

women than men, as does interstate migration, even though the mobility rates are quite similar for the sexes. That similarity does allow the use of a single "model of migration" for elderly men and women in the United States,[21] but it doesn't deny considerable differences in sex ratios in certain areas owing to sex selectivity in past migration. Because the elderly population is largely retired and their migration is not greatly affected by occupational considerations, it is less sex-selective than movement among younger people. In fact, economic factors of many kinds affect the migration of older people less than that of younger people, while non-economic factors such as climate and crime rates are more significant for the elderly.[22]

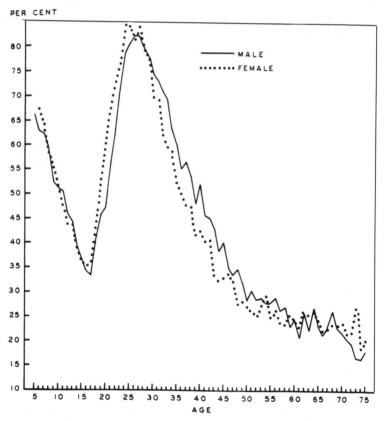

Figure 10-3. Percentages of American Males and Females Who Moved Between 1975 and 1980, by Single Years of Age in 1980
Source: U.S. Bureau of the Census, "Geographical Mobility: March 1975 to March 1980," *Current Population Reports,* P-20, no. 368 (1981), pp. 16; 17.

Differentials by Race

The migration of blacks out of the South, first to the industrial centers of the Northeast and North Central regions and later to the West, is legendary in the movement of Americans. It is also the background for considering the present migration of elderly black people.

The great movement actually began with the flight of slaves before the Civil War, picked up during the period of industrial expansion in the late

Table 10-1. Percentages of Persons Who Made Various Moves Between March 1975 and March 1980, by Sex and Selected Ages in 1980

Age and Sex	All Movers[a]	Same County	Different County, Same State	Different State
Male				
5+	45.7	25.8	10.4	9.5
20-24	59.6	32.7	14.6	12.3
25-29	76.3	40.2	18.9	17.2
55-59	25.9	14.5	6.7	4.7
60-64	23.5	12.6	6.0	4.9
65-69	22.7	12.7	5.4	4.6
70-74	18.9	9.9	4.8	4.2
75+	17.7	10.0	3.6	4.1
Female				
5+	44.4	25.7	9.9	8.8
20-24	69.7	39.6	16.6	13.5
25-29	78.1	42.6	19.1	16.4
55-59	24.2	14.2	5.8	4.2
60-64	24.2	12.4	7.0	4.8
65-69	22.5	12.6	5.4	4.5
70-74	22.2	13.6	4.2	4.4
75+	19.9	11.9	4.4	3.6

Source: U.S. Bureau of the Census, "Geographical Mobility: March 1975 to March 1980," Current Population Reports, P-20, no. 368 (1981), table 5.

[a]Includes movers from abroad.

1800s and early 1900s, and assumed large proportions when the Northern factories needed workers during World War I. (See Table 10-2.) The black migration from the South was slowed and finally stopped briefly by the Great Depression, which made poverty agriculture in the region a better survival alternative to industrial unemployment in the North. But the movement resumed after New Deal legislation in the early 1930s provided more relief provisions for urban populations than for farm people. A large share of Southern blacks fell into the latter category, and they migrated to urban centers in pursuit of the new if still meager assistance opportunities. So did great numbers of poor-white farm tenants, sharecroppers, wage laborers, marginal farm owners, and even some middle-class owners. Most of these groups contributed to the mass transfer of poverty from farms to cities, especially its shift from the South to other regions. The labor demands of World War II also swelled the movement out of the South and off the poorer farms elsewhere in the nation, and between 1933 and 1970, when movement from farms nearly exhausted the supply of potential migrants, about 55 million people left agriculture for the cities. Blacks were an unusually large share of that group.[23]

The exodus of blacks from the rural South resembled most other long-distance migrations, in that it consisted largely of young adults and their children, while people aged 65 and over were a very small share — probably less than 5 per cent. In 1949-1950, for example, which ended the decade of the largest black net migration from the South, 26 per cent of the blacks who left the region were aged 20-24 and 72 per cent were under age 35; only 3.5 per cent were 65 and over. But the blacks in the early exodus have now become an elderly population. Some of them are part of the new return migration to the South, though that movement consists largely of younger urban-born black people seeking economic opportunities away from the depressed industrial centers of the Northeast and North Central regions; even the West, which is still experiencing net gains of blacks by migration, is doing so at a decresing rate. Moreover, the migration to the South is a movement to metropolitan centers and suburbs, not a return to farms, and includes not just the poor and unemployed but also many highly paid and well-educated younger blacks as well as elderly persons returning home.

For many black elderly, who are a larger percentage of the return migration than elderly blacks were of the original exodus, a move to the South represents a move back to the extended family, which tends to be a more protective and integrative force in the lives of older blacks than of older whites. That is just now becoming apparent, however, because the strength and protective functions of the extended family, as well as the wide diversity of black family forms, have often been neglected by analysts who concentrated on the earlier mother-centered and frequently disrupted family of many blacks, especially the poor.[24] Therefore, the return to the security of the extended family by many elderly blacks helps modify the assumption of a single black family form and explains a significant share of the black movement back into the South. Other factors are at work, too, such as milder climate, nonfamily social contacts, occupational opportunities to supplement small pensions, better race relations, and the search for one's roots.

Nor are the patterns exclusive to blacks, for white people have also migrated to and from the South and other regions for many of the same reasons, and though whites were not the target of racial discrimination, many people of both races did share poverty as a motivation to leave originally. Therefore, the conditions that are drawing blacks to the South

Table 10-2. Net Migration of Blacks of All Ages, by Regions, 1870-1980

Period	Net Migration (1,000s)			
	South	Northeast	North Central	West
1870-1880	-60	+24	+36	....
1880-1890	-70	+46	+24	....
1890-1900	-168	+105	+63	....
1900-1910	-170	+95	+56	+20
1910-1920	-454	+182	+244	+28
1920-1930	-749	+349	+364	+36
1930-1940	-347	+171	+128	+49
1940-1950	-1,599	+463	+618	+339
1950-1960	-1,473	+496	+541	+293
1960-1970	-1,380	+612	+382	+301
1970-1975	+14	-64	-52	+102
1975-1980	+195	-175	-51	+30

Sources: U.S. Bureau of the Census, "The Social and Economic Status of the Black Population in the United States: An Historical View, 1790-1978," Current Population Reports, P-23, no. 80 (1979), table 8; "Mobility of the Population of the United States: March 1970 to March 1975," Current Population Reports, P-20, no. 285 (1975), table 28; "Geographical Mobility: March 1975 to March 1980," Current Population Reports, P-20, no. 368 (1981), table 42.

254

are also attracting whites, and in 1975-1980 that region gained more than 1.6 million whites of all ages by net migration, the West gained about half that number, and the Northeast and North Central regions each lost well over 1 million.

The overall migration rates of the races do not differ a great deal, for between 1975 and 1980 elderly blacks were only slightly less likely than older whites to have made a move of some kind. (See Table 10-3.) Furthermore, the moves that older blacks did make tended to be relatively short distance, because they were more inclined than whites to relocate within the same SMSA or same state. However, even though the rate of interstate migration among older blacks was only about two-thirds that of elderly whites, when blacks did change states they were much more likely to change regions as well, largely because of the movement back to the South. Thus, 83 per cent of the black interstate migrants went to another region in the process of moving, while only 60 per cent of the whites did so. Clearly, the regions that people felt offered the best opportunities earlier in the century seem less promising now, and to the extent net in-migration reveals the places where people feel their life chances are best, the South seems to offer more to elderly people of both races than do the other three regions.

Differentials by Marital Status

The choice to migrate is associated with marital status, though the presence or absence of children of particular ages is also a strategic variable in making that choice.[25] But while some elderly people may still have charge of older children or grandchildren, most lack that responsibility and the influence of marital status on their migration is little affected by children in the household. Even so, deciding whether or not to migrate is often influenced by the wish to be close to adult children who have established their own households, which is one reason why the migration rates of older people with offspring living nearby are especially low.

In general, elderly married people are less likely to move than are those who were never married or who are separated, widowed, or divorced. But there are some variations by sex, and marital status operates in the context of other personal, social, economic, and health circumstances that also promote or retard movement. Men are least likely to move if they are married, while single men are the most mobile, followed by those in the other marital categories. Women show similar but not identical migratory patterns by marital status: Married women are the least mobile, while those who are separated, widowed, or divorced are most likely to move. And since the nonmarried group consists largely of widows, the death of a husband affects many individual choices to move or stay put. For example, a great deal of elderly migration to the Sunbelt consists of married couples. But numerous husbands die after a few years in the new retirement areas and many of their widows then return to the communities they once left, while the Sunbelt populations are continually replenished by elderly married couples who migrate in. That helps explain why the 1980 sex ratio of elderly people was 76 in Florida and 79 in Arizona, compared with only 68 for the nation's older population as a whole, though the ratios in those states would be even higher if many women did not remain after being widowed.

Differentials by Level of Education

In the general population, educational attainment has a substantial effect on migration: Better-educated persons are most likely to change residence, while the poorly educated are considerably less mobile.[26]

Table 10-3. Percentages of Persons Aged 65 and Over in 1980 Who Made Specified Moves Between 1975 and 1980, by Race

Type of Move	White	Black
Same House (Nonmovers)	78.8	79.9
Total Movers within United States	20.9	20.1
Different House, Same SMSA	8.8	11.8
Different House, Different SMSA	3.3	2.0
Same State	16.6	17.2
Different State	4.3	2.9
Same Region	1.7	0.5
Different Region	2.6	2.4
Movers from Abroad	0.3	a

Source: U.S. Bureau of the Census, "Geographical Mobility: March 1975 to March 1980," Current Population Reports, P-20, no. 368 (1981), tables 36 and 40.

aLess than 0.1 per cent.

The same is true for the elderly, as shown in Table 10-4, though migration is affected by the interplay between education, occupation prior to retirement, and income. That is, the higher the level of one's education the better one's job is likely to have been, and the income and subsequent pension it produces make migration financially feasible.[27] In addition, new jobs are easier for well-educated people to find, and some older ones, especially men who retire relatively early, migrate to begin new careers.

Education also seems to have more impact than sex, race, and marital status on the distance older people move.[28] (See Table 10-4.) Thus, people with 0-8 years of schooling have the highest rates of movement from house to house within their counties, and the rates of local movement drop steadily as the level of schooling rises. This suggests that once they are established in a home or neighborhood, well-educated elderly people tend either to be more stable residentially or to go long distances if they move at all, while the poorly educated are more nomadic locally, mostly shifting between deteriorating sections of central cities in an effort to cope with high crime rates, frequent evictions, and other problems. Financial constraints keep most of them from escaping to another county or state or to the suburbs, and after retirement many even have to settle for worse conditions than they had known.

The people who move to another county within the same state and those who migrate to distant states tend to be relatively well educated. In fact, the rate of movement to noncontiguous states is more than two and a half times greater for people who attended college than it is for those who finished only eight grades or less. Long-distance movement is expensive and emotionally risky, and it is largely an activity of those whose educations and jobs provided them with enough income and psychological resources to move comfortably and safely. Long-distance migration is also dominated by the young-old, who are better educated as a group than are the old-old.

Finally, well educated or not, elderly people who are still in the labor force have significantly lower rates of migration than those who are retired, and when the working elderly of both sexes do move they tend to go short distances.[29] The basic reasons are the difficulty elderly people encounter in finding new jobs in new places and their reluctance to relinquish a present position for an uncertain employment future elsewhere. Even the wish to be employed part-time holds back some would-be migrants, though the need to work often reflects their inability to finance a move in the first place and the prospect of losing assistance from relatives, friends, and local agencies.

Table 10-4. Percentages of Persons Aged 65 and Over in 1980 Who Moved Within the United States Between 1975 and 1980, by School Years Completed

School Years	All Movers	Same County	Different County, Same State	Contiguous State	Noncontiguous State
All Levels	20.8	12.0	4.7	1.1	3.1
Elementary 0-8 Years	19.5	12.8	4.2	0.8	2.0
High School					
1-3 Years	21.3	12.7	4.4	1.5	2.7
4 Years	21.0	11.6	4.5	1.1	3.7
College					
1-3 Years	23.9	10.8	5.9	2.0	5.1
4 Years	22.2	9.1	5.5	1.4	6.2
5+ Years	22.0	7.5	7.9	1.3	5.1

Source: U.S. Bureau of the Census, "Geographical Mobility: March 1975 to March 1980," Current Population Reports, P-20, no. 368 (1981), table 24.

Metropolitan and Nonmetropolitan Migration

The Nonmetropolitan Revival

Since about 1960 the elderly have been part of the reverse spatial mobility that caused metropolitan areas to begin losing more people by migration than they gained, while nonmetropolitan places began to experience net gains.[30] Those older movers were joined later by many younger ones who were also fleeing central cities and even some suburbs for the towns, villages, and countrysides, some at considerable distance from the urban centers, though neither group moved back to agriculture. The nonmetropolitan movement was a revolutionary change, because virtually the entire history of the United States has been marked by greater urbanization and net migration gains in the cities, net losses in the rural areas.

We should be clear, however, that we are talking about *net gains and losses by migration,* for the reversal in metropolitan-nonmetropolitan growth rates by that process has not caused the absolute size of the metropolitan population to decrease. The opposite is true, because natural increase has so offset losses by net migration that in 1980 the 169.4 million Americans living in SMSAs were a larger number than ever before and their proportion (75 per cent) was also greater than at any prior time.[31] Even so, the populations in 29 of the 318 SMSAs identified in 1980 actually did decrease numerically during the 1970s. Moreover, Table 10-5 shows that the metropolitan population increased at a slower pace after 1960, while the nonmetropolitan segment grew at a faster rate, at least between 1960 and 1975; net migration losses by SMSAs and gains by nonmetropolitan areas were largely responsible. They almost caused the central cities collectively to stop growing in the 1970s, whereas the outlying parts of SMSAs — mostly suburbs — still increased, though at a slower rate than they had.

Just how long the movement to nonmetropolitan areas will last remains to be seen. Indeed, there is evidence that it reversed once again in the 1980s. But significant migration to the less urban sections is likely to continue until people perceive increases in the quality of urban life, or until the new attractions of the more rural areas stabilize or even wane; since 1978, for example, unemployment rates in those places have been higher than in the SMSAs.[32] As a result, the rate of net migration to nonmetropolitan places was lower between 1975 and 1980 than between 1970 and 1975, though it still produced significant gains there and substantial losses from the SMSAs (now called Metropolitan Statistical Areas - MSAs).

The participation of the elderly in these net gains and losses by migration during the 1970s is shown in Table 10-6, as is that of the population under age 65. For both groups, 1970-1975 was the peak period of net losses from metropolitan areas and net gains by the small towns and villages. In the following five years, the SMSAs still lost more migrants than they gained and the nonmetropolitan sections continued to gain, but the numbers and rates declined in both cases. Thus, between 1970 and 1975, nonmetropolitan areas gained 51 elderly perons for each 1,000 elderly nonmovers, but between 1975 and 1980 the ratio fell to 33. Conversely, the rate of loss from metroplitan areas slowed considerably and the ratio of elderly movers to nonmovers fell from 30 in 1970-1975 to 19 in the next half decade. As a result, the rate of net exodus from metropolitan areas, once higher for the elderly than for younger people, is now about the same for both groups, while older people are no more likely than younger ones to migrate to nonmetropolitan places. Some of the reasons include the higher costs of fuel to visit the cities, rising land prices and taxes in the less urbanized sections, reduced economic vigor and employment opportunities in many industries that located in rural areas, efforts by city governments to attract people back, and fewer of the recreational and "cultural" advantages to which urban people had grown accustomed.

Table 10-5. Percentage Increases in Metropolitan and Nonmetropolitan Populations of All Ages, 1950-1980

Area	1940 to 1950	1950 to 1960	1960 to 1970	1970 to 1980
United States	14.5	18.5	13.3	11.4
Metropolitan	22.0	26.4	16.6	10.2
In Central Cities	14.0	10.7	6.4	0.1
Outside Central Cities	35.5	48.6	26.8	18.2
Nonmetropolitan	6.1	7.1	6.8	15.1

Source: U.S. Bureau of the Census, 1980 Census of Population, Supplementary Reports, PC80-S1-5, Standard Metropolitan Statistical Areas and Standard Consolidated Statistical Areas: 1980 (1981), table B.

The combined effects of inflation and recession also make it financially impossible for some people to move, though the elderly are generally hurt more by inflation than by recession. Finally, when many elderly move to the Sunbelt, they seek out the SMSAs, not the more rural sections.

Though some elderly also move to nonmetropolitan parts of the Sunbelt, numerous others go to nonmetropolitan sections outside that band of states, seeking better environmental and recreational opportunities. Their destinations include the upper Great Lakes portions of several states, parts of the Ozarks and the Blue Ridge Mountains, some areas of the Rocky Mountains, and coastal parts of the Northeast and the Northwest.

Table 10-6. Metropolitan and Nonmetropolitan Migration of Persons in Two Age Groups, 1970-1980 (1,000s)

Area and Movement	5-64		65+	
	1970-75	1975-80	1970-75	1975-80
Metropolitan				
In-Migrants	4,928	5,736	198	257
Out-Migrants	6,229	6,857	492	481
Net Migration	-1,301	-1,121	-294	-224
Ratio to Nonmovers[a]	-22.8	-18.6	-30.1	-18.9
Nonmetropolitan				
In-Migrants	6,229	6,857	492	481
Out-Migrants	4,928	5,736	198	257
Net Migration	+1,301	+1,121	+294	+224
Ratio to Nonmovers[a]	+47.9	+39.3	+51.1	+32.6

Sources: U.S. Bureau of the Census, "Mobility of the Population of the United States: March 1970 to March 1975," Current Population Reports, P-20, no. 285 (1975), table 1; "Geographical Mobility: March 1975 to March 1980," Current Population Reports, P-20, no. 368 (1981), table 4.

[a]Number of net migrants per 1,000 nonmovers in each age group and residence area.

261

Many of these areas were long drained of rural people and have now been revitalized by the migration turnaround. Other sections, however, are still losing elderly people, including the Great Plains and central Midwest, large parts of Appalachia, sparsely settled areas of the West, and even some sections of the South, especially the Mississippi Delta.[33] It is important to recall, too, that most counties with the highest percentages of elderly have lost significant shares of their younger people, but have had little if any net in-migration of older persons.

Movement within SMSAs

Metropolitan movement includes more than just net losses to nonmetropolitan areas, because the shifts between central cities and suburbs within SMSAs are also substantial, as are movements inside the central cities. The bulk of the former migration is from the urban core to the outlying sections, but there is also a smaller reverse movement, and the elderly participate in both. The overall result is a slow increase in the segregation of the elderly in or near central cities, though it is still far less than the segregation of blacks of all ages in those areas.[34] At the same time, the numbers and proportions of older people are also increasing in the suburbs for several reasons: Suburban birth rates have fallen significantly; some younger people have moved to nonmetropolitan areas outside the suburban portions of SMSAs; original suburban populations are growing older; and more elderly persons are migrating to suburbs than are leaving them.

Because of these dynamics, the central cities of SMSAs are still losing people of all ages by net migration, including the elderly, while the outlying parts of SMSAs are gaining in the exchange within given SMSAs, between them, and between nonmetropolitan and metropolitan areas. Not all of the SMSA population outside central cities consists of suburbanites, but they do make up the large majority. Consequently, there is still a substantial flow of the elderly to suburbs from central cities, though as with any type of migration, their proportional representation is less than that of younger people; but the flow that does exist is helping to "age" some suburbs appreciably. That is particularly true of certain relatively low-density, low-cost ones in the more rural and often unincorporated parts of SMSAs.[35] Most of the elderly who move to these areas, as well as those who go to nonmetropolitan communities, are retired and free to seek places in which their reduced incomes will provide a more satisfactory quality of life or at least prevent its deterioration, and for them migration is an adjustment mechanism.[36]

There is also considerable movement of people within central cities and within outlying territory, and the elderly participate in those flows. Some of the shifts lead to further age segregation, basically because older people with similar social and economic backgrounds tend to be thrown together, not because they necessarily seek out each other. On the other hand, some older people do prefer housing especially for them, often at high rents in the urban fringe. Most elderly do not live in rigidly age-segregated neighborhoods, however, and those who do are often the residue of youthful out-migration; large proportions of them are relatively poor.

Interregional and Interstate Migration

Streams of Movement

Though local movement accounts for most of the spatial mobility among all age groups, significant numbers of people, including the elderly, do go from one major region to another. In the process they disperse in particular ways to states and counties, creating net migration gains in some and losses in others, while leaving still others virtually unchanged. The percentages of people of all ages who have relocated to another region in the process of interstate migration increased especially significantly after 1940, and even though the elderly are less likely than younger groups to migrate, the rates of increase in interregional migration have been about the same for both age groups.

Moreover, the elderly tend to concentrate at a smaller number of destinations, though they have a wide range of origins,[37] and they are particularly likely to seek areas that will make retirement more satisfying. That generally translates into the large movements from the Northeast and North Central regions to the South, as well as the smaller net flow to the West. Younger people also tend to be heading in most of the same general directions, though they go to a larger number of states and counties. Furthermore, blacks and whites follow many of the same migration routes, but between 1975 and 1980 older blacks produced net migration gains only in the South, whereas older whites did so there and in the West, largely because of their movement to California and Arizona. Elderly blacks and whites are deserting the North Central region at the highest rate and are leaving the Northeast, particularly the Middle Atlantic states and southern New England, at a pace that is only slightly slower.

The currents of interregional migration among the nation's elderly, as well as those aged 5-64, appear in Table 10-7, which shows the volume of migration to and from each major region. Together the streams that move in opposite directions are *gross migration,* while the difference between them is *net migration.* [38] The stream into the South is heavily dominated by the large-scale migration of elderly people to Florida, which is responsible for well over half of the total net gain of elderly people in all of the states with increases by migration. Within the South, sizable numbers also go to Texas, North Carolina, Mississippi, Tennessee, Arkansas, Alabama, Georgia, and South Carolina. Outside the South, Arizona and California acquire many more older people than they lose by migration, and there are also important net flows to some other parts of the West and

Table 10-7. Interregional Migration of Two Age Groups, by Race, 1975-1980 (1,000s)

Region and Movement	5-64		65+	
	White	Black	White	Black
Northeast				
In-Migrants	958	99	38	0
Out-Migrants	2,106	262	165	12
Net Migration	-1,148	-163	-127	-12
North Central				
In-Migrants	1,729	166	64	4
Out-Migrants	2,688	203	212	18
Net Migration	-959	-37	-148	-14
South				
In-Migrants	3,464	382	282	33
Out-Migrants	2,076	214	99	6
Net Migration	+1,388	+168	+193	+27
West				
In-Migrants	2,381	183	177	10
Out-Migrants	1,661	152	85	11
Net Migration	+720	+31	+92	-1

Sources: U.S. Bureau of the Census, "Geographical Mobility: March 1975 to March 1980," Current Population Reports, P-20, no. 368 (1981), table 40; 1980 Census of Population, Supplementary Reports, PC80-S1-1, Age, Sex, Race, and Spanish Origin of the Population by Regions, Divisions, and States: 1980 (1981), table 2; PHC80-S1-1, Provisional Estimates of Social, Economic, and Housing Characteristics (1982), table P-5.

even a few sections of New England. But no other state has more than a small fraction of Florida's proportional growth of elderly by net migration.

Characteristics of Sunbelt Migrants

Older people who migrate to the Sunbelt tend to be the young-old and are also likely to be married, to maintain independent households, to have relatively high incomes, and to derive those incomes from nonwork sources.[39] At least in the short run, therefore, the elderly migrants help the Sunbelt areas economically. If they don't return to the Snowbelt as they grow older, however, in the long run they tend to increase the demand for nursing homes, medical care, and other services for the old-old, though those functions also provide jobs and help boost local economies. But even if they do migrate back to where they grew up, the old-old join the poorer elderly they originally left behind, and the two groups together can impose relatively heavy demands on the public welfare services of their local areas,[40] for by the time they return to the Snowbelt, the migrants are apt to have lost a spouse and to be more dependent than they were at the time of the earlier move. Thus, not only are people who remain in the Snowbelt less advantaged on the average than those who move to the Sunbelt, but the ones among the latter who return to their old home areas tend to be less advantaged than the ones who remain in the Sunbelt. Because of these variations, services for the elderly have to account not just for their number in a state or local area, but also for their income, marital status, age, and the other characteristics that affect their level of dependence.[41]

Finally, the movement of elderly people to the Sunbelt includes not only those who seek permanent residence, but also many seasonal migrants. Some arrive in travel-trailers, spend the winter months, and drive home; others participate in time-sharing plans for a few weeks or months annually; still others rent rooms or other housing. The most affluent open their winter homes for "the season." Sometimes the seasonal move is a prelude to permanent migration after retirement, while for the wealthier elderly it is a way to enjoy the best of two climates. But most of the seasonal group is not included in the data on migration, so its size and specific destinations are not fully known. As part of the Sunbelt phenomenon, however, these elderly "snowbirds" deserve mention, for their numbers seem considerable even though their impact on the receiving areas is known only impressionistically.[42]

Some Reasons for Migration

Elderly people do not migrate for most of the same reasons that motivate younger ones. Job-related factors are less important to most elderly, and while some who migrate are still in the labor force,[43] retirement frees the large majority from having to live where work opportunities are the best. Instead, the decisions that older people make about moving are influenced by family and other social attachments, housing, climate, recreational facilities, present and prospective social environments, and levels of income and education.[44] For the elderly, migration generally represents a reduction in responsiblities, not a search for new ones, though some of it is motivated by tragedy, as in the case of widows who move closer to adult children when their husbands die. In short, a significant change in one's life situation, such as retirement, loss of a spouse, or illness, often precipitates migration,[45] which suggests that the reasons elderly people move are highly diverse. Even so, those reasons can be aggregated into a few categories that represent the characteristics of the migrants and the events on which they base their migration decisions.[46] Such a synopsis needs to distinguish between local and long-distance moves, because the two groups decide to change residence for some but not all of the same reasons.

The Decision-making Process

Like anyone else, elderly persons have variable needs and their lives are shaped by certain constraints, and these realities all influence the decision to move. They have to combine into a relatively powerful force, however, in which "push" factors encourage the decision to leave one place and "pull" factors influence the decision to enter another. Otherwise, sheer inertia will tend to prevent migration. Other things also stand in its way, such as poor health or poverty that force people to stay where they are, but for them the question of whether or not to move isn't debatable. In addition, most elderly are reasonably satisfied with their surroundings and choose not to leave, though that is also a decision. For those individuals and couples who do consider migration a possibility, however, the decision-making process has the following components:

1. Precipitating factors. These include retirement or other changes that free people to move as they enter a new stage of the life cycle; dissatisfaction with housing, climate, crime rates, and other conditions that tend to push people out; and the vision of better conditions elsewhere that pulls them toward particular areas. Other push factors are personal tragedies, especially the loss of a spouse, and the decline of financial and physical independence, while other pull factors include the wish to be nearer family and friends, and favorable reports from others who migrated.

2. Variables that help people decide whether or not a move is possible and desirable. These include levels of income, the strength of local social ties, any prior experience with migration, and judgments about how a move is likely to turn out. Other influential factors are the cost of housing at the destination and the consequences of leaving present housing, the overall cost of living in the new area, and the social networks that seem available.

3. Alternatives a prospective migrant has in choosing how far to go and whether to move permanently or seasonally. By this stage the elderly person or couple must decide that the first two groups of components either favor a move or do not. Having contemplated the matter means that either choice will have advantages and disadvantages, or there would be no decision to make — they would go or stay.

4. Variables that affect the choice of a destination after the decision to move has been made. That part of the larger decision-making process is influenced by people's knowledge of prospective destinations, perhaps from prior visits, what they hope to find, and the presence of friends who can ease the adjustment. As was true of foreign immigration, prior migration to a particular place by acquaintances is a powerful pull factor for others; it helps account for the large flows to Florida and the Southwest, and so do the promotional efforts of local governments and other recruiters.

5. Various consequences of migration. These include the housing that one can actually find and afford, the extent to which the overall dream becomes real, the degree to which the move has severed old connections, and the problems that arise in the new area. In turn, these factors affect people's degree of satisfaction with their original choice and their decision to stay, return home, or move elsewhere.[47]

These components of the decision-making process may be involved no matter how far people move, but they are particularly strategic for long-distance migrants, especially the young-old who are most likely to move just after they retire. Those people must account for various amenities at the point of destination, the kinship bonds and other things they will have to leave behind, the prospect of being able to return to the place where one grew up after a spouse has died, and other factors. Widowhood produces considerable return migration, especially among very elderly women.[48]

Local Movers

Elderly people who move from house to house in the same county may also seek amenities in the form of better or cheaper housing, a safer neighborhood, improved social contacts, and a leisure life style that can be found locally. Some also want smaller homes after they retire. Along with these pull factors are those that push people out, especially a stressful environment caused by high crime rates or juvenile harassment, or eviction by landlords who are often quick to expel people for nonpayment of rent but slow to make repairs that would encourage them to pay promptly and to help look after the property. Moreover, most elderly people leaving such conditions are poor, and while they may escape the original stress, they often have to move into similar dwellings and neighborhoods with the same problems.

Some local movers must shift in order to obtain assistance from kin, nursing homes, or other sources, because their incomes are too low or their health is too poor for them to remain alone. Widows make up a large part of this group, but elderly local movers in general are poorer than interstate migrants and tend to become more dependent on other people. Finally, some poorer elderly people are simply forced to move because tenements and other housing are destroyed as cities attempt to regenerate their centers, usually replacing low-cost housing and rundown hotels with high-cost apartments, condominiums, and offices. For these and other reasons, some elderly become chronic movers, shifting from rental to rental and often continuing a pattern begun much earlier.[49] Thus, residential satisfaction is crucial in much elderly movement, whether long-distance or local, and it is also a factor for those older people who would like to move but cannot.[50] Within the broad category of residential satisfaction, housing is by far the single most important component. But one could infer from the relatively small percentages of the elderly who do move locally and the even smaller proportions who migrate long distances that older people are generally satisfied with their housing, social bonds, and familiar settings. In fact, many cannot afford to move, and some elderly who claim to be satisfied with a poor residential situation are merely expressing their adjustment to a hopeless situation, while others actually do want to stay put because the compensations outweigh the problems.[51]

Trends in Elderly Migration

The migration rate of people aged 65 and older appears to have been declining since the mid-1950s, because the proportions who changed residences during a five-year period fell from 30 per cent in 1955-1960 to 21 per cent in 1975-1980. (See Table 10-8.) Moreover, the mobility rate decreased for each of the single years of age that make up the elderly group, and for the ones aged 55-64 as well. The decreases are especially significant before age 62, when people tend to hang onto the jobs they have and to stay in one place, but the rates have even dropped for people who reach the retirement ages.

Table 10-8. Percentages of Persons 65 and Over Who Made Specified Moves, 1955-1960 to 1975-1980[a]

Mobility Status	1955 to 1960	1965 to 1970	1975 to 1980
Total Population	100.0	100.0	100.0
Same House (Nonmovers)	70.1	71.9	78.7
Different House	29.7	27.7	20.9
Same County	20.7	17.9	12.0
Different County	9.0	9.8	8.9
Same State	4.8	5.3	4.7
Different State	4.2	4.5	4.2
Contiguous	1.4	1.4	1.1
Noncontiguous	2.8	3.1	3.1
Movers from Abroad	0.2	0.4	0.4

Sources: U.S. Bureau of the Census, U.S. Census of Population: 1960, Subject Reports, Mobility for States and State Economic Areas (1963), table 3; U.S. Census of Population: 1970, Subject Reports, Mobility for States and the Nation (1973), table 2; "Geographical Mobility: March 1975 to March 1980," Current Population Reports, P-20, no. 368 (1981), table 5.

[a]Age designated for the latter year of each five-year period.

Table 10-8 also shows that the overall rate of elderly migration fell because of a significant decrease in the proportion of local movers, while the percentages of people who made long-distance moves of various kinds changed far less. In particular, the rate of migration to noncontiguous states rose somewhat between 1955-1960 and 1965-1970, and held at the same level in 1975-1980. Thus, among people who actually did move, migration to a distant state increased in popularity, not just for the whole group aged 65 and over, but for each single year of age as well. At the same time, the percentage of movers who shift from house to house in the same county has continued to fall. These two patterns represent a sorting mechanism in the movement of elderly people, for while the whole group is not as mobile as it was, those who do move consist even more heavily than ever of affluent and well-educated people better able to leave their home states for distant attractions. Their movement reflects the trend toward earlier retirement and the ability of many early retirees to change both life style and residence.

Several reasons seem to account for the decrease in local movement, though all need further study. (1) Much of the flurry of urban renewal that destroyed old tenements and other low-cost housing is over and the large displacement of elderly residents has decreased. Some of these places are also being rehabilitated while people continue to inhabit them. (2) Supplement Security Income and cost-of-living increases in Social Security payments may enable more urban people to pay their rents and avoid the ceaseless trek from one place to another, while others are better able to keep and pay taxes on the homes they bought much earlier. (3) The decreasing proportion of elderly people below the poverty level may allow more of those who want to move to go longer distances in search of a whole group of amenities, and thus may increase the relative importance of interstate migration while that of local movement falls. For example, this helps account for the groups of elderly people in many of Florida's cities who live very modestly but who still migrate from elsewhere. (4) More of the withdrawal from the labor force of people over age 50 may be involuntary because of unemployment rates, poor health, and retirement practices; more of those people may remain in local areas hoping for re-employment.[52] It is possible, though, that the high unemployment rates of the early 1980s also prompted moves by some of the elderly who had to continue working, just as it caused many younger job-seekers to leave the older industrial centers for high-technology opportunities in the South and West. (5) Some elderly people who would like to move are simply too poor to do so.

Whatever the reasons, the overall spatial mobility rate of the elderly has decreased, while long-distance migrants have become a larger percentage of those who do move, local ones a smaller share. The former make up a significant part of the movement to the Sunbelt, attractive nonmetropoli-

270

tan places, and other areas that promise substantial amenities, while many of the latter remain behind in central cities, aging suburbs, and poor rural areas. Sometimes the two groups mix, as in the case of the Blue Ridge Mountains where affluent migrants enter the same counties as the elderly poor whose families have lived there for generations. In addition, a portion of the interstate migration of the oldest people represents a return to the areas where they grew up, and in the late 70s and 80s the rate of movement exceeds that of the young-old.

Summary

The migration of elderly people is not new, though their rate of movement is far below that of young adults, because most elderly have formed bonds and established roots they don't wish to dislodge, but also because many cannot afford to move. Moreover, while some elderly migrants shift between counties in the same state and between states and major regions, the great bulk of internal migration is local and only about a fifth of those who move go to another state. Therefore, despite its publicity, the elderly movement to Sunbelt areas is comparatively small, and the older one gets the less likely one is to leave home. There are some temporary increases, however, at the customary retirement ages and again at the oldest ages when some people, especially widows, return home.

Elderly men and women move at about the same rates, partly because much interstate migration occurs among married couples, though the rate for women does rise after age 70, when many new widows move to be near adult children or to nursing homes. Older black women are especially likely to migrate to the extended family, and many are returning to the South for that reason. In general, though, blacks tend to mover shorter distances than whites. For both races, marital status is significantly associated with migration rates, and both men and women who are unattached are the most mobile. Married people, however, move less than other groups over short distances, but more over long ones, especially between noncontiguous states. Those long-distance moves also reflect the flows of affluent, relatively well-educated elderly people to popular retirement areas, especially Florida, Arizona, and California. Conversely, the elderly poor, with low average levels of schooling, tend to stay put or to shift from house to house in the same county.

The elderly were in the vanguard of the migration from metropolitan to nonmetropolitan areas, especially villages and small towns. That movement was greater between 1970 and 1975 than in the following five years, however, and is partly countered by continuing movements to SMSAs, especially suburbs.

The various interstate exchanges result in significant gains and losses of older people by the nation's four major regions. In the 1970s the South, which was a long-time net loser of migrants, led the four in net gains, followed by the West. Conversely, the Northeast and North Central regions lost heavily by net migration of all age groups, including the elderly. Many of the latter headed toward the Sunbelt states in the South and West, though they tended to concentrate at just a few destinations. Moreover, other places, such as the upper Great Lakes and coastal parts of the Northeast and Northwest, also gained. In fact, elderly migration is a complex social, psychological, and economic phenomenon that reflects many individual reasons, especially the search for climatic and recreational amenities, financial and emotional support from kin, safety from crime, and the wish to return to the place where they grew up. Its motivations also vary according to the distance covered.

Finally, the overall movement rate of elderly people is declining, but only because of significant decreases in short-distance relocations. Among those who do move, intracounty movers are a decreasing percentage, though still the majority, while migrants to noncontiguous states are a growing share. Many of them are well-educated, affluent people who can afford the luxuries of retirement areas, though others of modest means also move to those places. Many of the elderly poor left behind, however, still have serious problems they cannot afford to escape by migrating.

NOTES

1. Francoise Cribier, "A European Assessment of Aged Migration," in Charles F. Longino, Jr. and David J. Jackson, eds., *Migration and the Aged,* special issue of *Research on Aging,* 2 (1980): 255.

2. Jacob S. Siegel, "On the Demography of Aging," *Demography* 17 (1980): 354.

3. Beth J. Soldo, "America's Elderly in the 1980s," *Population Bulletin* 35 (1980): 13.

4. Some representative studies are Charles R. Manley, "The Migration of Older People," *American Journal of Sociology* 59 (1954): 324-331; Henry S. Shryock, *Population Mobility Within the United States.* Chicago: Community and Family Study Center, University of Chicago, 1964, chapter 11; Larry H. Long, "Migration Differentials by Education and Occupation: Trends and Variations," *Demography* 10 (1973): 243-258; Steve L. Barsby and Dennis R. Cox, *Interstate Migration of the Elderly.* Lexington, MA: Heath, 1975; and Longino and Jackson, *op. cit.*

5. Regina McNamara, "Migration Measurement," in John A. Ross, ed., *International Encyclopedia of Population.* v. 2. New York: Free Press, 1982, p. 448.

6. Deborah Sullivan and Sylvia A. Stevens, "Snowbirds: Seasonal Migrants to the Sunbelt," *Research on Aging* 4 (1982): 160.

272

7. For a discussion of the usefulness and limitations of migration data, see Henry S. Shryock and Jacob S. Siegel, *The Methods and Materials of Demography.* v. 2. Washington, DC: U.S. Government Printing Office, 1973, pp. 616-617. Cf. McNamara, *op. cit.,* pp. 448-450.

8. Norfleet W. Rives, Jr., "Researching the Migration of the Elderly," in Longino and Jackson, *op. cit.,* pp. 160-161.

9. Cribier, *op. cit.,* pp. 257-259.

10. For proposed investigations in these areas, see Stephen M. Golant, "Future Directions for Elderly Migration Research," in Longino and Jackson, *op. cit.,* pp. 271-278.

11. U.S. Bureau of the Census, "Geographical Mobility: March 1975 to March 1980," *Current Population Reports,* P-20, no. 368 (1981): 131.

12. For several of these definitions, see Shryock and Siegel, *op. cit.,* p. 618.

13. See R. Paul Shaw, *Migration Theory and Fact: A Review and Bibliography of Current Literature.* Philadelphia: Regional Science Research Institute, 1975, pp. 18-19.

14. Larry H. Long, "Migration Differentials," in U.S. Bureau of the Census, "Population of the United States, Trends and Prospects: 1950-1990," *Current Population Reports,* P-23, no. 49 (1974): 133.

15. Jean van der Tak, "U.S. Population: Where We Are; Where We're Going," *Population Bulletin* 37 (1982): 26.

16. Shryock, *Population Mobility...,* *op. cit.,* p. 352, Figure 11.1.

17. James M. Brockway, Tanya K. Brockway and Marcia A. Steinhauer, *Kentucky Demographics: Migration Patterns of Kentucky's Older Population.* Louisville, KY: Urban Studies Center, University of Louisville, 1980, p. 4. Cf. Calvin Goldscheider, "Differential Residential Mobility of the Older Population," *Journal of Gerontology* 21 (1981): 103-108.

18. Cynthia B. Flynn, "General versus Aged Interstate Migration, 1965-1970," in Longino and Jackson, *op. cit.,* p. 175.

19. Frances M. Carp, "Housing and Living Arrangements of Older People," in Robert H. Binstock and Ethel Shanas, eds., *Handbook of Aging and the Social Sciences.* New York: Van Nostrand, 1976, p. 255.

20. U.S. Bureau of the Census, "A Statistical Portrait of Women in the U.S.," *Current Population Reports,* P-23, no. 58 (1976): 10.

21. Barsby and Cox, *op. cit.,* p. 137.

22. Stephen J. Tordella, *Reference Tables, Net Migration of Persons Aged 0 to 64 and 65 and over for United States Counties, 1970 to 1975.* Madison, WI: Applied Population Laboratory, University of Wisconsin, 1980, p. 7.

23. For an account of the rural-urban migration, see T. Lynn Smith and Paul E. Zopf, Jr., *Demography: Principles and Methods.* 2nd ed. Port Washington, NY: Alfred, 1976, pp. 498-513. Cf. John Reid, "Black America in the 1980s," *Population Bulletin* 37 (1982): 18-20.

24. Reid, *ibid.,* p. 20.

25. Long, *op. cit.,* p. 139.

26. U.S. Bureau of the Census, "Geographic Mobility...," *op. cit.*, p. 3.

27. Barsby and Cox, *op. cit.*, p. 17.

28. Shaw, *op. cit.*, pp. 22-24.

29. Barsby and Cox, *op. cit.*, pp. 16-17.

30. For a discussion of the reversal, see Calvin L. Beale, *The Revival of Population Growth in Nonmetropolitan America.* Washington, DC: Economic Research Service, U.S. Department of Agriculture, 1975. See also David Brown and Calvin L. Beale, "Diversity in Post-1970 Population Trends," in Amos H. Hawley and Sara Mazie, eds., *Nonmetropolitan America in Transition.* Chapel Hill, NC: University of North Carolina Press, 1981, pp. 27-71.

31. U.S. Bureau of the Census, *1980 Census of Population, Supplementary Reports,* PC80-S1-5, *Standard Metropolitan Statistical Areas and Standard Consolidated Statistical Areas: 1980* (1981), p. 1.

32. Calvin L. Beale, "Internal Migration," in van der Tak, *op. cit.*, p. 42.

33. Glenn V. Fuguitt and Stephen J. Tordella, "Elderly Net Migration," in Longino and Jackson, *op. cit.*, pp. 199-200.

34. John M. Stahura and Sidney M. Stahl, "Suburban Characteristics and Aged Net Migration," *Research on Aging* 2 (1989): 3-4.

35. *Ibid.*, p. 19.

36. Tim B. Heaton, William B. Clifford and Glenn V. Fuguitt, "Changing Patterns of Retirement Migration," *Research on Aging* 2 (1980): 101.

37. Flynn, *op. cit.*, p. 166.

38. Rives, *op. cit.*, p. 156.

39. Jeanne C. Biggar, "Reassessing Elderly Sunbelt Migration," in Longino and Jackson, *op. cit.*, pp. 183-185.

40. Soldo, *op. cit.*, p. 15. See also Jeanne C. Biggar, Charles F. Longino, Jr. and Cynthia B. Flynn, "Elderly Interstate Migration: The Impact on Sending and Receiving States, 1965 to 1970," in Longino and Jackson, *op. cit.*, pp. 217-232.

41. Biggar, Longino and Flynn, *op. cit.*, p. 229.

42. Sullivan and Stevens, *op. cit.*, pp. 159-177.

43. Cribier, *op. cit.*, p. 257.

44. Barsby and Cox, *op. cit.*, p. 10.

45. Everett S. Lee, "Migration of the Aged," in Longino and Jackson, *op. cit.*, p. 132.

46. Robert F. Wiseman, "Why Older People Move: Theoretical Issues," in Longino and Jackson, *op. cit.*, p. 151.

47. Parts of these five components are adapted from Wiseman, *ibid.*, p. 145. See also Ralph R. Sell and Gordon F. De Jong, "Toward a Motivational Theory of Migration Decision Making," *Journal of Population,* 1 (1978): 313-335.

48. Anne S. Lee, "Return Migration in the United States," in Daniel Kubat, Anthony H. Richmond and Jerzy Zubrzycki, eds., *Policy and Research on Migration: Canadian and World Perspectives,* special issue of *International Migration Review* 8 (1974): 286-291. Cf. William J. Serow, "Return Migration of the Elderly in the U.S.A.: 1955-60 and 1965-70," *Journal of Gerontology* 33 (1978): 288-295.

49. Wiseman, *op. cit.*, pp. 150-151.

50. Carp, *op. cit.*, pp. 244; 255.

51. Kenneth F. Ferraro, ''Relocation Desires and Outcomes Among the Elderly,'' *Research on Aging* 3 (1981): 167-169.

52. Barsby and Cox, *op. cit.*, p. 3.

Chapter 11

Some Implications of
America's Aging Population

The preceding chapters have examined America's elderly population largely on the basis of data collected by federal agencies and essentially as a group, though with many subdivisions. The analysis should not imply that the elderly population is homogeneous, however, or ignore its tremendous variety. Yet the elderly do have things in common besides occupying the same age-category: The majority are women and many problems of the elderly are the problems of women;[1] older people share the consequences of the aging process itself, such as slower reaction times, a growing awareness of death, and changes in the circle of kin and friends. They also share various societal consequences of growing old in a youth-oriented society, though it is no more useful to deny the real effects of aging than it is to turn them into discriminatory stereotypes. Most elderly also want to remain as active as they can for as long as they can, and while that means a job or volunteer work for many, "active" has much more diverse meanings.

Therefore, despite certain broad similarities and shared concerns, the traits that are thought of as typically old, even by many elderly, differ widely from person to person. As in their younger years, the elderly are optimistic or pessimistic, well adjusted or poorly adjusted, gregarious or withdrawn, or anywhere between those extremes. There is no "typical" older person or experience with aging,[2] and policies for the elderly need to account much more than they do for individual differences. In that context we conclude the book with a look at the prospects of faster increases in the older population than are now expected, and at the impact of aging on the elderly and on American society.

Intervening in the Aging Process

Revolutionary Technologies

New technology promises to intervene in mortality and the aging process to the degree that significant increases could occur in life expectancy
and even the life span itself. As large as we now expect the elderly
population to be in the next century, projections of numbers and proportions could be dwarfed by the demographic results of such innovation; the
social, economic, and political consequences of an elderly population that
greatly exceeds present expectations would be tremendous. The possibility hinges on three types of biomedical research: (1) efforts to prevent,
diagnose, and treat more effectively the three major causes of death —
heart disease, cancer, and stroke; (2) research into the aging process itself
and the prospect to slow it down significantly; and (3) work designed to
uncover and manipulate the social conditions that affect aging and
death.[3] In turn, these efforts produce two categories of technology, both
of which will increase the numbers and percentages of the elderly.

Curve-squaring technologies. Successful efforts that would increase the
number of middle-aged people who live longer would add to the population in all of the older years, but especially the 80s and 90s, and would do
so in a relatively short time. The top half of Figure 11-1 shows how such
improvements would change the number of survivors among each 100,000
Americans in specific age groups and the nation's age distribution in
general. The solid line represents the current survival ratios and the
dotted line represents those that would result after full implementation of
the new life-saving technologies, which tend to square the curve before it
falls off sharply. The curve-squaring technologies are mostly efforts to
control the degenerative diseases and to increase the life expectancy of
older people, contrasted with earlier efforts to control infectious and
parasitic diseases and to allow a larger percentage of infants to survive to
the older ages. As a result, in 2025 life expectancy at birth may be as high
as 85 years and the number of elderly people will be larger than now
projected; so will their percentage if no new baby-boom occurs.[4]

These life-saving technologies include prevention, diagnosis, and treatment of the three major causes of death; the use of artificial organ
substitutes; and improvements in the environment, such as stress
management, dietary modifications, and reductions in the proportion of
smokers. Many specific aspects of these technologies are already well
advanced and will probably improve significantly by 2000;[5] the three
major causes of death may even be substantially overcome within 50
years. Indeed, as we saw in Chapter 9, the death rate from heart disease

has fallen steadily since 1960, while new research into the genetic ante-
cedents of cancer promises to uncover a common element among the
hundreds of types of that disease and possibly to bring it under control,
perhaps with a vaccine.[6]

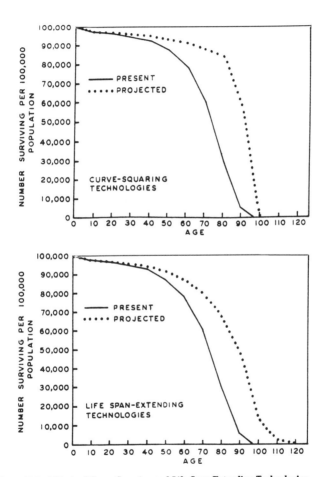

Figure 11-1. Effects of Curve-Squaring and Life Span-Extending Technologies
Source: Subcommittee on Human Services of the House Select Committee on Aging, *Future
Directions for Aging Policy: A Human Services Model,* Pub. no. 96-226. Washington, DC:
U.S.Government Printing Office, 1980, p. 110.

Life span-extending technologies. Another group of advances, which overlaps partly with the curve-squaring technologies, involves intervention in the process of aging itself and includes efforts to alter the ways that cells, organs, and whole bodily systems age, and to regenerate tissue. The lower half of Figure 11-1 shows how the number of survivors per 100,000 would increase at various ages as a result of these advances. The life span-extending technologies are more difficult to achieve than those directed primarily at disease control and prosthesis, and their principal demographic effects lie farther in the future.

Moreover, if such efforts are to extend the life *span* (as contrasted to life *expectancy*), they will have to be applied relatively early in life and not just when people have reached middle age. This is because they deal with the long-term effects of diet and temperature, the progressive breakdown of the immune system, the loss of tissue elasticity, the number of times cells can replicate, the gradual accumulation of cell substances that speed aging, the tendency for membranes to incur permanent damage, the process of abnormal oxidation, and other occurrences that influence human aging from the first day of life.[7]

It is not possible to conquer aging completely and make the human life span infinite, but much of the practical technology necessary to extend it significantly now exists or soon will. Therefore, the assumption that the life span is fixed at 100 years or so is outdated, and the advances that will probably come in the next century will lower the death rate even more and increase the numbers of elderly people, and most likely their percentages as well.

Effects of Increased Longevity

These technological breakthroughs are helping to age the nation's population and will speed that process even more in the future. At the same time, the financial resources necessary to meet the needs of the burgeoning elderly population are not keeping pace, as evidenced by problems with Medicare and the Social Security retirement fund crisis, which finally became serious enough to produce the compromise ameliorative legislation of 1983. The increases in life expectancy and the life span, on the one hand, and the unwillingness or inability to meet the needs of the elderly, on the other, represent a major dilemma for the United States and other developed countries now, and eventually they will do so for the entire world.

Demographically, the consequences will be profound. Projections made by the U.S. Bureau of the Census in 1977 anticipated that by 2025 elderly people would number about 51 million and be 17 per cent of the total population, but revisions in 1982 anticipated 59 million elderly by 2025 and that they would be almost 20 per cent of the total.[8] Those revisions account for the effects of curve-squaring technologies already operable, but if the technologies fulfill their potential, people aged 65 and older may well number 74 million and be 23 per cent of the total by 2025.[9] Recall, too, that by 2025 the large baby-boom generation will be aged 65 and over and that significant increases in their life expectancy will swell the ranks of the elderly very rapidly. In turn, the demographic changes may force us to raise retirement ages significantly, partly because many elderly will need to work, but basically because the employed population may be unable or unwilling to support a huge dependent group whose average retirement age is 62 or 65 or even 70, but who still have many years of life expectancy ahead.

As the elderly population grows and other changes occur, the nuclear family — already altered by divorce, migration, and other dynamics — may decline further in importance. But the significance of the modified extended family may increase and even be supplemented by quasi-families that provide intimate social bonds for the elderly outside the traditional family structure. The four-generation family may even become more commonplace, though the communication gap between the age extremes may prove unbridgeable, with middle-aged and young-old adults attempting to mediate between youth and the old-old. Two- and three-generation gaps may become common. Families will also experience higher health costs, because health needs increase with age and there will be more elderly, and because health care is a growth industry. Those costs may be offset some, however, if the needs are concentrated among the oldest people and the curve-squaring technologies make the young-old relatively healthy as a group.[10]

Some Basic Problem Areas

Some of the consequences of an aging population are not merely challenges for the nation, but are problems for older people themselves; they find many results real and immediate, not just the probable changes to be confronted in the next century. Many of the problems stem from prejudice, while others show that the nation was simply unprepared for the rapid increase in its elderly population. In our preoccupation with youth, we long studied and attempted to deal with the needs of the young, while until recently those of the elderly were neglected; in a throwaway society young people are perceived as a useful and envied commodity, whereas the elderly are thought to be used up and worn out. Because we also value change and deplore obsolescence, the past and the carriers of its culture seem irrelevant to the present and the future, so we isolate many elderly — a process that begins well before age 65. As a result of these realities, made more urgent by increases in the elderly population, some needs of older people are met less well than are those of younger ones. Consequently, while it is inaccurate to view old age *as* a social problem, it is a time *beset* by particular problems, many of which arise more from the social system than from the aging process itself.[*11*]

Income Maintenance

A decent level of living is probably the most urgent concern of the elderly, with health a close second, but the need for adequate income is poorly met for at least the quarter of all older people, who live below the poverty line or not far above it. The problem is especially acute for women and minorities, but on the average all elderly people suffer income reductions of at least a third when they retire, while many of their living costs do not fall. For many people, the resources available are far short of the 70 per cent or so of prior income that is necessary for most elderly to maintain a life style reasonably close to that of their preretirement years.

Moreover, Social Security, on which a large share of elderly persons depend heavily, still fails to prevent poverty or near-poverty for about a third of those who have little or no other income, while private pension plans cover only a minority of all elderly and provide low average benefits. Even the SSI program provides minimal amounts that barely enable survival, though it is really part of a more comprehensive package of provisions contained in the Older Americans Act of 1965 and its subsequent amendments. That Act created Medicare in 1965 to help with hospital expenses for Social Security recipients aged 65 and over and to provide a voluntary program, financed partly by participants' premiums, to help with doctors' fees and related costs; it also established Medicaid for those elderly who are too poor to pay Medicare premiums and deductibles.

SSI, financed from general revenues, also grew out of the Act in 1974 as a way to guarantee at least some income to people who are elderly, blind, or disabled, and federally provided amounts may be supplemented by the states. The Social Security Act has been amended to include disability payments, to raise the ceiling on the income one could earn and still receive full benefits, to lower to 62 the age at which one could begin to draw reduced benefits, to pay benefits to everyone aged 72 and older no matter what their income or former job status, to provide an income-floor for all elderly, and to guarantee periodic cost-of-living increases in benefits.[*12*] The federal government also makes grants to the states for public assistance, though not only for the elderly.

But the greatly expanded scope and cost of the programs, their failure still to provide enough income for the poorest people, and their tendency to oversubsidize the affluent are problems that coalesced into the Social Security financial crisis. The system simply ended up paying out far more than it took in, and the increased taxation of workers to "solve" that problem may soon prove to be prohibitively high.

The obsolete actuarial assumptions on which permissible retirement age is based are also part of the problem, and the system is even subject to considerable "leakage": Illegal aliens, for example, sometimes hold jobs covered by Social Security and may be able to receive benefits, while perhaps $100 million has been paid to dead people! Moreover, these difficulties may well become worse than was anticipated in the 1983 reforms, because the projected numbers of elderly people must certainly be revised upward. Life expectancy will surely rise, while the ratio of workers to retirees will continue to fall, especially if the trend toward early retirement resumes. It may not, however, because additional increases in the cost of living, even at a lower rate, will force some elderly people to continue working, provided they can get the jobs, and the Social Security crisis of the early 1980s will be seen as a mere prelude to the escalating costs of the various programs, especially retirement and Medicare. Private pension plans are unlikely to expand sufficiently, because even those already in force are paying out large sums that could go for wages; they are also used to prevent employee movement from company to company and are so plagued by paper work that small companies shun them.[13]

In short, the demographic trends, rising costs, and early retirement trend of the last several years may all conspire to reduce the average relative income of the elderly below present levels and further erode their economic well-being. Even the ameliorative efforts underway seem inadequate to prevent poverty for a significant share of the larger elderly population that will be with us in the first quarter of the next century.[14] This is one of the great challenges to the ingenuity of America's financial managers, and any policy to keep the elderly fully integrated in the society will be hampered if significant proportions lack adequate incomes.

The continuing reform of income-maintenance needs to address several questions: (1) How do incomes and expenditures actually change when one retires? (2) On what basis should retirement incomes be determined and how should they differ according to prior earnings, marital status, and other characteristics? (3) What level of living is reasonable and attainable for the elderly, assuming they are to have the same relative advantages as younger people? (4) Can and should income inequities be smoothed out, or should they continue to reflect the income disparities of people's earlier years? (5) How should other assets, such as paid-up home mortgages and help from family members, be weighed in assessing income adequacy for older people? (6) How can the taxation situation be improved for the elderly, especially real estate taxes and sales taxes on food and other necessities?[15]

These and other questions are not new and they have been addressed repeatedly. But none of them has been answered definitively, partly because policies for the elderly lack coordination and still permit many to become financial casualties. Significant numbers still fall close to or below the poverty line when they retire, and SSI and cost-of-living increases in Social Security benefits are not enough to prevent continuing financial erosion for many. Even the Older Americans Act has been amended to shift more responsibility to state and local governments, and finally back onto the elderly and their families. Thus, the basic causes of the financial problems of many elderly lie not in the lack of national resources, but in attitudes that still place the needs of older people too low on the list of national priorities, in forced retirement and limited work opportunities, and in a general view of the elderly as charity cases rather than as full participants in the socioeconomic system. Unless those attitudes change, income maintenance will continue to be a problem as the older population grows rapidly.[16]

Despite the deficiencies in income maintenance, in 1980 about $155 billion were allocated to Social Security, Medicare, and other federal programs primarily for the elderly. Therefore, the economic impact of the growing elderly population is tremendous, consisting largely of their withdrawals from rather than contributions to national funds. Figure 11-2 shows how federal expenditures were allocated in 1980, and emphasizes the overwhelming significance of retirement and health costs in the total picture; those expenditures now draw so heavily on public funds disbursed through Social Security taxes and general revenues, that they have become a serious problem of public finance and a huge burden for the working population.[17]

Health Care

The elderly are already the largest users of health resources, which they will continue to be as their numbers and proportions grow and higher percentages move into the old-old category, even if life expectancy is extended appreciably and most young-old remain healthy. Moreover, the elderly are increasingly likely to seek medical care, largely because they are better educated about health and more can afford the personal costs of help than could their parents. At present, they are half again as likely as middle-aged people to visit doctors and they appear disproportionately in the hospital population, account for 95 per cent of all nursing home residents, and have average medical costs that are about four times those of younger people. Moreover, the situation is complicated by the two contradictory goals of American health care policy — high quality care and cost containment — reflected in the periodic furor over "socialized medicine" and the mistrust of all care except that provided by highly trained physicians and registered nurses.

As a result, while Medicare and Medicaid are a boon to the elderly, Medicare especially is heavily biased toward institutions and provides poor coverage for people looked after at home. It thereby forces many elderly into nursing homes to receive benefits during convalescence, but even those benefits are relatively short term. And because the nation's whole health system is oriented to acute illness and dramatic intervention, it tends to treat elderly people with chronic illnesses by subsidizing institutionalization rather than home care. In turn, that raises the cost of care, from $6.5 billion for Medicare and Medicaid in 1967, the first full year those programs operated, to about $75 billion in 1983, or 9.5 per cent of all federal expenditures. The amount may be twice as high in 1988, despite rising deductibles and fewer hospital days that can be compensated. The emphasis on institutionalization in Medicare also deprives many elderly of the nurturing and support they would receive from family members or other caregivers at home. Proposed reforms are under consideration, including those that would make patients and the providers of care, such as hospitals, pay a larger share to head off serious Medicare

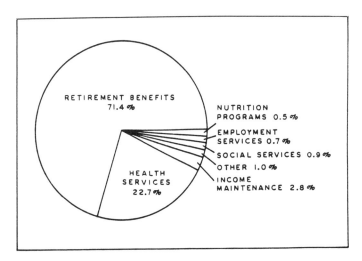

Figure 11-2. Allocation of the Federal Dollar Spent on Benefits for the Elderly
Source: Subcommittee on Human Services of the House Select Committee on Aging, *Future Directions for Aging Policy: A Human Services Model*, Pub. no. 96-226. Washington, DC: U.S. Government Printing Office, 1980, p. 31.

deficits. But if anything like the present practices continue, the cost of medical care for the growing elderly population will become even more formidable, or many will be forced to use up their own financial resources because of illness; some will be neglected entirely. Here again is the dilemma between care and costs.[18]

The degenerative diseases of old age often produce long, expensive periods of disability, especially for people aged 75 and older, and as in the case of income, poor health and the ability to pay for care are distributed unevenly throughout the elderly population. Those with the lowest social status are most affected by the degenerative illnesses, least likely to seek help, and least able to pay for it, though the Medicaid program for the elderly poor does help. But even with that program and Medicare, older people still bear relatively heavy personal health care expenses. Moreover, since only about 14 per cent of the noninstitutionalized elderly are completely free of chronic illnesses, such as arthritis, heart disease, hypertension, diabetes, arteriosclerosis, and Alzheimer's Disease,[19] the cost to them and the society is already large; it will grow much larger.

These realities argue for more physician's assistants, practical nurses, and others who can provide lower cost care for many illnesses and who can help with the activities of daily living; for careful monitoring of doctors, hospitals, and nursing homes to reduce overcharging; and for improved coverage of cost-effective hospice and home care. Home care also needs to be more innovative, however, because the proportion of women under age 65 who work is now so high that many elderly people cannot receive attention during the day from a member of the family. Better health education and information also are necessary for the elderly, so that more problems can be avoided or improved through diet, accident prevention, and reduced smoking, alcohol abuse, and misuse of medication. Proper nutrition is an especially acute problem for those who need financial assistance to buy better food and help to prepare it.[20]

In addition, we need more attention to mental health, especially malfunctions that strike because of organic bran damage from other problems, but also depression and other effects of widowhood, solitude, and the feeling of having been discarded. Such efforts are especially important for the dying, and in late 1983 Medicare regulations were broadened to provide new hospice benefits for them, 90 per cent of whom have cancer, though even those payments were below the levels proposed earlier.

Finally, because the elderly often require a special clinical approach, more physicians need to be trained in geriatric specialties. At present, less than half the medical schools offer elective courses in this field and few require them, partly because there is little federal assistance for geriatric programs,[21] but also because many doctors prefer to work with younger patients whose illnesses are more likely to be successfully treated.

Housing

About 70 per cent of the elderly own homes, but many of the houses are old and in need of repairs that some older people with reduced incomes cannot make. Therefore, more housing assistance is indicated, not just to repair dwellings but also to get many elderly out of high-crime areas and facilities that are inappropriate for those with physical disabilities. Moreover, many elderly people live alone in houses that are too large for their needs and carry high property taxes. As a result, a significant proportion of older people would probably live somewhere else if they had a choice, and many would rent if they could find decent, low-cost, relatively small apartments in safe neighborhoods.

If the trend for older people to migrate to nonmetropolitan places continues, more and better housing will be necessary in those villages and towns. In addition, widowhood and living alone call for more satisfactory group quarters, which should not always be nursing homes or retirement high-rises, but ought to include additional relatively small units in which quasi-families can develop. Older homes can be rehabilitated to house six or eight persons functioning as a social group. To provide the best atmosphere they probably should include people of both sexes, but given the low sex ratio in the older years, that probably would mean one or two men and several women. Such arrangements, which some elderly are already using, need to overcome prejudices, counterproductive moralizing, zoning restrictions, and other obstacles, because they are one way to solve several housing problems of the elderly. Those difficulties include the prohibitive costs of maintaining one-person households, the frailty that prevents many elderly from operating a home by themselves, and the need for care that many disabled persons have.

Quasi-family residences would keep many elderly in the community and out of institutions, and would even prevent their having to reside with adult children who cannot accommodate an aged parent. Congregate housing often does require outside social and health services, but those are more easily delivered to a group than to scattered individuals living alone, and the group arrangement is a better guarantee of proper nutrition, physical care, protection, and emotional support by others who share the experience of being elderly.[22] These needs are especially acute for elderly minority groups, women, and rural residents, who occupy a disproportionate share of the dilapidated housing.

There is already an extensive network of governmental programs designed to provide housing for the elderly, but many needs remain unmet. The 1974 Housing and Community Development Act, for example, is supposed to encourage builders to provide better rental units, including residential facilities for the elderly and the handicapped.[23] But only a small percentage of the elderly actually benefit from governmental housing programs, and almost a third live in "substandard, deteriorating or dilapidated housing."[24] Moreover, housing costs often take a disproportionately large share of the older person's total income, especially that of the elderly woman who lives alone and rents. Therefore, even the programs that do exist are insufficient to meet the housing needs of many elderly.

Work, Retirement, and Leisure

Despite the trend toward early retirement, more elderly would like to work, especially part time, than can find jobs. That is particularly true during times of substantial inflation, when one's planned retirement income proves inadequate and the level of living falls. But even when inflation rates are low, a truly full-employment economy would provide jobs for all who wished to work and who had or could acquire the necessary skills, and would ensure an adequate income, whether from work or other sources. In an economy with less than full employment, several questions arise that affect the elderly directly or indirectly: (1) Who is to get the scarce jobs and on what basis? (2) Should the elderly with modest retirement incomes be allowed jobs at all, presumably at the expense of younger people without nonwork income? (3) If the elderly who wish to work are not allowed to do so, at what level and for how long should the working population support them? (4) What is the most practical balance between a group of working elderly who take jobs that younger workers could hold, and a group of dependent elderly who take no jobs but who must be supported by the younger working population? Concomitantly, does the growing elderly population have to impose an increasing burden on younger people no matter which way the balance tips? (5) What obligations does society have to support its elderly and to supply housing, income, medical care, and other needs? What is the nature of the obligation, if one exists at all? (6) In a less than full-employment economy are the elderly expendable? By what criteria can their existence be justified if they don't produce?[25]

These and other questions are significant now but will become more so as the large baby-boom group reaches age 65 and must be supported by relatively small younger cohorts. Moreover, any significant increases in life expectancy and life span will make these questions some of the nation's most burning issues in the first quarter of the next century, when they will call for a major reappraisal of the work and retirement roles of the elderly. We are in a time when more nonworking elderly are living longer in retirement. In response the society can choose to shoulder a growing burden for their support; it can let more elderly people work longer at their present jobs, but thereby restrict the ascension of middle-aged workers to the positions held by some older ones; or it can force the elderly to take jobs no one else wants.

Each of these alternatives has obvious shortcomings for one group or another, but they represent the problems an aging population faces. They also underscore the situation in which the elderly are caught, the intergenerational clash that may intensify in the future, and the need for new work alternatives, such as more part-time jobs, flextime, and job sharing. Perhaps even old alternatives will be refurbished, such as one spouse limiting his/her labors to the home while the other works for wages, although the inflation that increased the number of two-earner couples in the first place would need to be eliminated for such an option to be realistic. If inflation were fully contained, however, the retirement incomes of more elderly people would suffice; fewer would compete for available jobs and the costs of Social Security would not escalate quite as fast as they do now. In any case, if we are to improve or merely maintain the economic situation of a rapidly growing elderly population and still not damage that of younger people, then work and other economic relations call for fundamental reorganization. Most urgently, the elderly need to know their incomes won't be ravaged by inflation or insolvency in the Social Security system, and that there will be more jobs for those who must work.[26]

The Question of Disengagement

The morale of the elderly is affected by the extent to which they remain full social participants, although participation is influenced far more by how a person spent his/her earlier life than by aging per se and is, therefore, highly individualized.[27] Consequently, the frequent notion that the elderly progressively withdraw — disengage — from society needs to be treated very cautiously, for it is sometimes a way to rationalize measures that exclude the elderly from social participation. Disengagement theory may also reinforce certain stereotypes about the elderly and help justify the view of them as a social problem.[28] That view keeps us from dealing constructively with the growing political involvement and power of the elderly, and with the probable intergenerational clash that lies ahead, for it falsely assumes older people will inevitably withdraw quietly into senescence. Instead, more elderly persons are rejecting the role of grateful beneficiary of policies allegedly created on their behalf by others, and are becoming directly involved in the development of those policies.[29] At that level, at least, they are more socially aware than ever.

But older people live their retirement years in a great variety of ways, and while some are social activists and others have essentially withdrawn into themselves, the majority range between these extremes.[30] Some disengage physically when activity becomes more difficult and energy wanes; others disengage psychologically by shifting their concern from the outer to the inner world of personal feelings and thoughts; still others disengage socially by withdrawing progressively from the social systems in which they participated. Furthermore, disengagement theory assumes that *most* elderly people go through these three processes; some of its proponents argue that disengagement enables the elderly to accept the inevitability of decline and death and of having their functions taken over by the young.[31]

In fact, older people do tend to withdraw gradually from *some* activities as they age, especially the work force, and their range of activities often grows smaller, though there are many individual exceptions. Many disengage from sex because of widowhood, declining health, boredom, and the fear of failure, though a significant number maintain or even increase their sexual activity. Moreover, other kinds of involvement do not decline, such as club memberships and church attendance, and the older person who becomes completely isolated is quite uncommon. Consequently, a certain degree of disengagement seems true for most elderly, but it is rarely total; significant minorities, such as the Gray Panthers, are anything but disengaged from the social and political systems and are even trying to change those systems. Moreover, since the elderly relate more to their own age cohort than to others, there is some tendency for an aged subculture to emerge, complete with group consciousness born of certain common experiences.[32] It is easy to carry that idea too far, however, and to see the elderly as a homogeneous mass. *Tendencies* among a majority of older persons do not demonstrate *universal characteristics;* nor should they deny the wide range of individuality and the plethora of minority contingents that pervade the total elderly population.

Victimization

Elderly people are not much more likely statistically to be the victims of crime than are other age groups, but this obscures the fact that many urban elderly are virtual prisoners in their homes because they fear street crime. In fact, a Harris survey commissioned by the National Council on the Aging found that nearly a quarter of all elderly people rate the fear of crime as a very serious problem that often caused their self-imposed isolation.[33] In that sense, abnormally large percentages of older people are victimized by the fear of assault, robbery, and other crimes, even though reported crimes against them may not seem disproportionately numerous. Moreover, we don't know how many older victims fail to report crimes and harassment because of threats of retaliation. Clearly, the fears and realities call for greater protection of the elderly, more efforts to compensate actual victims, and community action, such as watch programs and crime-prevention education. Some of the efforts should also be directed toward adolescents, who are the major perpetrators of crimes against vulnerable older people.[34] Some elderly also live in public or other housing where general crime rates are high, and they are easy prey to those who know their movements and when their pension checks arrive.

Elderly people are particularly susceptible to confidence games and frauds, because many living on fixed incomes are eager to increase their funds if possible, while some are too inexperienced or lonely to resist the overtures of friendly strangers. Many are simply too naive and trusting, while others desperately want cures for arthritis, other chronic illnesses, and even the cosmetic consequences of aging, and are victims of fad foods, elixirs, and gadgets. Moreover, those who are terminally ill are tempted to buy anything that promises life;[35] cancer-curing gimmicks are especially appealing. In short, many elderly, especially the poor and the less educated, are easy victims of hoodlums, confidence artists, and unscrupulous salespeople, and are unable to get protection or help after a crime occurs.

Political Consequences of an Aging Population

The difficulties encountered in reforming Social Security so as not to favor the well-to-do showed that certain large groups of elderly persons have considerable political power. Moreover, their strength has grown as the numbers and proportions of older people have increased, and as they have developed a more coordinated vested interest in preserving present privileges and obtaining new ones. Thus, while the elderly may be conservative on some issues, the politically active ones often espouse liberal positions on major issues. The mandatory retirement age was raised to 70, for example, because of the political power of certain elderly groups and their spokespeople, and even that limit may be swept away in another surge of "gray power." That power also kept the 1983 Social Security changes from significantly penalizing the present elderly and shifted the major impact onto relatively young working people, not onto those who are already old and beneficiaries of the system. In fact, the presumed conservatism of older people may actually reflect their defense of views and positions which were liberal or radical when the elderly were young, but which have become conservative only because new ideas and stances have come along.[36]

Politicians, always sensitive to where power and influence lie, can be expected to promote more favorable legislation for the elderly as the population ages, and may even fail to enact the most appropriate long-term Social Security reforms in their fear of gray power. They are virtually certain to divert funds from other programs as their constituencies become older and more vocal, and many politicians who assume that people grow more conservative as they age can be expected to sound more conservative themselves. But on many "bread-and-butter" issues the young and the elderly may disagree sharply, thus catching politicians in the middle. For example, the elderly are concerned to derive maximum benefits from the Social Security system, often without much heed to the burden they may place on people who are still working; the latter are concerned to contain the cost of supporting the elderly, though many also sympathize with the need for adequate programs, partly to protect their own parents and partly to prepare the way for their own retirement. Nonetheless, there is an incipient political conflict inherent in the variable vested interests of the two age groups, and it may become heated and overt if younger workers feel they are forced to carry an unfair burden. That burden can only become heavier if the growing elderly population has to be dependent because of mandatory retirement, restrictive hiring decisions, and other discrimination,[37] or if they choose to be so because of early and prolonged retirement.

It is unlikely that the elderly voting population will ever be a majority able to promote only their own interests, but they have enough potential power to influence many issues if their views are consolidated into bloc voting, especially if younger groups remain fragmented. In some cases, their votes could constitute a plurality. But whether they consolidate fully or not, the elderly have already grown more powerful and vocal politically and are fighting for more of their interests. Some concessions to them are long overdue and represent the gradual decline of discrimination. But the elderly also have the potential power to demand measures that younger people will oppose, especially on such national issues as pensions and in such retirement areas as Florida. Whether the clash of interests precipitates new discrimination will depend heavily on whether American society continues policies that keep most elderly dependent, or promotes new ones that foster greater independence without jeopardizing the positions of younger people. The directions of change will be quite different according to which approach dominates.

The impending choices also imply that it is pointless and even destructive to treat all elderly persons alike, which we tend to do, and that more attention should be paid to need as a criterion in providing benefits and less to age per se. Age, after all, is not a universally applicable index of health, productivity, adjustment, or financial well-being, and it has become an expensive decision-making criterion that American society probably can't afford in such a blanket fashion much longer.[38] At the very least, we need to distinguish between the needs of the affluent and the poor and the young-old and the old-old, though each of these groups is also far from homogeneous. Ultimately, the fundamental question in any set of changes and policies is: "What form should society take so that, in old age, a human being can still be a human being?"[39]

Public and Private Responsibilities

The growth of the elderly population in American society has generated growth in public programs on their behalf, and the Older Americans Act represents the role of the federal government in their well-being. Under the OAA the elderly are assumed to have the right to the following:

1. An adequate income.
2. The best possible physical and mental health.
3. Suitable housing.
4. Full restorative services.
5. Opportunity for employment with no age discrimination.
6. Retirement in health, honor, and dignity.
7. Pursuit of meaningful activity.
8. Efficient community services.
9. Immediate benefit from proven research knowledge.
10. Freedom, independence, and the free exercise of individual initiative.[40]

But we have seen that a significant share of the elderly population lacks some or even most of these things, and for them the ideals seem unattainable. In addition, the federal effort to realize the goals has grown so costly that its support network cannot possibly help all those elderly persons who are in slums, below the poverty level, or chronically ill. The Social Security payroll tax has already grown astronomically, from 5.2 per cent on maximum taxable earnings of $7,800 in 1971, to 6.7 per cent on a maximum of

$32,700 in 1982, to an already legislated 7.65 percent on a maximum of $66,900 in 1990, and wage earners face even greater increases after that in order to support the aging baby-boom population. The tax rate could rise to 15 per cent by the middle of the next century, and even that may not be enough to meet the need. The high costs of Medicare and other programs also add greatly to the burden, especially for people whose final days or months require expensive life-support systems and other costly heroic measures to prolong life or ease its ebb.

Furthermore, given the necessarily impersonal nature of governmental programs, they can do little to reduce loneliness, facilitate communication between the generations, or provide loving environments. Those functions, along with much financial responsibility for housing, health care, and other needs, lie with families, friends, churches, neighborhoods, and other small "natural" social groups that add meaning to the lives of older people. In fact, this informal network provides virtually all of the home care for the disabled elderly, solace during bereavement and loneliness, guidance in seeking formal assistance, and the feeling of continued significance even in old age.

Consequently, the future of America's growing elderly population will be shaped by a partnership of formal and informal support networks, each doing essentially different things, but all reasonably coordinated and mutually reinforcing. Even so, how many elderly people will we allow to fall between the cracks of this complex structure? The dozens of federal efforts already miss many of the elderly people, partly because the latter cannot deal with the maze of programs, regulations, and bureaucrats. Therefore, the delivery of services is not well coordinated and the things that are available are not always well used. Even the informal networks exclude many elderly persons, especially solitary women.

Some solutions to these problems lie in a more rational and comprehensive way to structure formal programs and deliver their services. The Comprehensive Older Americans Act Amendments of 1978 attempted some such reforms, though the major problems persist. The 1981 White House Conference on Aging also tried to bring more focus into the various programs, oriented around six major issues, and its efforts may produce significant improvements.

But the basic solution resides in changed attitudes about the elderly, so that they are seen as a valuable resource for the society rather than as its discards and charity cases. Negative stereotypes and attitudes about older people are still common and as emotionally nurtured as those about other groups forced into minority status. Therefore, we need more basic research to deal with a core problem: The source and nature of anti-elderly prejudice and discrimination.[41] Until basic attitudes change, we will patch at the problems of the elderly but won't solve them, and will continue to view the elderly themselves as a problem. The change calls for exactly the kind of consideration the rest of us want for ourselves, both in our younger years and when we reach the older ages.

Summary

The aging of America's population has powerful implications for the elderly, the younger population, and the nation and society as a whole. Moreover, because recent projections of the size of the elderly population seem certain to prove too low as curve-squaring and life span-extending technologies unfold, the impact of that aging will be greater than anticipated. Those technologies, which include efforts to control the major causes of death and to intervene in the aging process itself, will increase life expectancy by allowing more people to reach age 65 and by extending the average lifetime for persons already in that age group. The segment aged 75 and older will increase especially rapidly as we lengthen the average life span.

For the elderly themselves, the principal concerns of aging are income maintenance, health care, housing, and the relationship between work and leisure. In addition, the ability to live a meaningful existence, fully engaged in such social pursuits as they wish, is also fundamental. So is the fear of victimization, especially among poorer older people who live in high-crime-rate areas. The ways in which we now meet these concerns reflect a mixture of discrimination, benevolence, and hesitation, especially about the costs and the job prospects of younger people and their own aging.

One of the most pressing long-term problems is the huge and growing cost of the complex Social Security system, which now provides escalating retirement benefits to a rapidly growing older population; survivors' benefits to widows, widowers, and dependent children; disability benefits to various age groups; and Medicare and Medicaid benefits to those who are ill or disabled. There is urgent need for ongoing reforms to supplement the 1983 changes in the retirement system, but the proposals are influenced in certain ways by the dependent elderly, and in others by the working population and employers who must help finance the system. This generational clash of interests and the opposing political power it represents result in large part from other policies that have converted most of the elderly population into a nonworking one.

Thus, age discrimination and even the benevolence that accompanies it have had very expensive consequences, though even the reasons for the discrimination are complex. In a society which seems unable to sustain a full-employment economy, for example, there is certain justification to pension older workers so that young ones can enter the labor force and

294

middle-aged ones can move up. Nonetheless, those practices also show that we have not fulfilled our innovative potential to provide jobs for people of all ages who want and need them.

The aging of America's population, therefore, produces an intricate network of social, economic, and political consequences, many of which are serious social problems because the system is still poorly prepared to deal with such a large influx of older citizens and to balance humane concerns against practical realities.

NOTES

1. Mary Barberis, "America's Elderly: Policy Implications," *Population Bulletin* 35 (1981): 5.

2. Judith Murphy and Carol Florio, "Older Americans: Facts and Potential," in Ronald Gross, Beatrice Gross and Sylvia Seidman, eds., *The New Old: Struggling for Decent Aging.* Garden City, NY: Doubleday, 1978, p. 54.

3. Theodore J. Gordon, "Prospects for Aging in America," in Matilda White Riley, ed., *Aging from Birth to Death.* Boulder, CO: Westview Press, 1979, p. 183.

4. Subcommittee on Human Services of the House Select Committee on Aging, *Future Directions for Aging Policy: A Human Services Model,* Pub. no. 96-226. Washington DC: U.S. Government Printing Office, 1980, pp. 109-110.

5. *Ibid.,* pp. 111-112.

6. See Sharon McAuliffe and Kathleen McAuliffe, "Closing In on Cancer," *Reader's Digest* (March, 1983): 59-64.

7. Gordon, *op. cit.,* p. 186.

8. For the data, see U.S. Bureau of the Census, "Projections of the Population of the United States: 1977 to 2050," *Current Population Reports,* P-25, no. 704 (1977), table 11; "Projections of the Population of the United States: 1982 to 2050," (advance report), *Current Population Reports,* P-25, no. 922 (1982), table 2.

9. Gordon, *op. cit.,* p. 189.

10. These potential impacts are from *ibid.,* pp. 191-195.

11. Paul B. Horton and Gerald R. Leslie, *The Sociology of Social Problems.* 7th ed. Englewood Cliffs, NJ: Prentice-Hall, 1981, pp. 178-179.

12. Organisation for Economic Co-operation and Development, *Socio-economic Policies for the Elderly.* Paris: OECD, 1979, pp. 141-142.

13. J. John Palen, *Social Problems.* New York: McGraw-Hill, 1979, p. 398.

14. Subcommittee on Human Services.., *Future Directions..,* *op. cit.,* pp. 99-101.

15. Several of these questions are adapted from OECD, *Socio-economic Policies...,* *op. cit.,* pp. 157-158.

16. Carroll L. Estes, "Social Policy Alternatives: A Redefinition of Problems, Goals, and Strategies," in Harold Cox, ed., *Aging.* 3rd ed. Guilford, CT: Dushkin, 1983, p. 211.

17. Jacob S. Siegel, "Prospective Trends in the Size and Structure of the Elderly Population, Impact of Mortality Trends, and Some Implications," in U.S. Bureau of the Census, *Current Population Reports,* P-23, no. 78 (1979): 20.

18. Beth J. Soldo, "America's Elderly in the 1980s," *Population Bulletin,* 35 (1980): 40-41.

19. Barberis, *op. cit.,* pp. 7-8.

20. National Council on the Aging, *Perspective on Aging* 9 (1980): 37-38.

21. Subcommittee on Human Services, *op. cit.,* p. 106.

22. Several of the points in this section are from *ibid.,* pp. 91-94.

23. OECD, *Socio-economic Policies...,* *op. cit.,* pp. 145-146.

24. Barberis, *op. cit.,* p. 7.

25. Subcommittee on Human Services, *op. cit.,* pp. 94-95.

26. Joseph J. Spengler, *Population and America's Future.* San Francisco: Freeman, 1975, p. 108.

27. Kurt W. Back and Kenneth J. Gergen, "Cognitive and Motivational Factors in Aging and Disengagement," in Ida Harper Simpson and John C. McKinney, eds., *Social Aspects of Aging.* Durham, NC: Duke University Press, 1966, p. 303.

28. Estes, *op. cit.,* p. 212.

29. Palen, *op. cit.,* p. 412.

30. OECD, *op. cit.,* p. 158.

31. Erdman Palmore, *Social Patterns in Normal Aging: Findings from the Duke Longitudinal Study.* Durham, NC: Duke University Press, 1981, pp. 3-4.

32. For an analysis of this matter, see Charles F. Longino, Jr., Kent A. McClelland and Warren A. Peterson, "The Aged Subculture Hypothesis: Social Integration, Gerontophilia and Self-Confidence," *Journal of Gerontology* 35 (1980): 758-767.

33. Louis Harris & Associates, *The Myth and Reality of Aging in America. Washington, DC: National Council on the Aging, 1975, pp. 29; 30.*

34. National Council on the Aging, *Perspective on Aging, op. cit.,* p. 27.

35. Herman J. Loether, *Problems of Aging.* 2nd ed. Belmont, CA: Dickenson, 1975, pp. 112-113.

36. Ralph Thomlinson, *Population Dynamics: Causes and Consequences of World Demographic Change.* 2nd ed. New York: Random House, 1976, pp. 350-351.

37. Spengler, *op. cit.,* pp. 99-100.

38. On this question, see Bernice L. Neugarten, ed., *Age or Need? Public Policies for Older People.* Beverly Hills, CA: Sage, 1982.

39. OECD, *op. cit.,* p. 165.

40. Soldo, *op. cit.,* pp. 28-29.

41. Erdman Palmore, "Attitudes Toward the Aged: What We Know and Need to Know," *Research on Aging* 4 (1982): 333.

Bibliography

American Cancer Society, *Cancer Facts and Figures*, New York: American Cancer Society, 1983.

Anderson, Trudy B., "The Dependent Elderly Population: A Function of Retirement," *Research on Aging* 3 (1981): 311-324.

Angel, Ronald and Marta Tienda, "Determinants of Extended Household Structure: Cultural Patterns or Economic Need?" *American Journal of Sociology* 87 (1982): 1360-1383.

Apt, Patricia Harper and Roger Heimstra, "A Model for Learning Resource Networks for Senior Adults," *Educational Gerontology* 5 (1980): 163-173.

Atchley, Robert C., "The Process of Retirement: Comparing Women and Men," in Maximiliane Szinovacz, ed., *Women's Retirement*, Beverly Hills, CA: Sage, 1982, chapter 10.

Atchley, Robert C., "Retirement: Leaving the World of Work," *Annals of American Academy of Political and Social Science* 464 (1982): 120-131.

Atchley, Robert C., *The Sociology of Retirement*, Cambridge, MA: Schenkman, 1976.

Atchley, Robert C. and Judith L. Robinson, "Attitudes Toward Retirement and Distance from the Event," *Research on Aging*, 4 (1982): 299-313.

Back, Kurt W. and Kenneth J. Gergen, "Cognitive and Motivational Factors in Aging and Disengagement," in Ida Harper Simpson and John C. McKinney, eds., *Social Aspects of Aging*, Durham, NC: Duke University Press, 1966, chapter 18.

Back, Kurt W. and Carleton S. Guptill, "Retirement and Self-Ratings," in Ida Harper Simpson and John C. McKinney, eds., *Social Aspects of Aging*. Durham, NC: Duke Univerity Press, 1966, chapter 7.

Barberis, Mary, "America's Elderly: Policy Implications," *Population Bulletin*, 35 (1981).

Barsby, Steve L. and Dennis R. Cox, *Interstate Migration of the Elderly*, Lexington, MA: Heath, 1975.

Beale, Calvin L., "Internal Migration," in Jean van der Tak, "U.S. Population: Where We Are; Where We're Going," *Population Bulletin*, 37 (1982): 42.

Beale, Calvin L., *The Revival of Population Growth in Nonmetropolitan America*, Washington, DC: Economic Research Service, U.S. Department of Agriculture, 1975.

Beauvoir, Simon de, *Coming of Age*, New York: Putnam's Sons, 1972.

Belbin, R. Meredith, "Retirement Strategy in an Evolving Society," in Frances M. Carp, ed., *Retirement*, New York: Behavioral Publications, 172, chapter 6.

Berman, Phyllis W. and Estelle R. Ramey, eds., *Women: A Developmental Perspective*, Washington, DC: National Institutes of Health, 182.

Bernard, Jessie, *Remarriage,* New York: Dryden Press, 1956.

Biggar, Jeanne C., "Reassessing Elderly Sunbelt Migration," in Charles F. Longino, Jr. and David J. Jackson, *Migration and the Aged,* special issue of *Research on Aging,* 2 (1980): 177-190.

Biggar, Jeanne C., Charles F. Longino, Jr. and Cynthia B. Flynn, "Elderly Interstate Migration: The Impact on Sending and Receiving States, 1965 to 1970," in Charles F. Longino, Jr. and David J. Jackson, eds., *Migration and the Aged,* special issue of *Research on Aging,* 2 (1980): 217-232.

Binstock, Robert H. and Ethel Shanas, eds., *Handbook of Aging and the Social Sciences,* New York: Van Nostrand, 1976.

Bouvier, Leon F., "America's Baby Boom Generation: The Fateful Bulge," *Population Bulletin* 35 (1980).

Brickfield, Cyril F., "Rags to Riches — or Reality? Economic Prospects for the Elderly in the 1980s," in Kurt Finsterbusch, ed., *Social Problems 82/83,* Guilford, CT: Dushkin, 1982: 132-133.

Brockway, James M., Tanya K. Brockway and Marcia B. Steinhauer, *Kentucky Demographics: Migration Patterns of Kentucky's Older Population,* Louisville, KY: Urban Studies Center, University of Louisville, 1980.

Brody, Elaine M., "The Aging of the Family," *Annals of American Academy of Political and Social Science,* 438 (1978): 13-27.

Brody, Elaine M., statement in House Select Committee on Aging, "Families: Aging and Changing," June 4, 1980: 52-61.

Brown, David and Calvin L. Beale, "Diversity in Post-1970 Population Trends," in Amos H. Hawley and Sara Mazie, eds., *Nonmetropolitan America in Transition,* Chapel Hill, NC: University of North Carolina Press, 1981: 27-71.

Brubaker, Timothy H., ed., *Family Relationships in Later Life,* Beverly Hills, CA: Sage, 1983.

Butler, Robert N., "Ageism," in Kurt Finsterbusch, ed., *Social Problems 82/83,* Guilford, CT: Dushkin, 1982, pp. 125-131.

Calderone, Mary S., "Sex and the Aging," in Ronald Gross, Beatrice Gross and Sylvia Seidman, eds., *The New Old: Struggling for Decent Aging,* Garden City, NY: Doubleday, 1978: 205-208.

Califano, Jr., Joseph A., "The Aging of America: Questions for the Four-Generation Society," *Annals of American Academy of Political and Social Science* 438 (1978): 96-107.

Carp, Frances M., "Housing and Living Environments of Older People," in Robert H. Binstock and Ethel Shanas, eds., *Handbook of Aging and the Social Sciences,* New York: Van Nostrand, 1976, chapter 10.

Carp, Frances M., ed., *Retirement,* New York: Behavioral Publications, 1972.

Carp, Frances M. and Abraham Carp, "It May Not Be the Answer, It May Be the Question," *Research on Aging* 3 (1981): 85-100.

Clark, Robert L., Juanita Kreps and Joseph J. Spengler, "Aging Population: United States," in John A. Ross, ed., *International Encyclopedia of Population,* v. 1, New York: Free Press, 1982: 31-40.

Coale, Ansley J., "The Effects of Changes in Mortality and Fertility on Age Composition," *Milbank Memorial Fund Quarterly* 34 (1956): 79-114.

Coale, Ansley J., "How a Population Ages or Grows Younger," in Ronald Freedman, ed., *Population: The Vital Revolution,* Garden City, NY: Doubleday, 1964, chapter 3.

Collins, Glenn, "The Good News about 1984," *Psychology Today* 12 (1979): 34-48.

Congressional Budget Office, *Work and Retirement: Options for Continued Employment for Older Workers,* Washington, DC: U.S. Government Printing Office, 1982.

Cottrell, Fred, *Aging and the Aged,* Dubuque, IA: Wm. C. Brown, 1974.

Council on Environmental Quality and U.S. Department of State, *The Global 2000 Report to the President,* v. 2, *The Technical Report,* Washington, DC: U.S. Government Printing Office, 1980.

Cowgill, Donald O., "Residential Segregation by Age in American Metropolitan Areas," *Journal of Gerontology* 33 (1978): 446-453.

Cox, Harold, ed., *Aging,* 3rd ed., Guilford, CT: Dushkin, 1983.

Cribier, Francoise, "A European Assessment of Aged Migration," in Charles F. Longino, Jr. and David J. Jackson, eds., *Migration and the Aged,* special issue of *Research on Aging,* 2 (1980): 255-270.

Cumming, Elaine and William E. Henry, *Growing Old: The Process of Disengagement,* New York: Basic Books, 1961.

Datan, Nancy and Nancy Lohman, eds., *Transitions of Aging,* New York: Academic Press, 1980.

David Henry P., "Eastern Europe: Pronatalist Policies and Private Behavior," *Population Bulletin* 36 (1982).

Davis, Kingsley, "Population and Welfare in Industrialized Societies," *Population Review* 6 (1962): 17-29.

Davis, Kingsley and Pietronella van den Oever, "Age Relations and Public Policy in Advanced Industrial Societies," *Population and Development Review* 7 (1981): 1-18.

Dixon, J.C., ed., *Continuing Education in the Later Years,* Gainesville, FL: University of Florida Press, 1963.

Dono, John E., Cecilia M. Falbe, Barbara L. Kail, Eugene Litwak, Roger H. Sherman and David Siegal, "Primary Groups in Old Age," *Research on Aging* 1 (1979): 403-433.

Drake, Joseph, *The Aged in American Society,* New York: Ronald Press, 1958.

Duberman, Lucile, *Marriage and Its Alternatives,* New York: Praeger, 1974.

Easterlin, Richard A., "What Will 1984 Be Like? Socioeconomic Implications of Recent Twists in Age Structure," *Demography* 15 (1978): 397-421.

Eklund, Lowell, "Aging and the Field of Education," in Matilda White Riley, John W. Riley, Jr. and Marilyn E. Johnson, eds., *Aging and Society,* v. 2, *Aging and the Professions,* New York: Russell Sage Foundation, 1969, chapter 11.

Estes, Carroll L., "Social Policy Alternatives: A Redefinition of Problems, Goals, and Strategies," in Harold Cox, ed., *Aging,* 3rd ed., Guilford, CT: Dushkin, 1983: 210-220.

Fengler, Alfred P. and Nicholas Danigelis, "Residence, the Elderly Widow, and Life Satisfaction," *Research on Aging* 4 (1982): 113-135.

Ferrara, Peter J., *Social Security: Averting the Crisis,* Washington, DC: Cato Institute, 1982.

Ferrara, Peter J., *Social Security: The Inherent Contradiction*, Washington, DC: Cato Institute, 1980.

Ferraro, Kenneth F., "Relocation Desires and Outcomes among the Elderly," *Research on Aging* 3 (1981): 166-181.

Fingerhut, Lois A., "Changes in Mortality among the Elderly: United States, 1940-78," *Vital and Health Statistics* Analytical Studies, series 3, no. 22 (1982).

Fingerhut, Lois A., "Chartbook," in National Center for Health Statistics, *Health, United States, 1982*, PHS Pub. no. 83-1232 (1982): 6-37.

Fingerhut, Lois A. and Harry M. Rosenberg, "Mortality among the Elderly," in National Center for Health Statistics, *Health, United States, 1981*, PHS Pub. no. 82-1232 (1981): 15-24.

Finsterbusch, Kurt, ed., *Social Problems 82/83*, Guilford, CT: Dushkin, 1982.

Flynn, Cynthia B., "General versus Aged Interstate Migration, 1965-1970," in Charles F. Longino, Jr. and David J. Jackson, eds., *Migration and the Aged*, special issue of *Research on Aging*, 2 (1980): 165-176.

Folger, John K. and Charles B. Nam, *Education of the American Population*, Washington, DC: U.S. Government Printing Office, 1967.

Foner, Anne and Karen Schwab, *Aging and Retirement*, Monterey, CA: Brooks/Cole, 1981.

Freedman, Ronald, ed., *Population: The Vital Revolution*, Garden City, NY: Doubleday, 1964.

Fuguitt, Glenn V. and Stephen J. Tordella, "Elderly Net Migration," in Charles F. Longino, Jr. and David J. Jackson, eds., *Migration and the Aged*, special issue of *Research on Aging*, 2 (1980): 191-204.

Fullerton, Howard N., "The 1995 Labor Force: A First Look," in U.S. Bureau of Labor Statistics, *Economic Projections to 1990*, Bulletin 2121, Washington, DC: U.S. Government Printing Office, 1982: 48-58.

Gibson, Rose C., "Blacks at Middle and Late Life: Resources and Coping," *Annals of American Academy of Political and Social Science*, 464 (1982): 79-90.

Giesen, Carol Boellhoff and Nancy Datan, "The Competent Older Woman," in Nancy Datan and Nancy Lohman, eds., *Transitions of Aging*, New York: Academic Press, 1980, chapter 4.

Givens, Jr., Harrison, "An Evaluation of Mandatory Retirement," *Annals of American Academy of Political and Social Science* 438 (1978): 50-58.

Glick, Paul C., "Differential Mortality," in U.S. Bureau of Census, "Population of the United States, Trends and Prospects: 1950-1990," *Current Population Reports*, P-23, no. 49 (1974): 41-50.

Glick, Paul C., "The Future of the American Family," in U.S. Bureau of Census, *Current Population Reports*, P-23, no. 78 (1979): 1-6.

Golant, Stephen M., "Future Directions for Elderly Migration Research," in Charles F. Longino, Jr. and David J. Jackson, eds, *Migration and the Aged*, special issue of *Research on Aging*, 2 (1980): 271-278.

Golant, Stephen M., ed., *Location and Environment of the Elderly Population*, New York: Wiley, 1979.

Goldscheider, Calvin, "Differential Residential Mobility of the Older Population," *Journal of Gerontology* 21 (1981): 103-108.

Gordon, Theodore J., "Prospects for Aging in America," in Matilda White Riley, ed., *Aging from Birth to Death*, Boulder, CO: Westview Press, 1979, chapter 10.

301

Goudy, Willis J., "Antecedent Factors Related to Changing Work Expectations," *Research on Aging* 4 (1982): 139-157.

Graves, Edmund and Robert Pokras, "Expected Principal Source of Payment for Hospital Discharges: United States, 1979," in National Center for Health Statistics, *Advance Data from Vital and Health Statistics,* no. 75 (1982): 1-10.

Greenough, William C. and Francis P. King, *Pension Plans and Public Policy,* New York: Columbia University Press, 1976.

Gross, Ronald, "I Am Still Learning," in Ronald Gross, Beatrice Gross and Sylvia Seidman, eds., *The New Old: Struggling for Decent Aging,* Garden City, NY: Doubleday, 1978, pp.364-369.

Gross, Ronald, Beatrice Gross and Sylvia Seidman, eds., *The New Old: Struggling for Decent Aging,* Garden City, NY: Doubleday, 1978.

Grove, Robert D. and Alice M. Hetzel, *Vital Statistics Rates in the United States, 1940-1960,* Washington, DC: National Center for Health Statistics, 1968.

Hardy, Melissa A., "Social Policy and Determinants of Retirement: A Longitudinal Analysis of Older White Males," *Social Forces* 60 (1982): 1103-1122.

Harris, Charles S., *Fact Book on Aging: A Profile of America's Older Population,* Washington, DC: National Council on the Aging, 1978.

Harris, Louis & Associates, *The Myth and Reality of Aging in America,* Washington, DC: National Council on the Aging, 1975.

Harris, Louis & Associates, "Myths about Life for Older Americans," in Ronald Gross, Beatrice Gross and Sylvia Seidman, eds., *The New Old: Struggling for Decent Aging,* Garden City, NY: Doubleday, 1978, pp. 90-119.

Hauser, Philip M., "Aging and World-Wide Population Change," in Robert H. Binstock and Ethel Shanas, eds., *Handbook of Aging and the Social Sciences,* New York: Van Nostrand, 1976, chapter 3.

Heaton, Tim B., William B. Clifford and Glenn V. Fuguitt, "Changing Patterns of Retirement Migration," *Research on Aging* 2 (1980): 93-104.

Hicks, Nancy, "Life after 65," in *Social Problems 81/82,* Guilford, CT: Dushkin, 1981: 159-161.

Horton, Paul B. and Gerald R. Leslie, *The Sociology of Social Problems,* 7th ed., Englewood Cliffs, NJ: Prentice-Hall, 1981.

House Select Committee on Aging, "Families: Aging and Changing," Washington, DC: U.S. Government Printing Office, June 4, 1980.

International Labour Office, *Year Book of Labour Statistics, 1979,* Geneva: International Labour Office, 1979.

Jackson, Jacquelyne Johnson, "Death Rate Trends of Black Females, United States, 1964-1978," in Phyllis W. Berman and Estelle R. Ramey, eds., *Women: A Developmental Perspective,* Washington, DC: National Institutes of Health, 1982: 23-35.

Jackson, Jacquelyne Johnson, *Minorities and Aging,* Belmont, CA: Wadsworth, 1980.

Janson, Philip and Karen Frisbie Mueller, "Age, Ethnicity, and Well-Being," *Research on Aging* 5 (1983): 353-367.

302

Kalish, Richard A., "Death and Dying in Social Context," in Robert H. Binstock and Ethel Shanas, eds., *Handbook of Aging and the Social Sciences*, New York: Van Nostrand, 1976, chapter 19.

Kalish, Richard A., "Death and Survivorship: The Final Transition," *Annals of American Academy of Political and Social Science*, 464 (1982): 163-173.

Kalish, Richard A., *Late Adulthood: Perspectives on Human Development*, Monterey, CA: Brooks/Cole, 1975.

Kamerschen, David R., "On an Operational Index of 'Overpopulation'," *Economic Development and Cultural Change* 13 (1965): 169-187.

Keating, Norah and Judith Marshall, "The Process of Retirement: The Rural Self-Employed," *The Gerontologist* 20 (1980): 437-443.

Keyfitz, Nathan, "Age Distribution as a Challenge to Development," *American Journal of Sociology* 70 (1965): 659-668.

Keyfitz, Nathan and Antonio Golini, "Mortality Comparisons: The Male-Female Ratio," *Genus* 31 (1975): 1-33.

Kinsey, Alfred, Wardell Pomeroy and Paul Gebhard, *Sexual Behavior in the Human Female*, Philadelphia: Saunders, 1953.

Kinsey, Alfred, Wardell Pomeroy and Clyde Martin, *Sexual Behavior in the Human Male*, Philadelphia: Saunders, 1948.

Kleiman, Ephraim, "A Standardized Dependency Ratio," *Demography* 4 (1967): 876-893.

Kobrin, Frances E., "The Fall in Household Size and the Rise of the Primary Individual in the United States," *Demography* 13 (1976): 127-138.

Kreps, Juanita M., "The Economy and the Aged," in Robert H. Binstock and Ethel Shanas, eds., *Handbook of Aging and the Social Sciences*, New York: Van Nostrand, 1976, chapter 11.

Kubat, Daniel, Anthony H. Richmond and Jerzy Zubrzycki, eds., *Policy and Research on Migration: Canadian and World Perspectives*, special issue of *International Migration Review*, 8 (1974).

Lee, Anne S., "Return Migration in the United States," in Daniel Kubat, Anthony H. Richmond and Jerry Zubrzycki, eds., *Policy and Research on Migration: Canadian and World Perspectives*, special issue of *International Migration Review*, 8 (1974): 283-300.

Lee, Everett S., "Migration of the Aged," in Charles F. Longino, Jr. and David J. Jackson, eds., *Migration and the Aged*, special issue of *Research on Aging*, 2 (1980): 131-135.

Lee, Ronald D., "Demographic Forecasting and the Easterlin Hypothesis," *Population and Development Review* 2 (1976): 459-468.

Lerner, I.M., *Heredity, Evolution and Society*, San Francisco: Freeman, 1968.

Loether, Herman J., *Problems of Aging*, 2nd ed., Belmont, CA: Dickenson, 1975.

Lohman, Nancy, "Life Satisfaction Research in Aging: Implications for Policy Development," in Nancy Datan and Nancy Lohman, eds., *Transitions of Aging*, New York: Academic Press, chapter 2.

Long, Larry H., "Migration Differentials," in U.S. Bureau of Census, "Population of the United States, Trends and Prospects: 1950-1990," *Current Population Reports*, P-23, no. 49 (1974): 129-140.

Long, Larry H., "Migration Differentials by Education and Occupation: Trends and Variations," *Demography* 10 (1973): 243-258.

Longino, Jr., Charles F. and David L. Jackson, eds., *Migration and the Aged,* special issue of *Research on Aging,* 2 (1980): 131-280.

Longino, Jr., Charles F., Kent A. McClelland and Warren A. Peterson, "The Aged Subculture Hypothesis: Social Integration, Gerontophilia and Self-Conception," *Journal of Gerontology* 35 (1980): 758-767.

Lopata, Helena Znaniecki, "Loneliness: Forms and Components," *Social Problems* 17 (1969): 248-262.

Lopata, Helena Znaniecki, "The Widowed Family Member," in Nancy Datan and Nancy Lohman, eds., *Transitions of Aging,* New York: Academic Press, 1980, chapter 6.

Madigan, Francis C., "Are Sex Mortality Differentials Biologically Caused?" *Milbank Memorial Fund Quarterly* 35 (1957): 203-223.

Manley, Charles R., "The Migration of Older People," *American Journal of Sociology* 59 (1954): 324-331.

Manton, Kenneth G. and Eric Stallard, "Temporal Trends in U.S. Multiple Cause of Death Mortality Data: 1968 to 1977," *Demography* 19 (1982): 527-547.

Markle, Gerald E., "Sex Ratios at Birth: Values, Variance, and Some Determinants," *Demography* 11 (1974): 131-142.

Matras, Judah, *Introduction to Population,* Englewood Cliffs, NJ: Prentice-Hall, 1977.

McAuliffe, Sharon and Kathleen McAuliffe, "Closing in on Cancer," *Reader's Digest,* March, 1983: 59-64.

McCluskey, Neil G. and Edgar F. Borgatta, eds., *Aging and Retirement: Prospects, Planning, and Policy,* Beverly Hills, CA: Sage, 1981.

McNamara, Regina, "Migration Measurement," in John A. Ross, ed., *International Encyclopedia of Population,* v. 2. New York: Free Press, 1982, pp. 448-450.

McNamara, Regina, "Mortality Trends," in John A. Ross, ed., *International Encyclopedia of Population,* v. 2. New York: Free Press, 1982, pp. 459-461.

Metropolitan Life Foundation, *Statistical Bulletin* 63 (1982).

Michael, Robert T., Victor R. Fuchs and Sharon R. Scott, "Changes in the Propensity to Live Alone: 1950-1976," *Demography* 17 (1980): 39-56.

Morgenstern, Oskar, *National Income Statistics: A Critique of Macroeconomic Aggregation,* Washington, DC: Cato Institute, 1979.

Murphy, Judith and Carol Florio, "Older Americans: Facts and Potential," in Ronald Gross, Beatrice Gross and Sylvia Seidman, eds., *The New Old: Struggling for Decent Aging,* Garden City, NY: Doubleday, 1978, pp. 50-57.

Nam, Charles B. and Susan O. Gustavus, *Population: The Dynamics of Demographic Change,* Boston: Houghton Mifflin, 1976.

Nam, Charles B., Norman L. Weatherby and Kathleen A. Ockay, "Causes of Death which Contribute to the Mortality Crossover Effect," *Social Biology* 25 (1978): 306-314.

National Caucus on the Black Aged, "A Generation of Black People," in Ronald Gross, Beatrice Gross and Sylvia Seidman, eds., *The New Old: Struggling for Decent Aging,* Garden City, NY: Doubleday, 1978, pp. 281-283.

National Center for Health Statistics, "Advance Report of Final Mortality Statistics, 1979," *Monthly Vital Statistics Report* 31 (1982).

National Center for Health Statistics, "Advance Report of Final Mortality Statis-

304

tics, 1980," *Monthly Vital Statistics Report* 32 (1983).

National Center for Health Statistics, "Advance Report of Final Natality Statistics, 1980," *Monthly Vital Statistics Report* 31 (1982).

National Center for Health Statistics, "Annual Summary of Births, Deaths, Marriages, and Divorces: United States, 1981," *Monthly Vital Statistics Report* 30 (1982).

National Center for Health Statistics, "Final Mortality Statistics, 1978," *Monthly Vital Statistics Report* 29 (1980).

National Center for Health Statistics, *Health, United States, 1981,* PHS Pub. no. 82-1232 (1981).

National Center for Health Statistics, *Health, United States, 1982,* PHS Pub. no. 83-1232 (1982).

National Center for Health Statistics, *Vital Statistics of the United States, 1978,* v. 2, sec. 5, *Life Tables* (1980).

National Center for Health Statistics, *Vital Statistics of the United States, 1977,* v. 3, *Marriage and Divorce* (1981).

National Center for Health Statistics, *Vital Statistics of the United States, 1970,* v. 2, *Mortality,* part A (1974).

National Center for Health Statistics, *Vital Statistics of the United States, 1977,* v. 2, *Mortality,* part A (1981).

National Council on the Aging, *The Myth and Reality of Aging in America,* Washington, DC: NCOA, 1975.

National Council on the Aging, "NCOA Public Policy Agenda," *Perspective on Aging* 9 (1980): 12-39.

National Council on the Aging, *Perspective on Aging,* 9 (1980).

National Council on the Aging, "Special Concerns II," *Perspective on Aging* 9 (1980): 20-27.

Neugarten, Bernice L., "The Rise of the Young-Old," in Ronald Gross, Beatrice Gross and Sylvia, eds., *The New Old: Struggling for Decent Aging,* Garden City, NY: Doubleday, 1978, pp. 47-49.

Neugarten, Bernice L., ed., *Age or Need? Public Policies for Older People,* Beverly Hills, CA: Sage, 1982.

Norland, Joseph A., "Measuring Change in Sex Composition," *Demography,* 12 (1975): 81-88.

O'Gorman, Hubert, "False Consciousness of Kind: Pluralistic Ignorance among the Aged," *Research on Aging* 2 (1980): 105-128.

Omran, Abdel R., "The Epidemiologic Transition: A Theory of the Epidemiology of Population Change," *Milbank Memorial Fund Quarterly* 49 (1971): 509-538.

Organisation for Economic Co-operation and Development, *Socio-economic Policies for the Elderly,* Paris: OECD, 1979.

Palen, J. John, *Social Problems,* New York: McGraw-Hill, 1979.

Palmore, Erdman, "Attitudes toward the Aged: What We Know and Need to Know," *Research on Aging* 4 (1982): 333-348.

Palmore, Erdman, *Social Patterns in Normal Aging: Findings from the Duke Longitudinal Study,* Durham, NC: Duke University Press, 1981.

Pampel, Fred C., "Changes in the Propensity to Live Alone: Evidence from

Consecutive Cross-Sectional Surveys," *Demography* 20 (1983): 433-447.

Pampel, Fred C., *Social Change and the Aged*, Lexington, MA: Heath, 1981.

Patterson, George F., "Income," in U.S. Bureau of Census, "Population of the United States, Trends and Prospects: 1950-1990," *Current Population Reports*, P-23, no. 49 (1974): 163-172.

Petersen, William, *Population*, 3rd ed., New York: Macmillan, 1975.

Priebe, John A., "Occupation," in U.S. Bureau of Census, "Population of the United States, Trends and Prospects: 1950-1990," *Current Population Reports*, P-23, no. 49 (1974): 151-157.

Ramey, Estelle R., "The Natural Capacity for Health in Women," in Phyllis W. Berman and Estelle R. Ramey, eds., *Women: A Developmental Perspective*, Washington, DC: National Institutes of Health, 1982, pp. 3-12.

Reid, John, "Black America in the 1980s," *Population Bulletin*, 37 (1982).

Riley, Matilda White, ed., *Aging from Birth to Death*, Boulder, CO: Westview Press, 1979.

Riley, Matilda White, "Introduction: Life Course Perspectives," in Matilda White Riley, ed., *Aging from Birth to Death*, Boulder, CO: Westview Press, 1979, pp. 3-13.

Riley, Matilda White and Anne Foner, *Aging and Society*, v. 1, *An Inventory of Research Findings*, New York: Russell Sage Foundation, 1968.

Riley, Matilda White, Marilyn E. Johnson and Anne Foner, eds., *Aging and Society*, v. 3, *A Sociology of Age Stratification*, New York: Russell Sage Foundation, 1972.

Riley, Matilda White, John W. Riley, Jr. and Marilyn E. Johnson, eds., *Aging and Society*, v. 2, *Aging and the Professions*, New York: Russell Sage Foundation, 1969.

Rives, Jr., Norfleet W., "Researching the Migration of the Elderly," in Charles F. Longino, Jr. and David J. Jackson, eds., *Migration and the Aged*, special issue of *Research on Aging*, 2 (1980): 155-163.

Ross, John A., ed., *International Encyclopedia of Population*, 2 vols., New York: Free Press, 1982.

Schneider, Paula J. and Thomas J. Palumbo, "Social and Demographic Characteristics of the Labor Force," in U.S. Bureau of Census, "Population of the United States, Trends and Prospects: 1950-1990," *Current Population Reports*, P-23, no. 49 (1974): 142-151.

Schulz, James C., "Income Distribution and the Aging," in Robert H. Binstock and Ethel Shanas, eds., *Handbook of Aging and the Social Sciences*, New York: Van Nostrand, 1976, chapter 22.

Sell, Ralph R. and Gordon F. De Jong, "Toward a Motivational Theory of Migration Decision Making," *Journal of Population* 1 (1978): 313-335.

Serow, William J., "Return Migration of the Elderly in the U.S.A.: 1955-60 and 1965-70," *Journal of Gerontology* 33 (1978): 288-295.

Shanas, Ethel and Gordon F. Streib, eds., *Social Structure and the Family: Generational Relations*, Englewood Cliffs, NJ: Prentice-Hall, 1965.

Shanas, Ethel and Marvin B. Sussman, eds., *Family, Bureaucracy, and the Elderly*, Durham, NC: Duke University Press, 1977.

Shaw, R. Paul, *Migration Theory and Fact: A Review and Bibliography of Current Literature*, Philadelphia: Regional Science Research Institute, 1975.

306

Sheldon, Henry D., *The Older Population of the United States*, New York: Wiley, 1958.

Sheppard, Harold L., "Aging and Manpower Development," in Matilda White Riley, John W. Riley, Jr. and Marilyn E. Johnson, eds., *Aging and Society*, v. 2, *Aging and the Professions*, New York: Russell Sage Foundation, 1969, chapter 6.

Sheppard, Harold L., "The Issue of Mandatory Retirement," *Annals of American Academy of Political and Social Science*, 438 (1978): 40-49.

Sheppard, Harold L., "Work and Retirement," in Robert H. Binstock and Ethel Shanas, eds., *Handbook of Aging and the Social Sciences*, New York: Van Nostrand, 1976, chapter 12.

Shryock, Henry S., *Population Mobility within the United States*, Chicago: Community & Family Study Center, University of Chicago, 1964.

Shryock, Henry S. and Jacob S. Siegel, *The Methods and Materials of Demography*, 2 vols., Washington, DC: U.S. Government Printing Office, 1973.

Siegel, Jacob S., "On the Demography of Aging," *Demography* 17 (1980): 345-364.

Siegel, Jacob S., "Prospective Trends in the Size and Structure of the Elderly Population, Impact of Mortality Trends and Some Implications," in U.S. Bureau of the Census, *Current Population Reports*, P-23, no. 78 (1979): 7-22.

Simpson, Ida Harper and John C. McKinney, eds., *Social Aspects of Aging*, Durham, NC: Duke University Press, 1966.

Simpson, Ida Harper, Kurt W. Back and John C. McKinney, "Work and Retirement," in Ida Harper Simpson and John C.McKinney, eds., *Social Aspects of Aging*, Durham, NC: Duke University Press, 1966, chapter 2.

Simpson, Ida Harper, Richard L. Simpson, Mark Evers and Sharon Sandomirsky Poss, "Occupational Recruitment, Retention, and Labor Force Cohort Representation," *American Journal of Sociology* 87 (1982): 1287-1313.

Sirrocco, Al, "An Overview of the 1980 National Master Facility Inventory Survey of Nursing and Related Care Homes," in National Center for Health Statistics, *Advance Data from Vital and Health Statistics*, no. 91 (1983):1-5.

Smith, T. Lynn and Paul E. Zopf, Jr., *Demography: Principles and Methods*, 2nd ed., Port Washington, NY: Alfred, 1976.

Soldo, Beth J., "America's Elderly in the 1980s," *Population Bulletin* 35 (1980).

Spengler, Joseph J., *Population and America's Future*, San Francisco: Freeman, 1975.

Spengler, Joseph J., "Some Economic and Related Determinants Affecting the Older Worker's Occupational Role," in Ida Harper Simpson and John C. McKinney, eds., *Social Aspects of Aging*, Durham, NC: Duke University Press, 1966, chapter 1.

Stahura, John M. and Sidney M. Stahl, "Suburban Characteristics and Aged Net Migration," *Research on Aging* 2 (1980): 3-22.

Stimson, Ardyth, Jane F. Wise and John Stimson, "Sexuality and Self-Esteem among the Aged," *Research on Aging* 3 (1981): 228-239.

Streib, Gordon F., "Social Stratification and Aging," in Robert H. Binstock and Ethel Shanas, eds., *Handbook of Aging and the Social Sciences*, New York: Van Nostrand, 1976, chapter 7.

Streib, Gordon F. and Clement J. Schneider, *Retirement and American Society*, Ithaca, NY: Cornell University Press, 1971.

Subcommittee on Human Services of the House Select Committee on Aging, *Future*

Directions for Aging Policy: A Human Services Model, Pub. no. 96-226, Washington, DC: U.S. Government Printing Office, 1980.

Sullivan, Deborah and Sylvia A. Stevens, "Snowbirds: Seasonal Migrants to the Sunbelt," *Research on Aging* 4 (1982): 159-177.

Sussman, Marvin B., "An Analytical Model for the Sociological Study of Retirement," in Frances M. Carp, *Retirement,* New York: Behavioral Publications, 1972, chapter 2.

Thomlinson, Ralph, *Population Dynamics: Causes and Consequences of World Demographic Change,* 2nd ed., New York: Random House, 1976.

Tordella, Stephen J., *Reference Tables, Net Migration of Persons Aged 0 to 64 and 65 and Over for United States Counties, 1970 to 1975,* Madison, WI: Applied Population Laboratory, University of Wisconsin, 1980.

Treas, Judith and Vern L. Bengston, "The Demography of Mid- and Late-Life Transitions," *Annals of American Academy of Political and Social Science* 464 (1982): 11-21.

Uhlenberg, Peter, "Demographic Change and Problems of the Aged," in Matilda White Riley, ed., *Aging from Birth to Death,* Boulder, CO: Westview Press, 1979, chapter 8.

United Nations, *Demographic Yearbook, 1979,* New York: United Nations, 1979.

United Nations, *Demographic Yearbook, 1980,* New York: United Nations, 1980.

United Nations, *Demographic Yearbook, 1981,* New York: United Nations, 1981.

U.S. Bureau of the Census, "America in Transition: An Aging Society," *Current Population Reports,* P-23, no. 128 (1983).

U.S. Bureau of the Census, *1980 Census of Population, General Population Characteristics,* reports for states, 1981.

U.S. Bureau of the Census, *1980 Census of Population, Supplementary Reports,* PC80-S1-1, *Age, Sex, Race, and Spanish Origin of the Population by Regions, Divisions, and States: 1980,* 1981.

U.S. Bureau of the Census, *1980 Census of Population, Supplementary Reports,* PC80-S1-5, *Standard Metropolitan Statistical Areas and Standard Consolidated Statistical Areas: 1980,* 1981.

U.S. Bureau of the Census, *1980 Census of Population, Supplementary Reports,* PHC80-S1-1, *Provisional Estimates of Social, Economic, and Housing Characteristics,* 1982.

U.S. Bureau of the Census, "Characteristics of the Population below the Poverty Level: 1980," *Current Population Reports,* P-60, no. 133 (1982).

U.S. Bureau of the Census, "Demographic Aspects of Aging and the Older Population in the United States," *Current Population Reports,* P-23, no. 59 (1978).

U.S. Bureau of the Census, "Educational Attainment in the United States: March 1979 and 1978," *Current Population Reports,* P-20, no. 35 (1980).

U.S. Bureau of the Census, "Estimating After-Tax Money Income Distributions Using Data from the March Current Population Survey," *Current Population Reports,* P-23, no. 126 (1983).

U.S. Bureau of the Census, "Farm Population of the United States: 1980," *Current Population Reports,* P-27, no. 54 (1981).

U.S. Bureau of the Census, "Geographic Mobility: March 1975 to March 1980," *Current Population Reports,* P-20, no. 368 (1981).

U.S. Bureau of the Census, "Illiteracy in the United States: November 1969," *Current Population Reports*, P-20, no. 217, (1971).

U.S. Bureau of the Census, "Marital Status and Living Arrangements: March 1980," *Current Population Reports*, P-20, no. 365 (1981).

U.S. Bureau of the Census, "Mobility of the Population of the United States: March 1970 to March 1975," *Current Population Reports*, P-20, no. 285 (1975).

U.S. Bureau of the Census, "Money Income of Households, Families, and Persons in the United States: 1980," *Current Population Reports*, P-60, no. 132 (1982).

U.S. Bureau of the Census, *Negroes in the United States, 1920-32*, Washington, DC: U.S. Government Printing Office, 1935.

U.S. Bureau of the Census, "Persons of Spanish Origin in the United States: March 1980," (advance report) *Current Population Reports*, P-20, no. 361 (1981).

U.S. Bureau of the Census, "Population of the United States, Trends and Prospects: 1950-1990," *Current Population Reports*, P-23, no. 49 (1974).

U.S. Bureau of the Census, "Projections of the Population of the United States: 1977 to 2050," *Current Population Reports*, P-25, no. 704 (1977).

U.S. Bureau of the Census, "Projections of the Population of the United States: 1982 to 2050," *Current Population Reports*, P-25, no. 922 (1982).

U.S. Bureau of the Census, *Sixteenth Census of the United States: 1940, Characteristics of the Population, U.S. Summary*, 1943.

U.S. Bureau of the Census, *Sixteenth Census of the United States: 1940. The Labor Force, U.S. Summary*, 1943.

U.S. Bureau of the Census, "The Social and Economic Status of the Black Population in the United States: An Historical View, 1790-1978," *Current Population Reports*, P-23, no. 80 (1979).

U.S. Bureau of the Census, "Some Demographic Aspects of Aging in the United States," *Current Population Reports*, P-23, no. 43 (1973).

U.S. Bureau of the Census, *State and Metropolitan Area Data Book, 1982*, Washington, DC: U.S. Government Printing Office, 1982.

U.S. Bureau of the Census, *Statistical Abstract of the United States: 1960*, Washington, DC: U.S. Government Printing Office, 1960.

U.S. Bureau of the Census, *Statistical Abstract of the United States: 1979*, Washington, DC: U.S. Government Printing Office, 1979.

U.S. Bureau of the Census, *Statistical Abstract of the United States: 1981*, Washington, DC: U.S. Government Printing Office, 1981.

U.S. Bureau of the Census, *Statistical Abstract of the United States: 1982-83*, Washington, DC: U.S. Government Printing Office, 1982.

U.S. Bureau of the Census, "1976 Survey of Institutionalized Persons: A Study of Persons Receiving Long-Term Care," *Current Population Reports*, P-23, no. 69 (1978).

U.S. Bureau of the Census, *U.S. Census of Population: 1950, Detailed Characteristics, U.S. Summary*, 1953.

U.S. Bureau of the Census, *U.S. Census of Population: 1960, Characteristics of the Population, U.S. Summary*, 1964.

U.S. Bureau of the Census, *U.S. Census of Population: 1960, Detailed Characteristics, U.S. Summary*, 1964.

U.S. Bureau of the Census, *U.S. Census of Population: 1960, Subject Reports, Mobility for States and State Economic Areas*, 1963.

U.S. Bureau of the Census, *U.S. Census of Population: 1970, Detailed Characteristics, U.S. Summary*, 1973.

U.S. Bureau of the Census, *U.S. Census of Population: 1970, General Population Characteristics, U.S. Summary*, 1972.

U.S. Bureau of the Census, *U.S. Census of Population: 1970, General Population Characteristics*, reports for states, 1971.

U.S. Bureau of the Census, *U.S. Census of Population: 1970, Subject Reports, Mobility for States and the Nation*, 1973.

U.S. Bureau of Labor Statistics, *Economic Projections to 1990*, Bulletin 2121, Washington, DC: U.S. Government Printing Office, 1982.

U.S. Bureau of Labor Statistics, *Handbook of Labor Statistics, 1980*, Washington, DC: U.S. Government Printing Office, 1980.

U.S. Bureau of Labor Statistics, *Labor Force Statistics Derived from the Current Population Survey: A Databook*, 2 vols., Washington, DC: U.S. Government Printing Office, 1982.

U.S. Census Office, *Ninth Census of the United States, Vital Statistics of the United States*, 1872.

van der Tak, Jean, "U.S. Population: Where We Are; Where We're Going," *Population Bulletin*, 37 (1982).

Voss, Paul R., "The Increasing Ranks of Elderly Veterans: Where They Will Be in 1990," paper presented to the Southern Regional Demographic Group, Greensboro, NC, October 6-8, 1982.

Webber, Irving L., "The Educable Aged," in J.C. Dixon, ed., *Continuing Education in Later Years*, Gainesville, FL: University of Florida Press, 1963, pp. 14-25.

Weeks, John R., *Population: An Introduction to Concepts and Issues*, 2nd ed., Belmont, CA: Wadsworth, 1981.

Wiseman, Robert F., "Why Older People Move: Theoretical Issues," in Charles F. Longino, Jr. and David J. Jackson, eds., *Migration of the Aged*, special issue of *Research on Aging*, 2 (1980): 141-154.

World Health Organization, *Manual of the International Statistical Classification of Diseases, Injuries, and Causes of Death, Ninth Revision*, Geneva: WHO, 1977.

Zopf, Jr., Paul E., *Population: An Introduction to Social Demography*, Palo Alto, CA: Mayfield, 1984.

Zopf, Jr., Paul E., *Sociocultural Systems*, Washington, DC: University Press of America, 1978.

Zopf, Jr., Paul E., "Variations in Support Burdens as Measured by the Dependency Ratio," *Greek Review of Social Research*, no. 19-20 (1974): 29-43.

Indexes

Author and Source Index

Subject Index

318